THE ONCOGENE
FactsBook

Other books in the FactsBook Series:

A. Neil Barclay, Albertus D. Beyers, Marian L. Birkeland, Marion H. Brown,
Simon J. Davis, Chamorro Somoza, Alan F. Williams
The Leucocyte Antigen FactsBook

Rod Pigott and Christine Power
The Adhesion Molecule FactsBook

Ed Conley
The Ion Channel FactsBook

Shirley Ayad, Ray P. Boot-Handford, Martin J. Humphries, Karl E. Kadler and
C. Adrian Shuttleworth
The Extracellular Matrix FactsBook

Steve Watson and Steve Arkinstall
The G-Protein Linked Receptor FactsBook

Robin Callard and Andy Gearing
The Cytokine FactsBook

Grahame D. Hardie and Steven Hanks
The Protein Kinase FactsBook:
Serine Kinases,
and Tyrosine Kinases

THE ONCOGENE
FactsBook

Robin Hesketh
Department of Biochemistry
University of Cambridge, UK

Academic Press
Harcourt Brace & Company, Publishers
LONDON   SAN DIEGO   NEW YORK   BOSTON
SYDNEY   TOKYO   TORONTO

ACADEMIC PRESS LIMITED
24–28 Oval Road
LONDON NW1 7DX

U.S. Edition Published by
ACADEMIC PRESS INC.
San Diego, CA 92101

This book is printed on acid-free paper

Copyright © 1995 by
ACADEMIC PRESS LIMITED

A catalogue record for this book is available from the British Library

ISBN 0–12–344550–7

Typeset by Columns Design and Production Services Ltd, Reading
Printed and bound in Great Britain by Mackays of Chatham PLC, Chatham, Kent

Contents

Section I THE INTRODUCTORY CHAPTERS

Section II THE ONCOGENES

Section III   TUMOUR SUPPRESSOR GENES

Section IV   DNA TUMOUR VIRUSES

Preface

Much of the material in this book is derived from its predecessor The Oncogene Handbook and I remain deeply grateful to those colleagues around the world whose comments and suggestions I acknowledged in that book. However, The Oncogene FactsBook is essentially a completely new book, designed to be more concise and to focus particularly on protein function and associations with human cancers. As such I hope that undergraduates and clinicians as well as research scientists will find it helpful and informative. They will undoubtedly have suggestions for improvements and may detect errors and omissions: any of these I encourage them to forward to me.

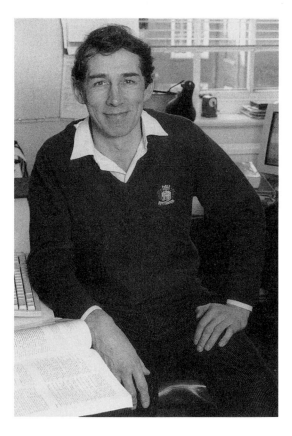

Robin Hesketh

Abbreviations

Ab-MuLV	Abelson murine leukemia virus
ABML	Abelson virus-induced myeloid lymphosarcoma
ADPRT	ADP-ribosyltransferase inhibitor
AEV	Avian erythroblastosis virus
ALL	Acute lymphoblastic leukaemia
ALV	Avian leukosis virus
AML	Acute myeloid leukaemia
AMV	Avian myeloblastosis virus
ANLL	Acute nonlymphocytic leukaemia
APL	Acute promyelocytic leukaemia
ARE	AU-rich element
ASV	Avian sarcoma virus
B-CLL	Chronic B cell lymphocytic leukemia
BDNF	Brain-derived neurotrophic factor
bHLH	Basic helix–loop–helix
BNU	Butylnitrosourea
CAR	Cell adhesion regulator
CBF	Core binding factor
CDK	Cyclin-dependent kinase
C/EBP	CCAAT/enhancer binding protein
CEF	Chick embryo fibroblast
CHRPE	Congental hypertrophy of the retinal pigment epithelium
CIN	Cervical intraepithelial carcinoma
CML	Chronic myelogenous leukaemia
Con A	Concanavalin A
CRE	cAMP response element
CSF	Cytostatic factor
DMBA	Dimethylbenzanthracene
DSE	Dyad symmetry element
EBV	Epstein–Barr virus
EGF	Epidermal growth factor
ENU	Ethylnitrosourea
ERK	Extracellular signal-regulated kinase (also called MAP kinase)
ES	Embryonic stem
ESV	Esh sarcoma virus
ETF	Epidermal growth factor (EGF) receptor transcription factor
FAP	Familial adenomatosis polyposis
FeLV	Feline leukaemia virus
FeSV	Feline sarcoma virus
FGF	Fibroblast growth factor
FIRE	*Fos* intragenic regulatory element
FMTC	Familial medullary thyroid carcinoma
FSH	Follical stimulating hormone
FSV	Fujinami sarcoma virus
FUSE	Far upstream element

GADD	Growth arrest on DNA damage
GAP	GTPase activating protein
GM-CSF	Granulocyte-macrophage colony stimulating factor
GNRP	Guanine nucleotide release protein
GRB	Growth factor receptor (protein)
GRF	Growth hormone-releasing factor
GRP	Gastric releasing peptide
GVBD	Germinal vesicle breakdown
HBGF	Heparin-binding growth factor
HBV	Hepatitis B virus
HCC	Hepatocellular carcinoma
HCP	Haematopoietic cell phosphatase (also called PTP1C)
HCP	Haematopoietic cell phosphatase
HGF	Hepatocyte growth factor
HIV	Human immunodeficiency virus
HLH/LZ	Helix–loop–helix/leucine zipper
HMBA	Hexamethylene bisacetamide
HOB1, HOB2	Homology box 1, 2
HPV	Human papilloma virus
HTLV	Human T cell leukaemia/lymphoma virus
HZ2-FeSV	Hardy–Zuckerman 2 feline sarcoma virus
IL	Interleukin
JNK	JUN N-terminal kinase
LDL	Low-density lipoprotein
LFA-1	Lymphocyte function-associated antigen-1
LPS	Lipopolysaccharide
LRM	Leucine-rich motif
LTR	Long terminal repeat
MAG	Myelin-associated glycoprotein
MAP kinases	Mitogen-activated protein kinases (also called ERK1, ERK2)
MAP	Microtubule associated protein
MAP2	Microtubule-associated protein 2
MAPKK	Mitogen-activated protein kinase kinase
MBR	Major breakpoint region
Mbcr	Major breakpoint cluster region
MCR	Minor cluster region
MDR	Multidrug resistance
MDV	Marek disease virus
MEN	Multiple endocrine neoplasia
MGF	Mast cell growth factor
MHC	Major histocompatibility complex
MMP	Matrix metalloproteinase
MMTV	Mouse mammary tumour virus
MNNG	N-methyl-N'-nitro-N-nitrosoguanidine
Mo-MSV	Moloney murine sarcoma virus
Mo-MuLV	Moloney murine leukaemia virus

Mo-MuSV	Molony murine sarcoma virus
MPF	Maturation promoting factor
MSV	Murine sarcoma virus
MTC	Major translocation cluster
MuLV	Murine leukaemia virus
NAF	NEU protein-specific activating factor
NCAM	Neural cell adhesion molecule
NDF	NEU differentiation factor
NDP	Nucleoside diphosphate
NFAT-1	Nuclear factor of activated T cells
NF1	Neurofibromatosis type 1
NF2	Neurofibromatosis type 2
NGF	Nerve growth factor
NMU	Nitrosomethylurea
NRE	Negative regulatory element
ODN	Oligodeoxynucleotide
OMGP	Oligodendrocyte-myelin glycoprotein
OPN	Osteopontin
ORD	Oncogene responsive domain
ORF	Open reading frame
PA	Plasminogen activator
PAI	Plasminogen activator inhibitor
PAF	Platelet activating factor
PCR	Polymerase chain reaction
PCNA	Proliferating cell nuclear antigen
PDGF	Platelet derived growth factor
PHA	Phytohaemagglutinin
PK-C	Protein kinase C
PKR	RNA-activated protein kinase
PLCγ	Phospholipase Cγ
PP2A	Protein phosphatase 2A
PTC	Papillary thyroid carcinoma (also called TPC)
PtdIns	Phosphatidylinositol
PTP1B	Protein tyrosine phosphatase 1B
PTP1C	Protein tyrosine phosphatase 1C (also called SH-PTP1, SHP or HCP)
PTP1D	Protein tyrosine phosphatase 1D (also called SYP, SH-PTP2, PTP2C or SH-PTP3)
RAR	Retinoic acid receptor
RCE	Retinoblastoma control element
REV	Reticuloendotheliosis virus
RSV	Rous sarcoma virus
SAP	SRF accessory protein
SCC	Squamous cell carcinoma
SCF	Stem cell factor
SCLC	Small cell lung carcinoma
SM-FeSV	Susan McDonough feline sarcoma virus

SRE	Serum response element
SRE BP	SRE binding protein
SRF	Serum response factor
SSV	Simian sarcoma virus
STK1	Stem cell tyrosine kinase 1
SV40	Simian vacuolating virus 40
T ALL	Acute T cell leukaemia
T_3	Triiodothyronine
TBP	TATA binding protein
TCR	T cell receptor
TGF	Transforming growth factor
THR	Thyroid hormone receptor
TIL	Tumour infiltrating lymphocyte
TIMP	Tissue inhibitor of metalloproteinase
TNF	Tumour necrosis factor
TPA	12-*O*-tetradecanoylphorbol-13-acetate (also called PMA)
TRE	TPA response element
UTR	Untranslated region
VCR	Varian cluster region
VDEPT	Virally directed enzyme prodrug therapy
VEGF-VPFR	Vascular endothelial growth factor
VSMC	Vascular smooth muscle cell

Introduction

ORGANIZATION

Section I begins with a summary of the principal developments in our understanding of oncogenes, together with a discussion of patterns of oncogene expression in human tumours (Chapters 1, 2 and 3). Chapter 4 lists genes that have been associated with metastasis and discusses major examples. Chapter 5 summarizes the present position with regard to gene therapy for human cancers. Chapter 6 comprises summary tables of the major categories of oncogenes and tumour suppressor genes. In Section II a constant format has been adopted for each entry, which includes the following (with minor modifications for individual genes as appropriate): Identification, Related genes, Table of properties (Nucleotides, Chromosome, Protein molecular mass), Cellular location, Tissue distribution, Protein function (including sections on Cancer, Transgenic animals, In animals and *In vitro*), Gene structure, Transcriptional regulation, Protein structure, Protein sequence, Domain structure, Database accession numbers, References (with Reviews indicated by bold type). The Tumour Suppressor Genes and DNA Tumour Viruses are considered in Sections III and IV. In the tables of properties the nucleotide entries indicate the size of the genomic region over which the cellular gene is distributed and the size of the complete viral genome. The panels at the left-hand side of the text in Sections II, III and IV contain an appropriate logo when the information in the accompanying text refers exclusively to one species.

The minimum number of references has been included compatible with giving the reader rapid access to the literature in the key areas of structure and function of each gene and its product. Thus the emphasis has been on listing the most up-to-date reference(s) for a particular topic, rather than providing an extensive bibliography.

For a more detailed discussion and comprehensive references the reader is referred to *The Oncogene Handbook* by Robin Hesketh, Academic Press, 1994.

NOMENCLATURE

The recommendations of the International Standing Committee on human gene nomenclature have been followed. Thus human genes are written in italicized capitals, their gene products in non-italicized capitals [1]. For genes of other species the nomenclature recommended for murine genes has been followed. Thus genes are italicized with an initial capital letter followed by lower case letters: the corresponding proteins are written in non-italicized capitals [2]. In the individual genes entries (Section II) the official designation is given at the outset but for some genes the commonly accepted form is used thereafter to avoid confusion. These are human *ABL1* (*ABL*), the avian *Erb* genes (*ErbA* and *ErbB*), *EPHT* (*EPH*), *TP53*/TP53 (*P53*/p53) and *NME1*/*NME2* (*NM23*). The designations *TGFβ*, *TCRα*, *TCRβ*, *TCRδ* and *TCRγ* are also used, rather than *TGFB*, *TCRA*, *TCRB*, *TCRD* and *TCRG*.

Viral oncogenes are referred to by trivial names of the form v-*onc* (e.g. v-*myc*), that is, the names do not imply target cell specificity or function [3]. The prefixes "p", "gp", "pp" or "P" followed by the molecular mass in kilodaltons indicate "protein", "glycoprotein", "phosphoprotein" or "polyprotein" respectively. An additional italicized superscript indicates the gene encoding the protein (e.g. p105*RB1*). Hyphenated superscripts denote polyproteins derived from two genes (e.g. gp180*gag-src*). Suffixes -a, -b, etc. denote inserts in the same virus that can code for different proteins via distinct RNAs (e.g. *Erba*, *Erbb*).

References

[1] Shows, T.B. et al. (1987) Cytogenet. Cell Genetics 46, 11–28.
[2] Lyon, M.F. (1984) Mouse News Lett. 72, 2–27.
[3] Coffin, J.M. (1981) J. Virol. 40, 953–957.

THE INTRODUCTORY CHAPTERS

Oncogenes are genes that cause cancer and it now seems probable that the interplay between the products of oncogenes is central to the development of most, if not all, cancer cells. Cellular oncogenes may be defined as genes which, under certain conditions, are capable of inducing neoplastic transformation of cells. Cellular oncogenes arise by the modification through mutation or change in the control of expression of a normal gene, referred to as a "proto-oncogene". In addition to oncogenes that arise within the cellular genome, some viruses carry oncogenes as part of their genome. The oncogenes of tumorigenic RNA viruses are derived from cellular proto-oncogenes: such viruses can rapidly transform cells in culture and induce tumours in appropriate host animals. Some DNA viruses are also tumorigenic but in general there is no evidence that the oncogenes that they express are derived from cellular progenitors.

The notion that cancer might be caused by genetic abnormality originated in the early nineteenth century when it was noted that predisposition to cancer seemed to run in families. By the turn of the century it had been observed using light microscopy that the chromosomes from cancer cells were frequently of abnormal length or shape when compared with those from normal cells. More recent discoveries have shown that there is a connection between susceptibility to cancers and an impaired ability of cells to repair damaged DNA and that the mutagenic potential of a substance is related to its carcinogenicity, all of which is consistent with the general concept that cellular genes (proto-oncogenes) in another form (oncogenes) cause neoplastic growth.

The *in vitro* paradigm of the neoplastic cancer cell is the transformed cell. The derivation of transformed cells from normal cells in culture is generally thought to involve "immortalization" of the cells so that they escape the limitation on growth of a finite number of division cycles. Such "established cell lines" are assumed to be partially transformed and a variety of carcinogenic agents can cause them subsequently to undergo full transformation to a state of unregulated growth resembling that of cancer cells. Transformed cells may be distinguished morphologically and by their decreased dependence on exogenous growth factors and are generally, although not invariably, tumorigenic when transplanted into immunologically compatible animals. There are presently about 100 known oncogenes that, under certain conditions, can release cells from the normal controls of growth, mortality and location to cause neoplastic transformation. It is probable that the majority of genes that possess oncogenic potential have now been identified and this figure of approximately 100 proto-oncogenes from about 30 000 functional human genes thereby sets an upper limit to the number of points at which the biochemical pathways controlling normal cell growth might be subverted by oncoproteins. The actual number of general mechanisms is probably much smaller, however, as oncoproteins fall into groups of similar activity (e.g. tyrosine kinases, guanine nucleotide binding, etc., see Table 1 on page 13), each of which is presumed to act at the same point in a pathway. In the main, oncogene activation is the result of somatic events (i.e. what we do to ourselves) rather than genetic causes. It is, in other words, a consequence of evolution (mutation and selection) within the body of one animal.

1 Tumour viruses and the identification of oncogenes

Oncogenes were first directly identified in viruses capable of inducing tumours in animals or of transforming cells *in vitro*. Many such viruses have RNA genomes and this family of "retroviruses" replicate through a DNA intermediate in infected cells (e.g. avian leukosis virus (ALV) and mouse mammary tumour virus (MMTV)). The oncogenes carried by such viruses are strongly homologous in sequence to normal cellular genes (proto-oncogenes) that are themselves highly conserved in evolution. Many DNA viruses are also oncogenic (e.g. SV40, polyoma, adenovirus and papillomavirus) although, as noted above, their transforming genes have not yet been shown to have proto-oncogene homologues within the normal genome, save for the presence of *BCL2* sequences in the Epstein–Barr virus *BHRF1* gene (see **DNA Tumour Viruses, EBV**).

Retroviruses are usually weakly pathogenic or apathogenic (e.g. ALV) although they are associated with a variety of chronic diseases. Productive infection has little effect on the host cell and progeny virus particles are released by budding from the plasma membrane without cell lysis. The basic genomes of retroviruses contain three genes (Fig. 1).

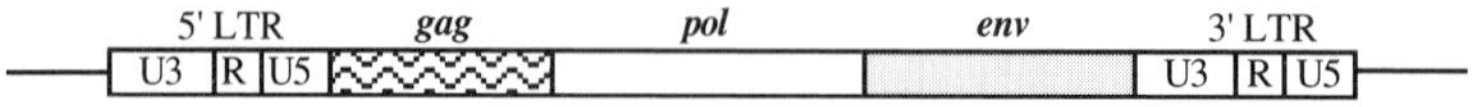

Figure 1. *Structure of a typical DNA provirus. U3, R and U5 within the long terminal repeat (LTR) regions refer to sequences derived from the 3' and 5' ends of the viral genome. gag (encoding group-specific antigens: viral capsid proteins), pol (reverse transcriptase and integrase) and env (the viral envelope proteins) are the three major structural and replicative genes. The lines indicate cellular DNA.*

Those retroviruses that can cause rapid neoplasia in infected organisms do so because they have acquired genes derived from normal cellular counterparts and the inappropriate expression of these transduced genes (or oncogenes) perturbs the normal regulation of cell growth. However, despite the fact that retroviruses induce cancers in a wide range of mammals and birds, no retrovirally borne gene has yet been demonstrated to be directly oncogenic in humans, including those in the genomes of the HIV and HTLV families.

For all retroviruses that have been studied, with the exception of some strains of Rous sarcoma virus (RSV), the acquisition of an oncogene disrupts the sequence of one or more of the *gag*, *pol* or *env* genes, rendering the virus replication defective. Replication of such defective viruses occurs in the presence of a helper virus that expresses complete *gag*, *pol* and *env* genes.

THE IDENTIFICATION OF ONCOGENES

The major steps in the experimental analysis of tumour viruses that led to the exposure of cancer genes began with the demonstration by Rous that cell-free filtrates of chicken sarcomas gave rise to sarcomas when inoculated into normal birds [1]. As Rous himself observed, "The...transmission of a true neoplasm by means of a cell-free filtrate assumes exceptional importance". Similar experiments at about this time had shown that avian leukaemia could be transmitted horizontally by cell-free preparations, although leukosis was not at that time recognized as a cancer.

Very little further progress occurred until the late 1950s, when the development of electron microscopic techniques enabled the infectious agent in these experiments to be recognized as a virus. In 1965 Fried [2], by treating polyoma virus with nitrous acid, derived a conditional mutation that was temperature-sensitive in its ability to transform normal hamster cells to neoplastic cells *in vitro*. This was a remarkable achievement, but DNA tumour viruses have subsequently proved difficult to work with in this context because their oncogenes may be involved in the expression and replication of viral DNA and they kill the cells in which they replicate.

The crucial retroviral experiment was performed by Martin [3] (1970) who used the chemical mutagen *N*-methyl-*N'*-nitro-*N*-nitrosoguanidine (MNNG) to obtain a temperature-sensitive mutant of RSV. With this mutant Martin was able to show that chick fibroblasts could be transformed to a fully neoplastic state by the expression of part of the viral genome alone and that sustained expression was required to maintain that state – an experiment that Bishop [4] has described as ushering in the "age of oncogenes". We now know that in RSV a single gene, *src*, is responsible for rapid oncogenesis.

Perhaps the most remarkable observation of the whole story came from screening total DNA in chickens when it emerged that the *Src* gene was not viral after all but is present in the normal genome [5]. These results led the way to the conclusion that highly conserved proto-oncogenes are present in normal cellular DNA in low copy number in virtually all members of the animal kingdom. This finding implied, although did not establish, the unification of the fields of retroviral research and cancer: if a normal gene misbehaving was responsible for retrovirally transmitted cancers in animals, then perhaps the same kind of mechanism might be involved in human tumours that arose spontaneously or were chemically induced and that apparently were not in any way caused by viruses. This was particularly encouraging in that neither at that time nor since has any evidence accumulated that retroviruses directly cause cancers in humans.

Further evidence that genes that had been normal at one time could become determinants of transformation came in the late 1970s from experiments in which the transfection of DNA from cell lines transformed by chemical carcinogens into normal cells gave rise to transformed phenotypes [6]. Shortly thereafter oncogenes began to be identified by transfection of cells *in vitro* with DNA taken from human tumours. The transfected cells were tumorigenic when injected into syngeneic animals and the genes responsible were shown to be homologous to the transforming genes of retroviruses, as first shown by Der and his colleagues [7] for *RAS*. During this period, Erikson and his colleagues [8] were able to show that the *Src* gene product, $pp60^{src}$, is a tyrosine kinase and that normal cells express low levels of the same protein. This was a striking finding because tyrosine phosphorylation is rare in cells: only 1 in 2000 of the phosphate groups linked to proteins are attached to tyrosine residues. Since then it has become clear that many other oncogenes encode kinases, several of which are tyrosine-specific (Table 1, page 13) and when activated increase total cellular phosphotyrosine content by up to tenfold. $pp60^{src}$ has subsequently been shown to act on many substrates but those that are essential mediators of transformation remain to be unequivocally identified (see **SRC**).

The observation that confirmed the normal origins of oncogenes was made in 1983 when Waterfield and his colleagues [9] showed that the transforming gene of simian sarcoma virus (v-*sis*) encodes a protein that is almost identical to the N-terminal 109 residues of the B chain of platelet-derived growth factor (PDGF).

PDGF is a normal growth factor secreted by platelets that stimulates the proliferation of fibroblasts. This discovery indicated that the v-*sis* viral oncogene was derived from a normal growth factor gene. The simplest explanation for the evolution of v-*sis* is that cells infected with simian sarcoma virus will continuously produce an autocrine growth factor. Shortly thereafter it was shown that the v-*erbB* gene codes for part of the epidermal growth factor (EGF) receptor, that other oncogenes (v-*fms* and v-*ros*, *MET* and *TRK*) are similarly derived from normal transmembrane receptors and that *THRA/ErbA* encodes a high-affinity thyroid hormone receptor.

HOW ARE PROTO-ONCOGENES ACTIVATED BY RETROVIRUSES?

Two general mechanisms account for the way in which transduced retroviral genes might promote cancers, even though they are derived from normal cellular genes:

1 The integration of viral DNA is potentially mutagenic: it can damage cellular genes directly or influence their expression by bringing them under the control of powerful regulatory elements in the viral genome (sometimes called "insertional mutagenesis") [10]. Both types of event are examples of *cis* activation. A further version of insertional mutagenesis may occur when the inserted provirus encodes a protein (i.e. viral) that can regulate transcription of a cellular gene – a form of *trans* activation independent of the respective locations of the proviral integration site and the normal gene within the host genome.

   Proviral insertion may occur anywhere in the host cell genome but, for a number of viruses, groups of preferred integration sites have been identified (Fig. 2). Such sites are sometimes adjacent to the loci of known proto-oncogenes but may also lie in proximity to previously unidentified genes. Genes that have been detected through being targets for insertional activation or mutation by viruses include *Ahi-1*, *Evi-1*, *Evi-2*, *Fli-1*, *Mlvi-1*, *Mlvi-2*, *Mlvi-3* and *Pvt-1* and for each of these common integration sites there is a significant frequency of double viral integration.

2 Recombination between retroviral and cellular genomes can insert a cellular gene in the viral genome, the cellular gene thus becoming oncogenic. This process is called "transduction". Because the cellular gene is now regulated by viral promoters its expression is independent of the site of proviral integration within chromosomal DNA. The oncoprotein expressed may consist of cellular information (usually altered) or may be a viral–cellular fusion protein.

As a consequence of insertional mutagenesis the action of viral promoters beyond the control of the cell may cause sustained overexpression of a normal host gene, leading to neoplastic growth. Most proto-oncogenes can transform established cell lines (although not primary explants of normal cells) when they are expressed at high levels. This was first observed in chicken lymphomas in which *Myc* was activated by retroviral DNA inserted upstream, within, or downstream of the gene (Fig. 2). Proviral insertion of ALV into the chicken genome is nearly always in the same transcriptional orientation as *Myc*, giving rise to promoter insertion in which transcription of the gene is initiated from the viral promoter. Insertions in the opposite orientation or 3' of the coding sequences are presumed to activate transcription by the ALV LTR functioning as a *cis* enhancer. In mammals infected by murine leukemia virus (MuLV) the converse situation

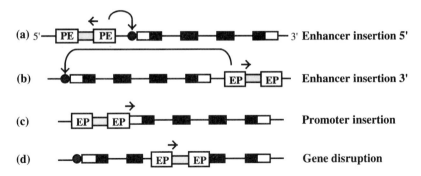

Figure 2. *Proviral activation of a cellular gene. E and P represent the viral enhancer and promoter elements within the LTR of the provirus. (a) insertion 5' to the cellular gene in the opposite orientation such that E is in close proximity to the cellular gene promoter (circle). (b) 3' insertion minimizing the distance between E and the cellular promoter. (c) Replacement of the cellular gene promoter by that of the virus. (d) Proviral integration within the cellular gene [11]. Potential avian or rodent oncogenes affected by viral insertion include, in addition to Myc and Wnt-1, ErbB, Hst, Int-2, Mos, Myb, Hras-1, RMO-Wnt-1, Pim-1 and Raf (see Table 2, Chapter 6). During the induction of erythroleukaemia by insertional mutagenesis of ALV, the ErbB gene (encoding the receptor for epidermal growth factor, EGFR) is truncated at the N-terminus, giving rise to a gene closely similar to v-erbB that arises from transduction. Integration sites regulating Myb expression occur in introns both 5' and 3' of the exons homologous to v-myb and Wnt-2 and Hst expression is altered by integration in 5' or 3' non-coding sequences.*

occurs: over 90% of viral insertions are in the opposite orientation to the gene with the viral sequences acting as an enhancer.

It is evident, therefore, that genes activated by viral insertion can mediate tumorigenesis but it seems certain that additional, undefined factors are involved. Thus, MMTV insertion can activate the *Wnt-1, Wnt-2, Wnt-3, Wnt-4* or *Hst* genes, of which only *Wnt-2* and *Hst* reside on the same chromosome. However, in MMTV-induced tumours that are histologically identical these genes may be activated collectively or only individually.

During transduction genes usually acquire mutations that can convert proto-oncogenes into oncogenes. Capture of cellular DNA by retroviruses generally involves trimming of either end of the gene. This may be critical in allowing enhanced expression (see **SRC** for comparison of v-*src* and *Src*). In some cases single point mutations are sufficient to activate oncogenic potential, for example, in *Ras* and *Neu*.

Retroviral infection is often harmless (if the viral genome lacks an oncogene) but even retroviruses that do not carry oncogenes can induce disease in susceptible hosts. However, they act more slowly and do not readily transform cells *in vitro*. Such viruses work by insertional activation of cellular proto-oncogenes. Known genes can be examined by Southern blot analysis to determine whether they are rearranged by viral integration in tumours. Novel genes can be detected by searching for proviral integration sites common to independent tumours: since retroviruses integrate into a large number of sites in the host genome, the probability of two such tumours having identical proviral integrations is very low.

The long latency of most neoplasms suggests that multiple steps are involved in the development of the disease. This concept is illustrated by the finding that in a number of retroviral infections distinct transforming genes (detectable by transfection of DNA into NIH 3T3 cells) are activated. Thus ALV-induced chicken lymphomas express *Blym-1* in addition to *Myc* and MMTV-induced mouse mammary carcinomas express *Hst-1* and combinations of the *Int* and *Wnt* families. Activated transforming genes have now been detected in a wide variety of primary tumours and derived cell lines of avian, rodent and human origin. The involvement of multiple genes in human cancers is discussed in Chapter 3.

Much of our understanding of the molecular biology of oncogenes has come from the study of tumour viruses and yet the variety of behaviour attributable to the oncoproteins that they express remains bewildering. Some tumour viruses are oncogenic *only* in animals *not* their host in nature whilst others are oncogenic in their natural host. Some do not transform cells in culture and yet are powerful oncogenes in animals. As will be discussed in the following sections, there is also great diversity in the oncoproteins synthesized by DNA and RNA tumour viruses: oncoproteins may act in the nucleus, cytoplasm or at the plasma membrane (see Chapter 3) but, although their cellular location may be known and specific protein functions are gradually being revealed, for the most part the manner in which the expression of multiple oncogenes integrates to cause cancers is not understood. From what is known, no correlation can be drawn between how proteins act and the nature of the tumour induced.

HOW ARE PROTO-ONCOGENES ACTIVATED IN HUMANS?

In normal cells proto-oncogene activation may occur by mutation, DNA rearrangement or oncogene amplification (Fig. 3). Point mutations may arise from the action of chemicals or radiation. For example, the transfection experiments that revealed activated *RAS* genes in human tumours led to the finding that, for *RAS*, the transformation from normal proto-oncogene to oncogene was due to substitution of a single base, resulting in the exchange of valine for glycine or glutamine for lysine at residues 12 or 61 respectively (see **RAS**).

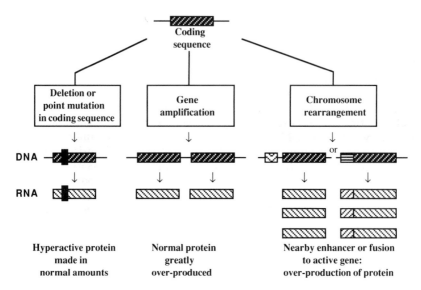

Figure 3. *Schematic representation of mechanisms of oncogene activation*

The mechanisms of chromosome translocation and amplification can provide a novel promoter for the cellular gene. The exchange of genetic material can occur between homologous or non-homologous chromosomes and can either be a balanced, reciprocal event or can involve loss of material from one or both junctions. Alternatively, inversion of segments within a chromosome may occur without net loss, or interstitial deletions may give rise to shortened chromosomes. Burkitt's lymphoma and human chronic myeloid leukaemia are characterized by chromosome exchange between non-homologous chromatids. In some B cell leukaemias the proto-oncogene comes under the control of an immunoglobulin promoter and enhancer. In Burkitt's lymphoma the gene involved is *MYC* and this releases transcription of *MYC* from normal controls so that it may be expressed at inappropriate times as well as being overexpressed. Damage to the translocated gene may also increase mRNA stability.

Gene amplification, thought to play a role in later stages of cancer, frequently involves proto-oncogenes. The process expands the number of copies of a gene which can lead to excess production of oncogene message and protein. Amplification of *MYC* and *MYCL* has frequently been observed in small cell carcinoma of the lung. Amplified genes may also have undergone mutation and, for *KRAS2* at least, there is evidence that amplification of the normal gene may occur in parallel with mutation of that gene.

DNA TUMOUR VIRUSES

The double-stranded DNA viruses of the adenovirus, herpesvirus, poxvirus and papovavirus families possess oncogenic potential. Most adenoviruses are tumorigenic in newborn rodents and will transform cells from such animals *in vitro*. The papovaviruses polyoma virus and simian vacuolating virus 40 (SV40) are also highly tumorigenic in rodent cells whereas in monkey cells (permissive cells) they enter the lytic cycle that leads to lysis of the infected cells and release of progeny viruses. A major difference between DNA viruses and retroviruses is that the former replicate autonomously without being integrated into the host chromosome. DNA viral genes, including those with oncogenic potential, have therefore evolved to encode proteins that are essential for the continuation of the life cycle of the virus. Hence the oncogenes of DNA viruses differ from those of retroviruses, possession of which confers no advantage on the virus.

In the early phase of SV40 infection the major proteins synthesized are the large T and small t antigens (see **DNA Tumour Viruses**). T antigen is the only viral protein necessary for viral DNA replication, achieved by its binding to and unwinding DNA and then interacting with DNA polymerase α. T antigen alone is a potent transforming agent whereas t antigen, although not necessary for either transformation or viral replication, enhances both processes. The polyoma locus encodes three early proteins, t antigen, middle t antigen and T antigen, of which middle t antigen is the strongest transforming protein. Adenoviruses encode two classes of early mRNA (E1A and E2B), from which alternative splicing patterns generate a range of proteins. Two E1A proteins of adenovirus 5 have been shown to act as transcription factors and to possess transforming activity. The E1B region does not possess transforming capacity but can promote that of E1A. As occurs with the proto-oncogene transcription factors (see Nuclear Oncoproteins below), most of these DNA tumour virus proteins can immortalize primary cells and cooperate with other oncoproteins (typically RAS) to transform. The general mechanism by which these different viral proteins cause transformation is by forming complexes with host cell proteins. Thus both E1A proteins and SV40 and polyoma T antigens form specific complexes with the retinoblastoma tumour suppressor gene product (p105^{RB1}) and these and other viral proteins share a sequence motif essential for interaction with p105^{RB1} (see **Tumour Suppressor Genes**). SV40 T antigen also forms complexes with the product of the tumour suppressor gene *P53* at a site separate from that binding p105^{RB1} and p53 also associates with E1B. These observations suggest that the transforming potential of SV40 T antigen lies in its capacity to bind to and inactivate p105^{RB1} and p53, both of which regulate the proliferation of normal cells. Human papilloma virus proteins E6 and E7 also bind to p53 and p105^{RB1}, respectively. The polyoma antigens do not bind p53 but it is probable that the increasing number of proteins being detected in complexes with these and other DNA viral antigens will include tumour suppressor gene products that are presently unknown (see **DNA Tumour Viruses**).

References

[1] Rous, P. (1911) J. Exp. Med. 13, 397–411.
[2] Fried, M. (1965) Proc. Natl Acad. Sci. USA 53, 486–491.
[3] Martin, G.S. (1970) Nature 227, 1021–1023.
[4] **Bishop, M.J. (1985) Cell 42, 23–38.**
[5] Stehelin, D. et al. (1976) Nature 260, 170–173.
[6] Shih, C. et al. (1979) Proc. Natl Acad. Sci. USA. 76, 5714–5718.
[7] Der, C.J. et al. (1982) Proc. Natl Acad. Sci. USA. 79, 3637–3640.
[8] Collett, M.S. et al. (1981) Nature 285, 167–169.
[9] Waterfield, M.D. et al. (1983) Nature 304, 35–39.
[10] **Kung, H.J. et al. (1991) Curr. Top. Microbiol. Immunol. 171, 1–25.**
[11] **Peters, G. (1991) Semin. Virolol. 2, 319–328.**

2 Normal cell growth and the functions of oncoproteins

ACTIVATION OF NORMAL CELL GROWTH

The stimulation of normal cell proliferation occurs as a consequence of the activation of biochemical pathways by growth factors (or mitogens) interacting with their receptors on the plasma membrane (Fig. 4). There are many different growth factors (e.g. PDGF, EGF, insulin, bombesin) and a single cell often possesses a variety of types of receptor. There are, however, only four known intracellular second messengers that can be activated by the interaction of a growth factor with its receptor:

1. Cyclic AMP, produced by the action of adenylate cyclase, a membrane-bound enzyme stimulated by many different signal–receptor complexes (e.g. prostaglandin E_2). Cyclic AMP-dependent protein kinases regulate many cellular processes.
2. Cyclic GMP, produced by the action of guanylate cyclase (e.g. cyclic GMP concentrations are modulated in retinal cells in response to light). Cyclic GMP directly regulates membrane cation channels in photoreceptor cells and mediates other processes including the relaxation of smooth muscle.
3. Elevation of the free, intracellular concentration of Ca^{2+} ($[Ca^{2+}]_i$), usually caused by the action of inositol 1,4,5-trisphosphate released during the hydrolysis of phosphatidylinositol 4,5-bisphosphate (PtdIns(4,5)P_2). Many growth factors cause PtdIns(4,5)P_2 hydrolysis when they activate their specific receptors on the cell surface (e.g. PDGF, bombesin, anti-T cell receptor antibody).
4. Activated protein tyrosine kinases. These enzymes, often intrinsic to the receptor molecule, are activated by many growth factors (e.g. EGF, PDGF).

One growth factor may recognize both receptors that activate adenylate cyclase and receptors that cause elevation of $[Ca^{2+}]_i$: such receptors are often, but not invariably, on different types of cell. Furthermore, the activation of tyrosine kinase(s) may be coupled to a mechanism for increasing $[Ca^{2+}]_i$.

The activation of second messengers causes the enhanced transcription of ~100 genes within 6 h. Of these, the "immediate early response genes" are activated within the first hour and include ornithine decarboxylase, the overexpression of which may cause transformation (see Table 1), and the proto-oncogene families of *JUN* and *FOS*. The proto-oncogenes *MYC* and *MYB* are also transcriptionally activated, approximately 2 h and 6 h, respectively, after cell stimulation.

In normal, untransformed cells the consistent pattern of a correlation between the early stages of proliferation and the expression of the proto-oncogenes *ETS*, *FOS*, *JUN* and *MYC* clearly suggests that these proto-oncogenes function as essential mediators of the biochemical pathways that regulate proliferation and that their corresponding oncogenic forms may act via sustained perturbation of normal growth control mechanisms.

It should also be noted that normal growth factors synthesized in an appropriate setting may act as "promoters" in the early stages of the development of cancers. Gastric releasing peptide (GRP or mammalian bombesin) functions as an autocrine growth factor in small cell lung cancer: these tumour cells produce large amounts of the peptide which causes PtdIns(4,5)P_2 hydrolysis and an increase in $[Ca^{2+}]_i$ [4], characteristic responses of cells entering the cell cycle. In this situation the growth factor may act selectively to promote the proliferation of a clone of tumour cells.

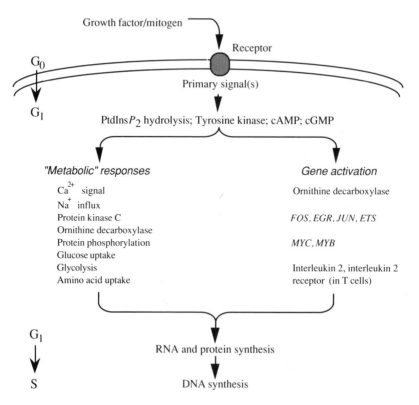

Figure 4. *Biochemical events during proliferation in eukaryotic cells. The interaction of growth factors with their receptors on the cell surface causes quiescent, somatic cells to leave G_0, traverse G_1 and enter S phase, whereupon cells are normally committed to at least one round of the cell cycle. Following the generation of one or more primary signals a sequence of "metabolic" events occurs that includes ionic changes, increased ornithine decarboxylase activity, protein phosphorylation and enhanced glycolytic flux. In parallel with and independent of these events the coordinated transcription of ~100 genes is activated [1,2]. The "immediate early response genes" activated within approximately 1 h include ornithine decarboxylase, ETS1 and ETS2, the JUN family (JUN, JUNB and JUND), the FOS family (FOS, FRA1, FRA2 and FOSB), serum response factor (SRF), the steroid hormone receptors Nurk77, N10, NGFI-B, T1, TIS1 and the early growth response family (EGR1, EGR2, EGR3 and EGR4), TIS11, TTP, Nup475, fibronectin, fibronectin receptor β subunit, β-actin, α-tropomyosin, NGFI-A, CEF-4 (or 9E3, related to IL-8), CEF-5 d-2, c25, rIRF-1, p27, Mtf, the glucose transporter, KC, N51, JE, TIS10, Cyr61, PC4, TIS7, Snk (serum-inducible kinase) and Pip92 [3]. In HTLV-1-infected T cells the Tax1 protein activates the JUN and FOS families, EGR1 and EGR2, ICP82 and 225 and other genes involved in proliferation.*

WHAT DO ONCOPROTEINS DO?

The gene products of *ETS*, *FOS*, *JUN* and *MYC* and their oncogenic equivalents function as nuclear transcription factors. In addition to controlling mRNA synthesis, only three basic ways are known by which the products of oncogenes can interfere with normal cell function (Table 1) [5]: (1) protein phosphorylation (Tyr, Ser, Thr), (2) metabolic regulation via G proteins, (3) modulation of DNA repair and replication. The DNA tumour viruses participate in replication but there is no evidence that oncogenes derived from proto-oncogenes work in this way.

Table 1. *Functional classification of oncogene products*

Class 1. Growth factor related proteins:
   PDGFB/SIS, INT2, HSTF1/HST-1

Class 2. Tyrosine kinases:
   Receptor-like tyrosine kinases: EPH, EGFR/ERBB, FMS, KIT, MET, HER2/NEU, RET, TRK
   Non-receptor tyrosine kinases: ABL, FPS/FES
   Membrane-associated non-receptor tyrosine kinases: SRC, FGR, FYN, HCK, LCK, YES

Class 3. Receptors lacking protein kinase activity:
   MAS

Class 4. Membrane-associated G proteins:
   HRAS, KRAS2, NRAS, GSP, GIP2

Class 5. Cytoplasmic protein serine kinases:
   BCR, MOS, PIM1, RAF/MIL

Class 6. Protein serine-, threonine- and tyrosine kinase:
   STY

Class 7. Cytoplasmic regulators:
   CRK

Class 8. Cell cycle regulators:
   MTS1, cyclin D1

Class 9. DNA binding proteins (transcription factors) or proteins located mostly in the nucleus:
   ETS1, ETS2, FOS, JUN, MYC, MYB, P53, RB1, REL, THRA/ERBA

Class 10. DNA repair enzymes:
   MLH1, MSH2

Class 11. Mitochondrial membrane factor:
   BCL2

Class 12. Function unknown:
   LCO

This table is a selected list of prominent oncoproteins: for complete lists see Table 5 in Chapter 6.

Class 1 (Table 1) includes the v-*sis* gene product referred to earlier, that appears to function as an autocrine growth factor providing sustained activation of proliferation via a normal plasma membrane receptor. v-*sis* encodes the B chain subunit of PDGF and in some cells a v-*sis* homodimer of PDGF is released that has a structure and activity similar to that of PDGF-BB. Hence, one possibility is that the cells proliferate indefinitely by an autocrine mechanism, although no increase in tyrosine phosphorylation corresponding to that caused by activation of the PDGF receptor has yet been detected. There are three possibilities that could account for the fact that v-SIS but not PDGF causes transformation: (i) it has abnormal activity compared with PDGF, (ii) it causes the receptor to be processed abnormally, (iii) it acts at an anomalous site within the cell. There is some evidence for (iii) in that the v-*sis* product may not need to leave the cell to evoke neoplastic growth but may combine with an intracellular receptor.

In addition to v-SIS and the transcription factors, oncogene products may be located in or attached to the plasma membrane or in the cytosol (Fig. 5). Thus, in principle, oncogenesis may occur as the result of perturbation at any point on the normal biochemical pathways that control proliferation.

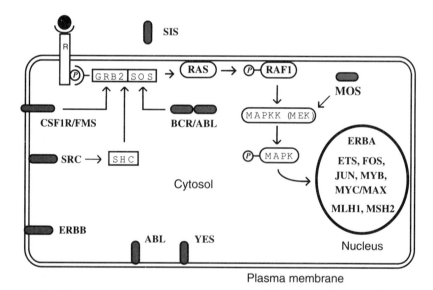

Figure 5. *Cellular location of some oncogene products*

In Fig. 5 the locations of a variety of oncoproteins are represented to illustrate that they may act as extracellular growth factors (SIS), as ligand-independent membrane-associated proteins (ERBB, SRC, FMS, RAS, YES), as cytosolic factors (ABL, MOS, RAF) or in the nucleus as transcription factors (ERBA, ETS, FOS, JUN, MYB, MYC) or DNA repair enzymes (MLH1, MSH2). One of the signal transduction pathways by which growth factors or oncoproteins may cause the activation of mitogen-activated protein serine/threonine kinases (MAPKs or extracellular signal-regulated kinases (ERKs)) is also shown. In this pathway, growth factor-activated receptors (R) or oncoproteins (SRC, BCR/ABL) interact with SH2 domain adaptor proteins (SHC, GRB2, SOS) to activate RAS. Activated RAS then causes the initiation of a cascade of protein phosphorylation by serine/threonine kinases including RAF, MAPKK (or MEK (_MAP_ kinase or _E_RK _k_inase)) and MAPKs [6]. In germ cells MOS activates MAPKK by serine phosphorylation.

In addition to these oncoproteins, the overexpression of various seven transmembrane spanning receptors or of a mutated $G_{\alpha q}$ protein renders some cultured cells tumorigenic [7].

Oncogenes that encode tyrosine kinase receptor-like proteins are generally considered to exert their effects through the sustained activation of their kinase domain. All tyrosine-specific protein kinases share sequence homology over ~300 amino acids although some (e.g. PDGFR, KIT, CSF1R/FMS) contain an insert region (Fig. 6).

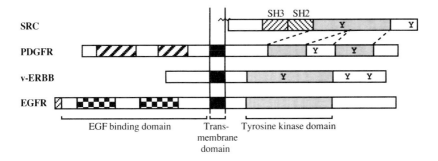

Figure 6. SRC, v-ERBB _and the transmembrane receptors for epidermal growth factor (EGF), and platelet-derived growth factor (PDGF). The kinase domains are homologous but that of the_ PDGF _receptor is divided by a kinase insert region._ v-ERBB _is homologous to the_ EGF _receptor but truncated at both ends, resulting in the loss of the ligand binding region and of a C-terminal regulatory tyrosine residue._

The transforming activity of avian erythroblastosis virus (AEV) arises from v-_erbB_ which encodes a truncated form of the EGFR that has lost the ligand binding domain and remains active as a protein tyrosine kinase, independent of EGF. v-ERBB has also lost a C-terminal region that includes an autophosphorylation site, presumed important for normal function. It is, however, difficult to show that v-ERBB has sustained tyrosine kinase activity. The major substrate for the activated EGFR is a 42 kDa protein, detected in some but not all cells transformed by oncogenes encoding a tyrosine kinase. In general, little is known about protein substrates for the EGFR or v-ERBB. Nevertheless, it would appear that the oncogenic action of v-ERBB is due to: (i) sustained tyrosine kinase activity, and (ii) absence of downregulation of the receptor on account of the missing EGF binding site.

In general, for the cytoplasmic and plasma membrane oncoproteins (e.g. v-RAS, v-SRC, v-ERBB, etc.) it appears that mutation in the cellular genes releases the translation products from the normal allosteric controls. As exemplified by v-ERBB, however, specific phosphorylation targets for the oncogenic tyrosine kinases that are involved in cell transformation remain largely undiscovered (see individual sections on **SRC, RAS** and **THRA/ErbA, EGFR/ErbB-1, HER2/ErbB-2/Neu, HER3/ErbB-3** and **HER4/ErbB-4**).

NUCLEAR ONCOPROTEINS

The early response proto-oncogenes that encode transcription factors are of particular interest in that they may regulate, either positively or negatively, genes that are directly involved in growth control. Although much is known about the interactions of these proteins with DNA *in vitro* (Table 2), their function *in vivo* remains largely obscure. The following is a general summary of what is currently known of the effects on transcription of the major nuclear oncoproteins FOS, JUN, ETS, MYB, MYC, REL and ERBA. The individual sections should be consulted for details and references relating to specific proteins.

Table 2. *Oncoproteins that act as transcription factors*

Gene family	Transcription factors	DNA target sequence
ETS	ETS1, ETS2	$GC^C/_GGGAAGT$
FOS	FOS, FOSB, FRA1, FRA2	$TGA^C/_GTCA$ (AP-1)
		TGACGTCA (CRE)
JUN	JUN, JUNB, JUND	$TGA^C/_GTCA$ (AP-1)
MYB	MYB	$C^A/_CGTT^A/_G$
MYC	MYC/MAX	CACGTG
REL	REL/NF-κB	$GGG^A/_GNT^T/_CT^T/_CCC$
THRA/ErbA	THRA/ERBA/T_3	TCAGGTCATGACCTGA

The ETS family of transcription factors show strong homology in their DNA binding domains across a wide range of species. Their expression is modulated by growth stimuli during differentiation and from their distribution it appears that they are tissue-specific regulators of gene expression. ETS1 and ETS2 activate transcription through the PEA 3 motif (CACTTCCT) that is present in the oncogene responsive domain (ORD) of the polyoma enhancer, where it overlaps an AP-1 site (GTTAGTCA). Transcriptional activation of the HTLV1 LTR requires the synergistic action of ETS1 and SP1 and, in general, ETS family proteins appear to function as components of transcription factor complexes to regulate the expression of viral and cellular genes.

The members of the *FOS* and *JUN* families are the major components of the transcription factor AP-1. Cellular expression (by transfection) of several oncogenes (*Fos*, *Mos*, *Ras*, *Raf*, *Src* or polyoma middle T) induces AP-1 activity and AP-1-binding enhancer elements occur in the *cis* control regions of a number of genes that are strongly expressed in transformed cells, including collagenase, metallothionein IIA and stromelysin. FOS cannot dimerize with itself and dimerization between FOS and JUN or between members of the JUN family is necessary for DNA binding. Eighteen different dimeric combinations can thus be formed from within the FOS and JUN families. DNA binding occurs by interaction between the leucine zipper regions (see *JUN*) of the proteins that lie next to basic DNA binding domains. JUN proteins also bind with high affinity to the cAMP response element (CRE) and JUN, but not FOS, proteins dimerize with some members of the CREB family, the dimers formed binding preferentially to the CRE. The capacity of JUN to interact with cAMP signalling pathways by forming JUN/CREB dimers thus provides an additional group of transcription factors. The basic and leucine zipper regions are present in both the normal and oncogenic forms of FOS and JUN and mutations that prevent dimerization decrease the transforming potential of v-FOS and v-JUN. In fibroblasts that have been stimulated by serum all the products of the *Fos* and *Jun* gene families coexist but the extent and temporal pattern of expression varies. These genes are also differentially expressed during development. This suggests that these proteins have distinct functions that are probably mediated by the wide range of affinities for AP-1 sites of the different dimeric forms. Thus JUN dimers have a tenfold greater affinity for AP-1 than JUNB or JUND: in JUN/FOS dimers the affinity and the half-life of interaction with DNA depends on the specific FOS protein involved (FOSB>FRA1>FOS). Furthermore, single base substitutions in the regions immediately flanking the AP-1 sequence (or the CRE element) can cause a tenfold change in binding affinity. These *in vitro* determinations of relative affinities are consistent with the finding that *Jun* with *Hras-1* is a more potent transforming combination than *JunB* and *Hras-1* and that *JunB* expressed at high levels inhibits the transforming potential of *Jun*.

The principal difference between the oncogenic form of JUN and the cellular form is the loss of a 27 amino acid N-terminal region (δ) that is not well conserved in JUNB and JUND. The δ region appears to facilitate or stabilize the interaction of an inhibitor protein present in some cells with the A1 transcription activation domain of JUN. v-JUN and JUN bind equally well to the AP-1 site but in HeLa cells that express the inhibitory protein, v-JUN is a much stronger transcriptional activator. Thus the deletion of δ in v-JUN releases the oncoprotein from regulation by the inhibitory protein. However, JUN from which δ has been deleted is still less effective at activating transcription than v-JUN, indicating the importance of the three additional mutations present in v-JUN. JUN/FOS heterodimers do not appear to bind the inhibitory protein.

In the FOS family, although the leucine zipper and basic domains are essential for DNA binding, the regulation of transcription from AP-1 sites is also dependent on net negative charge in a C-terminal region, usually conferred by phosphorylation [8]. In both v-FOS and the truncated form of the normal protein FOS, FOSB2, the C-terminus is deleted: such proteins form dimers with JUN that bind to AP-1 but do not activate transcription from AP-1 promoters or suppress *Fos* transcription. Thus the effect of FOSB2 is to compete with normal FOS, thereby decreasing the concentration of active FOS/JUN dimers.

MYB contains transcriptional activation and negative regulatory domains as well as a domain that binds directly to the DNA sequence PyAAC$^G/_T$G to activate transcription. MYB DNA binding activity is negatively regulated via phosphorylation by casein kinase II. The cellular activity of this enzyme is increased by the action of some growth factors (e.g. insulin), although not by others (e.g. PDGF), suggesting that proliferation may involve the suppression of MYB-controlled genes. The casein kinase II phosphorylation site is in the N-terminal region of MYB but in all oncogenic forms of MYB N-terminal mutations cause the deletion of this site together with most of the negative regulatory domain. These changes result in DNA binding that is independent of a normal regulatory mechanism and in an enhanced level of transcription caused by loss of the inhibitory region. An alternative product of *Myb* (*Mbm-2*) encodes a truncated protein that retains the DNA binding and nuclear localization regions but has lost the regulatory regions required for transcriptional activation. Expression of normal *Myb* blocks differentiation whereas the effect of *Mbm-2* is to enhance differentiation. Similarly, FOSB2 possesses normal FOS binding functions but not *trans*-activation potential. Thus *Mbm-2* interferes with *Myb* function during mouse erythroid leukaemia cell differentiation and FOSB inhibits *trans*-activation by v-FOS, FOS or FOSB, acting effectively as a *trans*-negative regulator.

The MYC proteins (MYC, MYCN and MYCL) each contain basic helix–loop–helix and leucine zipper domains. Each forms heterodimers with the protein MAX (which also contains all three motifs) that bind specifically to DNA as *trans*-activating complexes. MAX expression is independent of MYC and MAX may thus regulate transcription of genes independently of MYC. The specificity of MYC–DNA interaction appears to arise from the fact that MAX is the only known helix–loop–helix protein that forms dimers with MYC. However, other leucine zipper proteins (MAD/MXI1) form heterodimers with MAX that repress transcription by binding to the MYC/MAX consensus sequence, and so the action of MYC/MAX may be regulated indirectly by the abundance of these proteins.

The DNA binding domains of the REL oncoproteins are strongly homologous to the DNA binding subunits of the NF-κB transcription factor family. v-REL thus appears to be a transcription factor but is unique in that it transforms cells equally effectively whether it is located in the cytoplasm or the nucleus. v-REL has, however, lost the strong transcription activating element in the C-terminus of REL and appears by itself to be a weak activator of transcription. C-terminal loss may promote movement to the nucleus (C-terminal removal does allow the protein to move to the nucleus but v-REL to which the C-terminus of REL has been attached remains cytoplasmic and yet still transforms). v-REL forms complexes with REL and with three proteins to which REL binds, two of which (p115/p124) may be precursors of NF-κB. Thus v-REL may deplete the cell of transcription factor precursors or bind directly to NF-κB or REL DNA target sequences. In any of these mechanisms v-REL would be acting as a dominant negative oncogene.

The v-*erbB* and v-*erbA* genes are both carried by the avian erythroblastosis virus AEV-ES4. v-*erbA* is the oncogenic homologue of *ErbA*, the thyroid hormone receptor (THR), and it increases the transforming potential of other oncogenes, including v-*erbB*. ERBA appears to be permanently bound to the THR response element. The physiological ligand for ERBA (triiodothyronine, T_3) stimulates transcription by over 50-fold. v-ERBA represses transcription to a level similar to that caused by ERBA but is insensitive to T_3. Thus v-ERBA causes sustained repression and thus apparently acts as a dominant negative oncoprotein. The N- and C-terminal truncations occurring in the conversion of *ErbA* to v-*erbA* affect only its hormone responsiveness, not its capacity to bind to DNA. An additional mutation removes a phosphorylation site from ERBA, the loss of which is essential for the effects of v-*erbA* on transformation.

SUMMARY

The nuclear proto-oncogenes fall into two major categories: those that only interact with DNA as complexes with other proteins (FOS/JUN, MYC and probably REL) and those that, in monomeric form, possess a high affinity for specific DNA sequences (ETS, MYB and ERBA). The activity as transcription factors of proteins in both of these categories can be regulated by phosphorylation, for example FOS, JUN, MYB and MYC/MAX, and this may well be a general mechanism. The modulation of the activity of relevant kinases (e.g. casein kinase II) by growth factors provides one mechanism by which transcriptional regulation mediated by these proto-oncogene products may be coupled to proliferation.

The FOS/JUN system, thus far unique in its resolved complexity, illustrates the way in which the transcriptional control exerted by various heterodimeric combinations may undergo subtle modulation during cell development or proliferation as the extent of transcription and translation of different members of the families changes.

The oncoprotein forms of many of these transcription factors have deleted C-terminal regions. This does not affect their DNA binding capacity but it invariably alters the effect that the bound protein can exert on transcription. Thus v-FOS and v-ERBA bind normally to promoter regions but v-FOS is unable to suppress *Fos* transcription and v-ERBA is insensitive to T$_3$. The effect of each is that of a dominant negative oncogene and resembles the dominant negative mutations that may occur in the tumour suppressor gene *P53* that causes the formation of complexes between mutant and wild-type p53, inhibiting the function of the latter.

It should be noted that structural modifications leading to altered transcriptional regulation are not confined to the products of oncogenes but occur during normal cell development, usually by alternative splicing. This provides a mechanism by which the biological function of a single gene can be expanded and many oncogenes and tumour suppressor genes (e.g., *Abl*, *Fos*, *Myb*, *Myc*, *APC* and *WT1*) generate more than one product by this means.

References

1 Almendral, J.M. et al. (1988) Mol. Cell. Biol. 8, 2140–2148.
2 Zipfel, P.F. et al. (1989) Mol. Cell. Biol. 9, 1041–1048.
3 **Herschman, H.R. (1991) Annu. Rev. Biochem. 60, 281–319.**
4 Minna, J.D. (1988) Lung Cancer 4, P6–P10.
5 **Hunter, T. (1991) Cell 64, 249–270.**
6 **Crews, C.M. et al. (1992) Science 258, 478–480.**
7 De Vivo, M. et al. (1992) J. Biol. Chem. 267, 18263–18266.
8 **Hunter, T. and Karin, M. (1992) Cell 70, 375–387.**

3 General consequences of oncogene expression

The epidemiology of cancer in populations strongly suggests that to drive a cell through the various stages preceding the production of a tumour *in vivo* requires the accumulation of several genetic lesions. *In vitro* cellular studies generally support the notion that transformation is at least a two-stage process, one oncogene being needed for immortalization and another for transformation. Thus, primary fibroblasts can often be transformed to a focal growth phenotype (anchorage-independent) by expression of a single oncogene (e.g. *Src*, *Ras*, *Raf*, *Mos*, *Trk*, *Fos*, *Sis* or SV40 large T antigen). Full transformation, however, generally requires the expression of two complementing oncogenes, typically *Ras* and *Myc*. For example, mutant *RAS* from human tumours only transforms embryonic rat cells when supplemented with other oncogenes in transfected cells, e.g. the E1A adenovirus gene, large T antigen of polyoma or cellular or viral *myc*. However, massive overexpression of a single gene can probably override this distinction, thus v-*myc* alone can transform embryonic cells.

In experimental animals the chemical induction of tumours generally requires the sequential application of two types of agent, an "initiator" and a "promoter". The initiator is usually a mutagen that has irreversible effects and must be administered before the promoter. These model systems indicate that the initiating event in tumorigenesis is mutation and that subsequent tumour progression may be mediated by either genetic or epigenetic mechanisms.

In humans the multi-step nature of neoplastic development may be readily distinguished in some forms of the disease. In cervical cancer the initiating event is probably infection with human papillomavirus. Subsequently cervical dysplasia (cervical intraepithelial neoplasia, CIN) may arise. CIN types I, II and III represent progressively more severe forms in the development of malignant cervical carcinoma. However, the development of an abnormal cell clone (CIN types I and II) is usually followed by its disappearance and only very infrequently does it give rise to a still more abnormal clone of fully invasive cells. The fact that smoking significantly increases the probability of cervical tumour progression indicates the importance of environmental factors that may not operate through genetic mechanisms.

Table 3. *Combinations of oncogenes frequently associated with some human cancers*

Affected loci	Tumour
APC, MCC, DCC, KRAS2, P53	Colorectal carcinoma
HRAS, MYC	Cervical carcinoma
MYB, MYC, EGFR, HER2, HRAS, P53, RB1, BRCA1, BCL1, HSTF1, INT2	Breast carcinoma
JUN, MYC, MYCN, MYCL, HRAS, RB1, P53, RAF1	Lung carcinoma
HRAS, P53, RAF1, INT2	Squamous cell carcinoma
MYC, BLYM	Burkitt's lymphoma
P53, (EGFR, MYC, MYCN, GLI, HER2, PDGFB, ROS)	Astrocytoma
ABL	Chronic myelogenous leukaemia

The detailed studies of malignant colorectal carcinomas indicate that they develop from benign adenomas in a process requiring mutation of at least four genes (Table 3) [1]. Prominent among the abnormalities that characterize colorectal carcinomas are the acquisition of mutations in *RAS* and deletions in chromosomes 5q, 18q and 17p. Although mutations in *RAS* and chromosome 17p usually appear at a relatively advanced stage of colorectal carcinoma development, the sequence in which they and the 5q (*APC* and *MCC*) and 18q (*DCC*) changes arise varies between different tumours. This fact has led to the suggestion that the development of malignant colorectal carcinoma requires an overall accumulation rather than a fixed sequence of somatic mutations. It may also be noted that, although the majority of colorectal carcinomas show mutations in *RAS* (50%), 17p (>75%) and 18q (>70%), this disease is typical of the vast majority of cancers in that there is no combination of genetic abnormalities that correlates absolutely with its development.

The region deleted in chromosome 17p in most colorectal neoplasms contains the tumour suppressor gene *P53*. Mutations in the single copy *P53* gene are the most frequent genetic changes yet shown to be associated with human cancers, and point mutations, deletions or insertions in *P53* occur in ~70% of all tumours. The rare, autosomal dominant Li–Fraumeni syndrome arises from *P53* mutations inherited through the germline [2]: 50% of the carriers develop diverse cancers by 30 years of age, compared with 1% in the normal population. In general, however, *P53* mutations are somatic and occur with high frequency in all types of lung cancer, in over 60% of breast tumours and in ~40% of brain tumours (astrocytomas), frequently in combination with the activation of other oncogenes (Table 3). Nevertheless, as observed previously and despite the high frequency of *P53* mutations, individual forms of cancer are not generally characterized by a specific combination of genetic defects.

The most notable exception to the pattern of variable expression of cancer genes in histologically identical tumours is provided by the retinoblastoma gene (*RB1*), both alleles of which are defective in all retinoblastomas. However, inactivation of this tumour suppressor gene also occurs in other neoplasms (Table 3), e.g. Wilms' kidney tumour, breast cancer and small cell lung carcinoma (SCLC), and individuals with retinoblastoma are particularly susceptible to the development of sarcomas. The frequency of *RB1* inactivation in tumours other than retinoblastoma varies widely. It is mutated with high frequency in SCLCs and most osteosarcomas and soft tissue sarcomas: in non-SCLCs (e.g. adenocarcinomas, squamous cell carcinomas or large cell carcinomas), however, *RB1* mutations are infrequent although some tumours of this type have been shown to be defective in both *RB1* and *P53*. *P53* mutations are common in some non-SCLCs (squamous cell carcinomas) but not in others (adenocarcinomas), whereas chromosomal deletions affecting *HRAS*, *RAF1* and *INT2* are relatively common (occurring in 18–50% of cases examined) in both these types of SCLC.

In breast cancer, bladder cancer and some other adenocarcinomas there is a correlation between the degree of *HER2* overexpression and tumour stage. In one study *HER2* expression has been shown to be inversely correlated with the expression of *MYB*. Overexpression of the EGF receptor (*EGFR*) has been reported to be associated with oestrogen-receptor negative breast tumours: thus *EGFR* and *MYB* expression provide indicators of a poor or good prognosis, respectively.

Deletion of genes is also relatively common in human breast cancer. Inactivation of the breast cancer gene *BRCA1* on chromosome 17q, a putative tumour suppressor gene, occurs in the majority of cases and the *RB1* gene is inactivated in ~20% of primary carcinomas. In ~65% of cases there is allelic loss of the *P53* gene on chromosome 17. The retained *P53* allele frequently contains point mutations although some tumours retain one normal allele. Between 20% and 50% of breast carcinomas contain non-random loss of heterozygosity for specific locations on chromosomes 1q, 3p or 11p at which specific genes have not been identified and virtually all chromosomes show some susceptibility to allelic imbalance either as an increase in allele copy number (~25%) or as loss of heterozygosity [3].

The *EGFR* gene is also amplified in cell lines derived from squamous carcinomas, glioblastomas and bladder carcinomas. *MYC*, *MYCL* and *MYCN* amplification is frequently associated with both breast carcinomas and lung tumours. In breast carcinomas the combination of enhanced *MYC* and *HER2* expression is indicative of a particularly poor prognosis. Amplification of *MYC* is almost invariably associated with the translocation occurring in Burkitt's lymphoma and is accompanied by the activation of the transforming gene *BLYM1*.

A variety of lymphoid neoplasms are frequently associated with chromosomal translocations where the breakpoints are adjacent to the *BCL* genes. The region containing *BCL1* is also amplified in approximately 20% of breast and squamous cell carcinomas. In breast carcinomas *BCL1* is usually co-amplified with *HSTF1* and *INT2* and, in a very small proportion of cases, with *SEA* which is located on the same chromosome. The proteins encoded by these genes have not been fully characterized, however, and evidence for their involvement in tumorigenesis remains circumstantial.

Table 4. *Individual proto-oncogenes activated in human cancers*

Proto-oncogene	Method of identification
Abl, ErbB-1, Myc, Hras-1, Kras-2, Src	Retrovirus
ABL, BEK, EGFR, HER2 , HER3, FGR, FLG, FPS, GLI, JUN, MET, MYB, MYC, MYCN, MYCL, PIM1, KRAS2, YES	Amplification
DBL, EPH, ETS1, FOS, FPS/FES, FYN, KIT, LCK, SEA	Overexpression
ABL, BCL1, BCL2, BCL3, BCR, BTG1, CAN, DEK, ETS1, ELK, ERG, FLI1, HOX11, LCK, LYL1, MLL, MOS, MYC, PML, PVT1, RBTN1, RBTN2, REL, SET, SIL, TAL1, TAL2, TAN1	Translocation
BLYM, HSTF1, LCA, MAS, MCF3, MET, HER2, RAF, NRAS, RET, TRK, TLM	Transfection
GSP, GIP2	Adenylyl cyclase activity

The chromosome translocation involving *ABL* occurs in over 95% of cases of chronic myelogenous leukaemia (CML) and in 25% of adult acute lymphocytic leukaemias. The translocation involves the loss of N-terminal ABL sequences (as happens during retroviral transduction when *Abl* is juxtaposed to viral *gag*) and the activation of the ABL protein tyrosine kinase. The *ABL* gene is also amplified tenfold in CML. There is clear evidence for the involvement of the *RAS* family (*HRAS, KRAS2* and *NRAS*) in a wide range of cancers. In all cancers the average incidence of *RAS* mutations is approximately 15% but in pancreatic carcinomas, for example, *KRAS2* mutations occur in 95% of tumours. In general, mutations in *RAS* reduce its GTPase activity, the oncogenic protein thus remaining in an active, GTP-bound state. One consequence of this would be the sustained activation of the RAF–MAP kinase pathway (see Fig. 2, page 14). *GSP* and *GIP2* are also genes the products of which regulate GTPase activity: for *GSP* and *GIP2*, however, oncogenic mutations cause a sustained elevation of cAMP that appears to promote thyroid carcinomas and ovarian tumours. Point mutations in *RET* (which encodes receptor tyrosine kinases) occur in familial medullary thyroid carcinoma and in multiple endocrine neoplasia types 2A and 2B. *RET* appears to be the first gene detected in which dominantly acting point mutations initiate human hereditary neoplasia.

All of the oncogenes included in Table 4 have been shown to be activated in at least one type of human tumour. However, with the exception of *ABL* in CML and *RET*, the frequency of their involvement varies widely and for a considerable number (e.g. *YES*) is confined to isolated reports.

References
1 **Fearon, E.R. and Vogelstein, B. (1990) Cell 61, 759-767.**
2 Srivastava, S. et al. (1990) Nature 348, 747-749.
3 Devilee, P. et al. (1991) Oncogene 6, 1705-1711.

4 Metastasis

A characteristic feature of malignant cells is their capacity to invade adjacent tissues. Subsequently, malignant tumours frequently spread to distant locations and this event, leading to the establishment of secondary tumours at sites remote from the primary tumour is known as metastasis. Not all invasive tumours metastasize but all metastatic tumours have developed via invasion. In addition to local invasion, crucial steps in the development of metastases include the detachment of cells from the primary tumour, their invasion of a blood vessel and their subsequent entrapment at secondary sites. The expression of a considerable number of genes in a variety of experimental systems has been shown to affect metastatic capacity (Table 5). However, it seems probable that many of these effects were indirect and attention has therefore focused on changes specific to tumour cells in the expression of cell surface adhesion molecules and of proteolytic enzymes that might be involved in degradation of the basement membrane. The major families of such proteins are (a) cadherins, (b) integrins, (c) tissue inhibitors of metalloproteinases (TIMPs) which, together with the serine, cysteine and aspartic proteinases and heparanase, regulate the activation of matrix metalloproteinases (MMPs), and (d) the putative metastasis-suppressor genes *NME1* and *NME2*.

Table 5. *Gene products modulating metastasis* in vivo *or* in vitro

Metastasis enhancement	Metastasis suppression
CD44, JUNB, FPS, MYC, RAS, NEU, TGFβ, Hepatocyte growth factor (HGF), HSTF1 Acidic fibroblast growth factor (aFGF),v-SRC, SV40 T Ag, HPV E6, HPV E7, Integrins	FOS, JUN, IL2, IL6, IFNγ, NME1/NME2, TIMPs, Plasminogen activator inhibitors (PAIs), Gelsolin, suramin, tropomyosin 1, Adenovirus 5 E1A (*Neu*-transformed cells), E-cadherin, Integrins

CADHERINS

Cadherins are a multigene family of transmembrane glycoproteins that mediate Ca^{2+}-dependent intercellular adhesion, cytoskeletal anchoring and signalling, and are thought to be essential for the control of morphogenetic processes, including myogenesis [1]. The family includes B-cadherin, E-cadherin (also known as uvomorulin (*UVO*), *Arc-1* or cell-CAM 120/80), EP-cadherin, M-cadherin, N-cadherin (A-CAM), P-cadherin, R-cadherin, T-cadherin, U-cadherin, cadherins 4–11 and L-CAM. Cadherin function is regulated by cytoplasmic proteins including a vinculin-like protein, α-catenin (or CAP102), and β-catenin, a homologue of plakoglobulin. Catenins undergo tyrosine phosphorylation in cells transformed by v-*src* that correlates with metastatic potential and may reflect the modulation of cell–cell adhesion [2]. Furthermore, the tumour suppressor gene product APC binds to the catenins and catenin–APC complexes may play a role in regulating cell growth and/or metastasis (see **Tumour Suppressor Genes: *APC*, *MCC***).

The loss of cell–cell adhesion caused by the selective downregulation of E-cadherin expression can cause de-differentiation and invasiveness of human carcinoma cells. Impaired E-cadherin expression has been detected in 53% of a sample of primary breast cancers [3]. Human cell lines derived from bladder, breast, lung and pancreatic carcinomas that have an epithelioid phenotype are non-invasive and express E-cadherin but those with a fibroblastoid phenotype are invasive and have lost E-cadherin expression. Invasiveness is blocked by transfection with E-cadherin cDNA and re-induced by treatment of the transfected cells with anti-E-cadherin monoclonal antibodies. The expression of E-cadherin-specific antisense RNA in non-invasive *RAS*-transformed cells with high endogenous E-cadherin expression renders the cells invasive. Furthermore, some invasive cells that retain E-cadherin on their surface appear to block its function by expressing enlarged proteoglycans [4]. E-Cadherin protein expression is also lost in primary hepatocellular carcinomas, metastatic squamous cell carcinomas and prostate cancers and mRNA levels are lower in squamous cell carcinoma lines than in normal keratinocytes, whereas P-cadherin levels are similar. In gastric carcinomas, however, P-cadherin expression is either downregulated or unstable whereas that of E-cadherin is normal. Expression of E-cadherin inhibits the migration of cells into three-dimensional collagen gels and, taken together, these observations suggest that E-cadherin and possibly other members of the family act as invasion suppressors.

INTEGRINS

The integrins are a family of cell-surface proteins that mediate cell–substratum and cell–cell adhesion [5,6]. Integrins are heterodimers of non-covalently linked α and β subunits, each of which is a transmembrane protein. Eleven α and six β subunits have been identified that give rise to at least 16 distinct integrins and, in addition, a single α or β subunit can associate with more than one β or α chain, respectively. Although no integrin has yet been shown to be a tumour suppressor gene, they mediate some of the processes involved in metastasis and changes in integrin expression accompany malignant transformation. Thus, loss of α_1, α_2 or α_3 expression and enhanced expression of α_v occur frequently in lung cancer and both loss and aberrant expression of various integrins has been detected in breast and colon cancers. However, thus far it has been difficult to discern correlations between altered patterns of integrin expression and tumorigenicity.

In some cells *in vivo* tumorigenicity is reduced by the expression of the $\alpha_5\beta_1$ integrin (fibronectin) receptor. However, the capacity of human lung adenocarcinoma cells to adhere to endothelial cells is increased when the latter are treated with IL1. This increases the expression of both the fibronectin receptor and the vitronectin receptor ($\alpha_v\beta_3$-integrin) and the latter appears to be responsible for the increased adhesiveness of the cells [7]. In lung carcinomas, particularly small cell lung carcinoma, upregulation of integrin α_{RLC}, which is closely related to integrin α_4, is a frequent occurrence [8].

Human melanoma cells are stimulated to proliferate by fibronectin acting *via* the $\alpha_5\beta_1$ receptor and the tumorigenicity of these cells correlates with the expression of $\alpha_v\beta_3$-integrin. The invasiveness *in vitro* of human melanoma cells is inhibited by antibody directed against $\alpha_v\beta_3$-integrin that also inhibits the adhesive activity of the receptor [9]. However, an anti-α_v antibody that does not affect adhesive capacity also promotes invasion, as does the ligand vitronectin. This suggests that ligation of the vitronectin receptor activates a cellular response that promotes invasion by melanoma cells through the basement membrane matrices, a conclusion consistent with the finding that these cells increase secretion of type IV collagenase in response to $\alpha_v\beta_3$ antibody.

In primary breast carcinomas the expression of $\alpha_6\beta_4$-integrin is either reduced or modulated such that the polarized pattern of distribution at the basolateral aspect of the epithelium occurring in normal tissue is lost [10]. However, increased expression of β_4 or loss of α_2, α_3 and α_6 has been detected in some squamous cell carcinomas [11]. The expression of a functional $\alpha_2\beta_1$-integrin receptor in rhabdomyosarcoma cells correlates with increased formation of metastatic tumours in nude mice [12] and there is evidence that the expression of β_3-integrin correlates with melanoma metastasis [13]. In contrast, reduced expression of $\alpha_2\beta_1$-integrins (and $\alpha_5\beta_1$) has been detected in severe cases of cervical intraepithelial neoplasia with HPV infection [14]. In human E1A-transformed tumour cells the overexpression of active TGFβ1 enhances the tumorigenicity of the cells in nude mice and causes increased adhesiveness *in vitro* that correlates with the increased expression of $\alpha_1\beta_1$-, $\alpha_2\beta_1$- and $\alpha_3\beta_1$-integrins, all of which recognize laminin [15]. TGFβ has also been shown to exert a less strong growth-inhibitory effect on melanoma cells than on normal melanocytes [16] and to stimulate normal fibroblasts to induce apoptosis of transformed counterparts [17].

The aggregation of platelets mediated by the binding of fibrinogen to $\alpha_{IIb}\beta_3$-integrin stimulates the tyrosine phosphorylation and kinase activity of p125^{FAK} and p125^{FAK} phosphorylation has been observed in a variety of other types of cells undergoing attachment to extracellular matrix proteins [18]. p125^{FAK} is also activated by v-*src* transformation and by a number of normal growth factors, including bombesin, vasopressin or endothelin [19] but not by oncogenic *Ras* [20]. Thus pp125^{FAK} and truncated forms of FAK termed FRNK (FAK-related non-kinase), both of which are localized in focal adhesions [21], may mediate signals initiated by integrin-dependent cell adhesion and by growth factors as well as providing a cytoplasmic target for tyrosine kinase oncoproteins.

TISSUE INHIBITORS OF METALLOPROTEINASES (TIMPS)

Cell lines with high metastatic capacity synthesize abnormally large amounts of matrix metalloproteinases (MMPs). The MMP family includes interstitial collagenase, type IV collagenase, gelatinases and stromelysins. These enzymes are secreted as zymogens and activated by plasmin. Activated MMPs are subject to regulation by TIMPs that are present in normal bone and cartilage cells and secreted by a variety of cells in culture. Plasmin is itself generated from its plasma zymogen by plasminogen activators, the two major forms of which are tissue plasminogen activator (t-PA) and urokinase-type plasminogen activator (u-PA), both being serine proteinases (Fig. 7).

The expression of t-PA shows no specific correlation with tumour or benign cells, whereas high expression of u-PA (and PAI-1) has been detected in a variety of malignant tissues, including breast tumours, brain tumours and melanomas, and blockade of the u-PA receptor has been shown to inhibit *in vivo* tumour cell invasiveness [22-26].

The 72 kDa and 95 kDa forms of gelatinase are synthesized by *RAS*-transformed human bronchial epithelial cells and other tumorigenic cells [27,28]. Stromelysins, that synergize with gelatinase in matrix degradation, are also synthesized by some

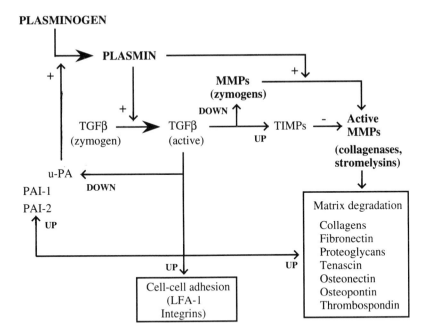

Figure 7. *Regulation of the activity of cell adhesion proteins by plasmin and transforming growth factor β. MMPs: matrix metalloproteinases; TIMPs: tissue inhibitors of metalloproteinases; u-PA: urokinase-type plasminogen activator; PAI: plasminogen activator inhibitor; LFA-1: lymphocyte function associated antigen 1; + = activator; – = inhibitor; UP = upregulation; DOWN = downregulation.*

tumour cells [29]. The observations appear consistent with the finding that the induction of plasminogen activator inhibitor 1 (PAI-1) by TGFβ is transient in carcinoma cells and sustained in normal cells, thereby leading to increased matrix dissolution by active MMPs secreted by the invasive cells [30].

TIMP-1 forms a stoichiometric inactivating complex with MMPs. TIMP-1 is expressed at elevated levels in some malignant non-Hodgkin's lymphomas, the amounts correlating with tumour aggressiveness [31]. The transfection of Swiss 3T3 fibroblasts with a vector conferring constitutive expression of TIMP antisense deoxyoligonucleotide renders the cells tumorigenic and metastatic in mice. Transfection of tumour cells with a vector expressing TIMP-2 decreases the activity of secreted MMPs and the growth rate of the cells *in vivo* as well as suppressing the invasive capacity of the cells for surrounding tissue [32,33]. However, the expression of TIMP also increases transcription of several proteinases, and of the Ca^{2+} binding proteins osteopontin (OPN), SPP and calcyclin [34]. Although the significance of these effects is unclear, OPN expression has been detected in TPA-treated epidermal cells and in *Ras*-transformed cell lines, the tumorigenicity of the latter being reduced by expression of antisense OPN DNA [35]. TIMP-3 promotes the detachment of cells from the extracellular matrix and may promote the development of the transformed phenotype [36].

The cysteine proteinases degrade matrix protein *in vitro* and there is evidence that one of these proteinases, cathepsin L, is overexpressed on metastatic melanoma cells compared with normal melanocytes and that carcinoma-derived cells can secrete mature forms of cathepsins L and B [37,38]. Cathepsin L is also highly expressed in *Ras*-transformed fibroblasts. The lysosomal aspartic proteinsase cathepsin D is overexpressed in most primary breast cancers, undergoing abnormal secretion as a pro-enzyme. Overexpression of the human gene increases metastasis in nude mice [39]. Heparanase, a heparan sulphate-specific endo-β–D-glucuronidase, is involved in metastasis of malignant melanoma cells and is inhibited by suramin [40].

NME1 AND NME2

NME1 (*non-m*etastatic cells 1, *e*xpressed) and *NME2* (formerly *NM23* (non-metastatic 23)) encode nucleoside diphosphate (NDP) kinases expressed on the cell surface. The concentration of NDP kinase A (encoded by human *NME1* and 88% identical to NDP kinase B (*NME2*)) increases in proliferating normal cells [41] and reduced *NM23* expression correlates with high metastatic potential in some tumours and cell lines. The transfection of human or murine *NME1* cDNA reduces primary tumour formation and metastasis *in vivo* [42]. However, *NM23* expression is increased in some neoplastic tissues, although in ductal breast carcinomas this increase does not appear to correlate with tumour size, oestrogen or progesterone receptor expression, lymph node metastases or other prognostic factors [43]. Amplification and overexpression of *NM23* has been detected in childhood neuroblastomas, but this is accompanied by a point mutation in the gene and mutations have also been detected in colorectal adenocarcinoma [44,45].

References
1 **Takeichi, M. (1991) Science 251, 1451–1455.**
2 Hamaguchi, M. et al. (1993) EMBO J. 12, 307–314.
3 Oka, H. et al. (1993) Cancer Res. 53, 1696–1701.
4 Vleminckx, K. et al. (1994) Cancer Res. 54, 873–877.
5 Hynes, R.O. (1992) Cell 69, 11–25.
6 Pigott, R. and Power, C. (1993) The Adhesion Molecule FactsBook, Academic Press, London.
7 Lafrenie, R.M. et al. (1992) Cancer Res. 52, 2202–2208.
8 Hibi, K. et al. (1994) Oncogene 9, 611–619.
9 Seftor, R.E.B. et al. (1992) Proc. Natl Acad. Sci. USA 89, 1557–1561.
10 Natali, P.G. et al. (1992) Br. J. Cancer 66, 318–322.
11 Waleh, N.S. et al. (1994) Cancer Res. 54, 838–843.
12 Chan, B.M.C. et al. (1991) Science 251, 1600–1602.
13 Albeda, S.M. et al. (1990) Cancer Res. 50, 6757–6764.
14 Hodivala, K.J. et al. (1994) Oncogene 9, 943–948.
15 Arrick, B.A. et al. (1992) J. Cell Biol. 118, 715–726.
16 Rodeck, U. et al. (1994) Cancer Res. 54, 575–581.
17 Jurgensmeier, J.M. et al. (1994) Cancer Res. 54, 393–398.
18 Lipfert, L. et al. (1992) J. Cell. Biol. 119, 905–912.
19 Zachary, I. et al. (1992) J. Biol. Chem. 267, 19031–19034.
20 Guan, J.-L. and Shalloway, D. (1992) Nature 358, 690–692.
21 Schaller, M.D. et al. (1993) Mol. Cell. Biol. 13, 785–791.
22 Jankun, J. et al. (1993) J. Cell. Biochem. 53, 135–144.

23 Montgomery, A.M.P. et al. (1993) Cancer Res. 53, 693–700.

24 Crowley, C.W. et al. (1993) Proc. Natl Acad. Sci. USA. 90, 5021–5025.

25 Landau, B.J. et al. (1994) Cancer Res. 54, 1105–1108.

26 **Blasi, F. (1993) BioEssays 15, 105–111.**

27 Collier, I.E. et al. (1988) J. Biol. Chem. 263, 6579–6587.

28 Yamagata, S. et al. (1989) Biochem. Biophys. Res. Commun. 158, 228–234.

29 Matrisian, L.M. et al. (1986). Proc. Natl Acad. Sci. USA 83, 9413–9417.

30 Keski-Oja, J. et al. (1988) J. Biol. Chem. 263, 3111–3115.

31 Kossakowska, A.E. et al. (1991) Blood 77, 2475–2481.

32 Curry, V.A. et al. (1992) Biochem. J. 285, 143–147.

33 DeClerck, Y.A. et al. (1992) Cancer Res. 52, 701–708.

34 Khokha, R. et al. (1992) J. Natl Cancer Inst. 84, 1017–1022.

35 Behrend, E.I. et al. (1994) Cancer Res. 54, 832–837.

36 Yang, T.-T. and Hawkes, S.P. (1992) Proc. Natl Acad. Sci. USA 89, 10676–10680.

37 Rozhin, J. et al. (1989) Biochem. Biophys. Res. Commun. 164, 556–561.

38 Maciewicz, R.A. et al. (1989). Int. J. Cancer 43, 478–486.

39 Liaudet, E. et al. (1994) Oncogene 9, 1145–1154.

40 Nakajima, M. et al. (1991) J. Biol. Chem. 266, 9661–9666.

41 Keim, D. et al. (1992) J. Clin. Invest. 89, 919–924.

42 Leone, A. et al. (1993b) Oncogene 8, 2325–2333.

43 Sastre-Garau, X. et al. (1992) Int. J. Cancer 50, 533–538.

44 Leone, A. et al. (1993a) Oncogene 8, 855–865.

45 Wang, L. et al. (1993) Cancer Res. 53, 717–720.

5 Gene therapy for cancer

The facility with which exogenous genes may be introduced into somatic cells offers in principle the possibility of effective treatment for most if not all cancers. Thus far the main approaches have utilized either (i) antisense oligode-oxynucleotides, (ii) drug targeting, (iii) the production of cytokines, or (iv) the introduction of genes the expression of which reverses the effects of dominant oncogenes or of mutated tumour suppressor genes [1]. Virtually all applications directed towards human cancers have utilized retroviral vectors for gene transduction [2]. This method uses non-infectious virions that can transfer exogenous genes with high efficiency (30–50%) and precise integration into the DNA of almost all types of eukaryotic cell. Four principal types of application employing these techniques have so far shown promise as forms of anti-cancer therapy: virally directed enzyme prodrug therapy, tumour infiltrating cells, antisense oligodeoxynucleotides and modulation of metastatic potential.

VIRALLY DIRECTED ENZYME PRODRUG THERAPY

The incorporation of specific promoters into retroviral vectors has led to the technique of virally directed enzyme prodrug therapy (VDEPT). This has been used, for example, to permit the expression of herpes simplex thymidine kinase specifically in hepatoma cells through the activation of the α-fetoprotein promoter [3]. The prodrug 6-methoxypurine arabinonucleoside (araM) is a good substrate for thymidine kinase and is converted to the cytotoxic metabolite araATP within the tumour cells.

TUMOUR INFILTRATING CELLS

Genetic modification of tumour infiltrating lymphocytes (TIL) has been accomplished by transduction of a retroviral vector expressing an active tumour necrosis factor (TNF) gene into cells from patients with melanoma [4]. TILs have been grown *in vitro* in the presence of IL2 from tumour cell samples from a wide variety of human cancers, including colon, breast, bladder, melanoma, renal, lymphoma and neuroblastoma. TILs infiltrate and accumulate within developing tumours and hence high local concentrations of synthesized, diffusible cytokine encoded by the vector are delivered to the site of the tumour without requirement for high systemic doses. The administration of TNF–TIL together with IL2 has been effective in causing tumour regression in patients with melanoma and this technique is clearly suitable for the introduction of other cytokines and agents of potential therapeutic value into TIL.

ANTISENSE OLIGODEOXYNUCLEOTIDES

Antisense oligodeoxynucleotides expressed from transduced retroviral vectors have been used to modulate the tumorigenicity or metastatic potential of a number of oncogenes including *ABL*, *MYB*, *MYC*, *MYCN*, *RAF1*, *RAS*, *SCL*, *Src*, HPV E7, *RB1* and *P53* (see individual oncogene sections).

MODULATION OF METASTATIC POTENTIAL

The expression of a variety of genes has been shown either to modulate the metastatic potential of transformed cells or to cause their reversion to a normal phenotype. Thus in some cells *in vivo* tumorigenicity is reduced by the expression from retroviral vectors of the *JE*/MCP-1 gene [5], *NM23* [6] or $\alpha_5\beta_1$-integrin (fibronectin receptor) [7]. *In vitro* invasiveness is decreased when the highly metastatic cell line B16-F10 is transfected with a plasmid expressing βm-actin [8]. Furthermore, the expression of antisense RNA directed against the cell adhesion molecule E-cadherin or against tissue inhibitors of metalloproteinases (TIMP) can confer metastatic capacity (see above). The expression of anti-sense oligodeoxynucleotide directed against human type I regulatory subunit (RIα) of the cAMP-dependent protein kinase arrests the growth of human and rodent cancer cells *in vitro* and antisense RIIα blocks cAMP-inducible growth inhibition and differentiation. Cell growth is also inhibited by retroviral vector expression of RIIβ [9].

Genes the expression of which induces reversion of transformed cells to a normal morphology include *Krev*-1/*rap*1 in *Kras-2* transformed cells (see **RAS**) and wild-type genes inserted to replace defective copies of the tumour suppressor genes *P53*, retinoblastoma, Wilms' kidney tumour or neurofibromatosis type 1 (see **Tumour Suppressor Genes**).

RIBOZYMES

In addition to these methods the design of ribozymes to cleave specific transcripts offers a further possibility for genetic therapy. This has been demonstrated by the ribozyme-mediated cleavage of *BCR–ABL* transcripts *in vitro* and by the elimination of P210$^{BCR\text{-}ABL}$ protein kinase activity in the chronic myelogenous leukaemia blast crisis cell line K562 [10].

References
1 **Gutierrez, A.A. et al. (1992) Lancet 339, 715–721.**
2 **Miller, A.D. (1992) Nature 357, 455–460.**
3 Huber, B.E. et al. (1991) Proc. Natl Acad. Sci. USA. 88, 8039–8043.
4 **Rosenberg, S.A. (1992) J. Clin. Oncol. 10, 180–199.**
5 Rollins, B.J. and Sunday, M.E. (1991) Mol. Cell. Biol. 11, 3125–3131.
6 Leone, A. et al. (1991). Cell 65, 25–35.
7 Giancotti, F.G. and Ruoslahti, E. (1990) Cell 60, 849–859.
8 Sadano, H. et al. (1990) FEBS Lett. 271, 23–27.
9 Cho-Chung, Y.S. et al. (1991) Life Sci. 48, 1123–1132.
10 Shore, S.K. et al. (1993) Oncogene 8, 3183–3188.

6 Summary tables

Table 1. *Oncogenes transduced by retroviruses*

Gene/locus	Activating virus	Associated tumours
Abl	Ab-MuLV/HZ2-FeSV	T lymphoid/sarcoma
Akt	AKT8	Thymoma
Cbl	Cas NS-1	B lymphomas
Cyl-1	MuLV	Lymphomas
Crk	ASV CT10	Sarcoma
ErbA/ErbB	AEV-ES4	Erythroid
ErbB	ALV/RPL25/RPL28	Erythroid
Ets	AEV E26	Erythroid
Fgr	GR-FeSV	Sarcoma
Fms	SM-FeSV and HZ5-FeSV	Sarcoma
Fos	FBJ and FBR MuSV	Sarcoma
Fps/Fes	FSV	Sarcoma
Jun	ASV 17	T lymphomas
Kit	HZ4-FeSV	Sarcoma
Maf	AS42	Sarcoma
Mos	Mo-MuSV	B lymphoid/sarcoma
Mpl	MyLV	Erythroid
Myc	ALV, MuLV, REV, FeLV	T and B cell lymphomas
Myb	MuLV, ALV	B lymphoid, myeloid
Raf/Mil/*Mht*	MuSV	Carcinoma/lymphoma
Hras	ALV	Nephroblastic
Kras	F-MuLV	Erythroid
Qin	ASV 31	Sarcoma
Rel	REV	B lymphomas
Ros	ASV UR2	Sarcoma
Ryk	RPL30	Sarcoma
Sea	AEV-S13	Erythroid/sarcoma
Sis	SSV	Glioblastoma
Ski	SKV	Carcinoma
Src	RSV	Sarcoma
Yes	Esh and Y73	Sarcoma

AEV: avian erythroblastosis virus; AKT8: leukaemia virus isolated from lymphomatous AKR mice; ALV: avian leukosis virus; ASV: avian sarcoma virus; FeLV: feline leukaemia virus; F-MuLV: Friend murine leukaemia virus; FSV: Fujinami sarcoma virus; GaLV: gibbon ape leukaemia virus; G-MuLV: Gross murine leukaemia virus; GR-FeSV: Gardner–Rasheed feline sarcoma virus; HZ4-FeSV: Hardy–Zuckerman 4 feline sarcoma virus; Mo-MuLV: Moloney murine leukaemia virus; MMTV: mouse mammary tumour virus; MuSV: murine sarcoma virus; MyLV: myeloproliferative leukaemia virus; REV: reticuloendotheliosis virus; RPL30: acute avian retrovirus; RSV: Rous sarcoma virus; SFFV: spleen focus forming virus; SKV: Sloan–Kettering virus; SM-FeSV: Susan McDonough feline sarcoma virus; SSV: simian sarcoma virus.

Genes shown in bold type are described in individual entries in Section II. For summaries/references for genes shown in plain type see R. Hesketh, *The Oncogene Handbook*, Academic Press, 1994.

Table 2. *Oncogenes activated by retroviral insertion*

Gene/locus	Chromosomal location	Activating virus/system	Associated tumours
A. Mouse mammary tumour virus			
Hst-1/kFGF	7	BR6	Mammary
Wnt-1 (*Int-1*) and *Int-2*	15	BALB/cfC3H; BR6; C3H; GR; GRf; C3Hf; *Mus cervicolor*	Mammary
Int-3	17	BR6; Czech II	Mammary
Wnt-3 (*Int-4*)	11	BALB/cfC3H; GR	Mammary
Int-5	9	BALB/c	Mammary
B. Murine leukaemia viruses			
Ahi-1	10	Mo-MuLV (Abelson)	Pre-B cell
Bla-1	?	Eµ-*myc* transgenics	B cell
Bmi-1/Bup	2	Eµ-*myc* transgenics	B cell
Pal-1	5	Eµ-*myc* transgenics	B cell
CSF-1	3	BALB/c eco	Monocytic
Dsi-1	4	Mo-MuLV (rat)	T cell
Evi-2	11	MuLV (BXH-2)	Myeloid
Fim-1	13	F-MuLV	Myeloid
*Fim-2/**Fms***	18	F-MuLV	Myeloid
Fim-3 (or *Evi-1* or *CB-1*)	3	F-MuLV	Myeloid
Fis-1 (or *Cyl-1*)	7	F-MuLV	Myeloid, lymphoid
Fli-1	9	F-MuLV	Erythroid
Gin-1	19	Gross A	T cell
Lck	4	Mo-MuLV	T cell
Mlvi-1 (or *Pvt, Mis-1* or *RMO-int-1*)	15	AKR; AKXD; Mo-MuLV (rat)	T cell
Mlvi-2, -3, -4	15	Mo-MuLV (rat)	T cell
Myb	10	Mo-MuLV (Abelson); Cas-Br-M	Myeloid NFS-60 cell line
Myc	15	AKR; AKXD; Gross A; MCF247; MCF69L1; Mo-MuLV (rat); Soule; Eµ-*pim-1* transgenics	T cell
Nmyc-1	12	MCF247; Mo-MuLV Eµ-*pim-1* transgenics	T cell
Pim-1	17	AKR; AKXD; MCF247; MCF1233; MCF69L1	T cell
		AKXD	Non-T cell
		ΔMo-MuLV + SV	B lymphoblastic
Pim-2	17	AKXD; Mo-MuLV; Transplanted	T cell
Hras	7	Mo-MuLV	T cell
Kras	6	F-MuLV	Myeloid
Sic-1	9	Cas-Br-E MuLV	Non-B, non-T cell
Spi-1	2	SFFV	Erythroid
P53	11	F-MuLV; SFFV	Erythroid
		Abelson MuLV	Lymphoid
*Tpl-1/**Ets-1***	9	Mo-MuLV	T cell
Vin-1	6	RadLV	T cell

Table 2. *Continued*

Gene/locus	Activating virus/system	Associated tumours
C. Avian retroviruses		
Bic	UR2AV + RAV-2	Lymphomas
Erbb	RAV-1	Erythroblastosis
Myb	RAV-1; EU-8;	Lymphomas
	UR2AV + RAV-2	
Myc	ALV; REV (CSV); RPV	B lymphomas
	RPV	Adenocarcinoma
	REV	T lymphoma
Nov	MAV1	Myeloblastosis
Hras	MAV	Nephroblastoma
Blym	ALV	B lymphoma
Rel	ALV	B lymphoma
D. Other systems		
Erythropoietin receptor	SFFV	Erythroid
Flvi-1	FeLV	T cell
His-1, His-2	CasBr Mo-MuLV (IL3-dependent)	Myeloid
Hox-2.4	IAP	WEHI-3B
IL2	GaLV	T cell line
IL3	IAP	WEHI-3B
IL2R	IAP	Lymphoma cell line
Mos	IAP	Plasmacytoma
Myc	IAP	Plasmacytoma
Myc	F-MuLV	T cell
Myc	Retrotransposon	Canine
Pim-1	F-MuLV	T cell

Source: Peters, G. (1990) Cell Growth Differ. 1, 503–510.

Abbreviations are given in the legend to Table 1 (RadLV: BL.VL3 radiation leukaemia virus; IAP: intracisternal A particle).

Genes shown in bold type are described in individual entries in Section II. For summaries/references for genes shown in plain type see R. Hesketh, *The Oncogene Handbook*, Academic Press, 1994.

Table 3. *Oncogenes at chromosomal translocations*

Gene (chromosome)	Translocation	Leukaemia
ABL (9q34.1) **BCR** (22q11)	(9;22)(q34;q11)	CML
ALK (2p23) [1] NPM (5q35)	(2;5)(p23;q35)	Non-Hodgkin's lymphoma
AML1 (21q22) [2,3] ETO (8q22) MTG8 (8)	(8;21)(q22;q22)	AML
AML1 (21q22) [4] EAP (3q26) EVI1 (3q26) [5]	(3;21)(q26;q22)	CML, Myelodysplasia
ATF1 (12q13) [6] EWS (22q12)	(12;22)(q13;q12)	Malignant melanoma of soft parts (MMSP)
BCL1 (11q13.3) IgH (14q32)	(11;14)(q13;q32)	B cell lymphomas, B-CLL, multiple myeloma
BCL2 (18q21.3) IgH (14q32)	(14;18)(q32;q21)	Non-Hodgkin's lymphoma
BCL3 (19q13.1) IgH (14q32)	(14;19)(q32;q13)	B-CLL
BCL6 (3q27) [7] IgH (14q32)	(3;14)(q27;q32) (3;22)(q27;q11)	Non-Hodgkin's lymphoma
BTG1 (12q22) [8] Deletion	(8;12)(q24;q22)	B-CLL
CAN (6p23) [9] DEK (9q34) SET (9q34) [10]	(6;9)(p23;q34)	AML
CBFB (16q22) [11] MYH11 (16p13.12–p13.13)	inv(16)(p13q22)	AML
ERG (21q22.3) EWS (22q12)	(22;21)(q12;q22)	Ewing's sarcoma
FLI1 (11q24) EWS (22q12)	(11;22)(q24;q12)	Ewing's sarcoma
HLF (17q22) [12] E2A (19p13.3)	(17;19)(q22;p13)	Pre-B ALL
HOX11 (10q24) [13] TCRD (14q11.2) TCRB (7q35)	(10;14)(q24;q11) (7;10)(q35;q24)	T-ALL
IL2 (4q26) [14] BCM (16p13)	(4;16)(q26;p13)	T cell lymphoma
IL3 (5q31) [15] IgH (14q32)	(5;14)(q31;q32)	Acute pre-B cell

Table 3. *Continued*

Gene (chromosome)	Translocation	Leukaemia
LCK (1p34) TCRB (7q35)	(1;7)(p34;q35)	T-ALL
LAZ3 (3q27) [16] IgH (14q32)	(3;14)(q27;q32) (3;4)(q27;p11)	Non-Hodgkin's lymphoma
LYL1 (19p13.2) [17] TCRB (7q35)	(7;19)(q35;p13)	T cell leukaemia line
LYT10 (NFκB2: 10q24) [18] IgH (14q32)	(10;14)(q24;q32)	B lymphoma T lymphoma Multiple myeloma
MLL /ALL1/HRX (11q23) [19] AF4 (4q21) [20]	(4;11)(q21;q23)	ALL
AF6 (6q27) [21]	(6;11)(q27;q23)	AML
AF9 (9q22)	(9;11)(q22;q23)	AML
AF-1p (1p32) [22]	(1;11)(p32;q23)	AML
ENL (19p13.3) [23]	(11;19)(q23;p13)	AML
RCK (11q23.3) [24]	(11;14)(q23;q32)	ALL
AFX1 (Xq13)	(X;11)(q13;q23)	ALL
MYC (8q24) IgH (14q32) Igλ (22q11) Igκ (2p12) TCRA (14q11) [25]	(8;14)(q24;q32) (8;22)(q24;q11) (2;8)(p12;q24) (8;14)(q24;q11)	Burkitt's lymphoma B cell lymphoma
MYC (8q24) [26] **BCL2** (18q21.3) IgH (14q32)	(8;14)(q24;q32) (14;18)(q32;q21)	ALL
PBX1/PRL (1q23) [27] E2A (19p13.3)	(1;19)(q23;p13)	Pre-B ALL
PDGFRB (5q33) [28] TEL (12p13)	(5;12)(q33;p13)	CML
PLZF (11q23) [29] RARA (17q21)	(11;17)(q23;q21)	APL
PML (15q22) [30] RARA (17q21.1)	(15;17)(q21;q22)	APL
RBTN1 (11p15) [31] RBTN2 (11p13) TCRD (14q11.2)	(11;14)(p15;q11) (11;14)(p13;q11)	T-ALL
TAL1 (1p32) TCRA (14q11)	(1;14)(p32;q11)	T-ALL
TAL2 (9q34) [32, 33] TCRB (7q35)	(7;9)(q34;q32)	T-ALL
TAN1 (9q34) [34] Deletion	(7;9)(q34;q34)	T-ALL

Table 3. *Continued*

Gene (chromosome)	Translocation	Leukaemia
c6.1A/c6.1B (Xq28) [35, 36] TCRA (14q11.2)	t(X;14)(q28;q11)	T-PLL
WT1 (11p13) [37] EWS (22q12)	(11;22)(p13;q12)	Desmoplastic small round cell tumour (DSRCT)
ERG (21q22.3) [38] TLS/FUS (16p11)	(16;21)(p11;q22)	CML
TLS/FUS (16p11) [39] CHOP (12q13)	(12;16)(q13;p11)	Myxoid liposarcoma
PAX3 (2q35) [40] FKHR/ALV (13q14)	(2;13)(q35;q14)	Alveolar rhabdomyosarcoma
PAX7 (1p36) [41] FKHR/ALV (13q14)	(1;13)(p36;q14)	Alveolar rhabdomyosarcoma
RET (10q11.2) Protein kinase A RIα (17q23)	(10;17)(q11.2;q23)	Papillary thyroid carcinomas
D10S170 (10q21) ELE1 (10)	(10;10)(q11.2;q21)	

ALL: acute lymphoblastic leukaemia; AML: acute myeloid leukaemia; APL: acute promyelocytic leukaemia (a subtype of AML); ANLL: acute non-lymphocytic leukaemia; B-CLL: chronic B cell lymphocytic leukaemia; CML: chronic myelogenous leukaemia; T-ALL: acute T cell leukaemia; T-PLL: T cell pro-lymphocytic leukaemia.

Genes shown in bold type are described in individual entries in Section II. For summaries and additional references for genes shown in plain type see R. Hesketh, *The Oncogene Handbook*, Academic Press, 1994.

References
1 Morris, S.W. et al. (1994) Science 263, 1281–1284.
2 Chang, K.-S. et al. (1993) Oncogene 8, 983–988.
3 Erickson, P.F. et al. (1994) Cancer Res. 54, 1782–1786.
4 Nucifora, G. et al. (1993) Proc. Natl Acad. Sci. USA 90, 7784–7788.
5 Mitani, K. et al. (1994) EMBO J. 13, 504–510.
6 Zucman, J. et al. (1993) Nature Genetics 4, 341–345.
7 Baron, B. W. et al. (1993) Proc. Natl Acad. Sci. USA 90, 5262–5266.
8 Roualt, J.-P. et al. (1992) EMBO J. 11, 1663–1670.
9 von Lindern, M. et al. (1992) Mol. Cell. Biol. 12, 3346–3355.
10 Adachi, Y. et al. (1994) J. Biol. Chem. 269, 2258–2262.
11 Liu, P. et al. (1993) Science 261, 1041–1044.
12 Hunger, S.P. et al. (1992) Genes Devel. 6, 1608–1620.
13 Dear, T.N. et al. (1993) Proc. Natl Acad. Sci. USA 90, 4431–4435.
14 Laabi, Y. et al. (1992) EMBO J. 11, 3897–3904.
15 Meeker, T.C. et al. (1990) Blood 76, 285–289.
16 Kerckaert, J.-P. et al. (1993) Nature Genetics 5, 66–69.
17 Visvader, J. et al. (1991) Oncogene 6, 187–194.
18 Fracchiolla, N.S. et al. (1993) Oncogene 8, 2839–2845.
19 Prasad, R. et al. (1993) Cancer Res. 53, 5624–5628.
20 Corral, J. et al. (1993) Proc. Natl Acad. Sci. USA 90, 8538–8542.

[21] Tkachuk, D.C. et al. (1992) Cell 71, 691–700.

[22] Bernard, O.A. et al. (1994) Oncogene 9,1039–1045.

[23] Nakamura, T. et al. (1993) Proc. Natl Acad. Sci. USA 90, 4631–4635.

[24] Akao, Y. et al. (1992) Cancer Res. 52, 6083–6087.

[25] Park, J. K. et al. (1989) Genes Chromosomes Cancer 1, 15–22.

[26] Kiem, H. P. et al. (1990) Oncogene 5, 1815–1819.

[27] Dedera, D.A. et al. (1993) Cell 74, 833–843.

[28] Golub, T.R. et al. (1994) Cell 77, 307–316.

[29] Chen, Z. et al. (1993) EMBO J. 12, 1161–1167.

[30] Perez, A. et al. (1993) EMBO J. 12, 3171–3182.

[31] Fisch, P. et al. (1992) Oncogene 7, 2389–2397.

[32] Xia, Y. et al. (1991) Proc. Natl Acad. Sci. USA 88, 11416–11420.

[33] Xia, Y. et al. (1994) Oncogene 9, 1437–1446.

[34] Ellisen, L.W. et al. (1991) Cell 66, 649–661.

[35] Fisch, P. et al. (1993) Oncogene 8, 3271–3276.

[36] Stern, M. H. et al. (1993) Oncogene 8, 2475–2483.

[37] Ladanyi, M. and Gerald, W. (1994) Cancer Res. 54, 2837–2840.

[38] Ichikawa, H. et al. (1994) Cancer Res. 54, 2865–2868.

[39] Crozat, A. et al. (1993) Nature 363, 640–644.

[40] Rabbitts, T.H. et al. (1993) Nature Genetics 4, 175–180.

[41] Galili, N. et al. (1993) Nature Genetics 5, 230–235.

[42] Davis, R.J. et al. (1994) Cancer Res. 54, 2869–2872.

Table 4. *Tumour suppressor genes detected in human tumours*

Gene	Chromosomal locus	Neoplasm
APC	5q21–q22	Familial adenomatosis polyposis (FAP)
CMAR/CAR	16q	Breast, prostate cancers
DCC	18q21	Colon carcinoma
MLH1	3p21.3–p23	Hereditary non-polyposis colon cancer (HNPCC)
MSH2	2p22–p21	Hereditary non-polyposis colon cancer (HNPCC)
MTS1 (CDK4 inhibitor)	9p21	Many cancers
NF1	17q11.2	Neurofibromatosis type 1
NF2	22q12	Neurofibromatosis type 2
NME1, NME2 (NM23)	17q21.3	Neuroblastoma, colon carcinoma
PHB	17q21	Breast carcinoma
P53	17p13.1	Sarcomas, gliomas, carcinomas
RB1	13q14	Retinoblastoma, sarcomas, carcinomas
VHL	3p25–p26	von Hippel–Lindau disease
WT1	11p12	Wilms' tumour
BCNS [1]	9q31	Medulloblastoma
BRCA1 [2]	17q21	Breast and ovarian carcinomas
BRUSH1 [3]	13q12–q13	Breast carcinoma
BWS [4]	11p15.5	Wilms' tumour
HRCA1 [5]	3p14	Hereditary renal carcinoma
NRC1 [6]	3p14–p12	Non-papillary renal carcinoma
LC1 [7]	3p14–p21	Lung carcinoma
MEN1 [8]	11q13	Parathyroid (?), pancreatic and pituitary tumours
MLM [9]	9p21	Melanoma

Table 4. *Continued*

Gene	Chromosomal locus	Neoplasm
MTS1/MTS2/CDK4I [10, 11]	9p21	Melanoma
NB1 [12]	1p36.1	Neuroblastoma, pituitary and adrenal cortex tumours
TSC1 [1]	9q34	Tuberous sclerosis
TSC2 [13]	16p13.3	Tuberous sclerosis
[14]	3p21.3	Lung carcinoma (?)
[15]	5q35–qter	Hepatocellular carcinoma (HCC) without cirrhosis
[16]	8p22, 10q24, 16q	Prostate cancer
[17]	13q14	B cell chronic lymphocytic leukaemia
IRF [18]	5q31.1	Leukemia

Genes shown in bold type are described in individual entries in Section II or the Introduction (*NM23*). With the exception of *BRCA1*, the remaining putative tumour suppressor genes have not been cloned.

References

[1] Bare, J.W. et al. (1993) Am. J. Hum. Genet. 53 (Suppl.), Abstract 274.
[2] Miki, Y. et al. (1994) Science 266, 66–71.
[3] Schott et al. (1994) Cancer Res. 54, 1393–1396.
[4] Koufos, A. et al. (1993) Am. J. Hum. Genet. 44, 711–719.
[5] Boldog, F.L. et al. (1993). Proc. Natl Acad. Sci. USA 90, 8509–8513.
[6] Sanchez, Y. et al. (1994). Proc. Natl Acad. Sci. USA 91, 3383–3387.
[7] Whang-Peng, J. et al. (1993) Genes Chromosomes Cancer 3, 168–188.
[8] Larsson, C. et al. (1993) Nature 332, 85–87.
[9] Walker, G.J. et al. (1994) Oncogene 9, 819–824.
[10] Nobori, T. et al., (1994) Nature 368, 753–756.
[11] Kamb et al. (1994) Science 264, 436–440.
[12] Biegel, J.A. et al. (1993) Am. J. Hum. Genet. 52, 176–182.
[13] Green, A.J. (1994). Nature Genetics 6, 193–196.
[14] Hibi, K. et al. (1994) Oncogene 9, 611–619.
[15] Ding, S.F., et al. (1993) Cancer Detect. Prev. 17, 405–409.
[16] Bova, G.S. et al. (1993) Cancer Res. 53, 3869–3873.
[17] Chapman, R.M. et al. (1994) Oncogene 9, 1289–1293.
[18] Tanaka, N. et al. (1994) Cell 77, 829–839.

Table 5. *Functions of oncoproteins*

Class 1 Growth factors

AIGF [1], **HSTF1/Hst-1**, **INT-2**, **PDGFB/SIS**, **WNT1**, **WNT2**, **WNT3**

Class 2. Tyrosine kinases
Receptor-like tyrosine kinases
EPH, (**ECK**, **EEK**, **ELK**, **ERK**, CEK, HEK, MEK, NUK, SEK), **EGFR/ERBB**, **FMS**, **KIT**, TYK1/LTK, **MET**, **HER2/NEU**, **RET**, **ROS**, EYK/RYK, **SEA**, TIE, **TRK**, UFO

Table 5. *Continued*

Class 2. *Continued*
  Non-receptor tyrosine kinases
    ABL1, (**ARG**), CSK/CYL, **FPS/FES**, (FER/TYK3), TKF
  Membrane-associated non-receptor tyrosine kinases
    SRC, SRC-related kinases: BLK, **FGR**, **FYN**, **HCK**, **LCK**, LYN/SYN, TKL, **YES**

Class 3. Receptors lacking protein kinase activity
  MAS, MPL

Class 4a. Membrane-associated G proteins
  HRAS, **KRAS**, **NRAS**, GSP, GIP2

Class 4b. Guanine nucleotide exchange proteins
  SDC25

Class 4c. GTPase-activating proteins
  GAP, NF1

Class 4d. RHO/RAC binding proteins
  BCR, DBL, ECT2, TIM^2

Class 5. Cytoplasmic protein serine kinases
  BCR, CLK (& NEK), EST/COT, **MOS**, **PIM1**, **RAF/MIL**, Protein kinase Cε

Class 6. Protein serine-, threonine- and tyrosine kinase
  STY

Class 7. Cytoplasmic regulators
  BCL1, **CRK**, NCK, ODC1, PEM, PKR

Class 8. Cell Cycle regulators
  MTS1 (CDK4 inhibitor: see Table 4), cyclin D1 (see **BCL1**)

Class 9. Transcription Factors
  BCL3, CBL, ERBA, ETS, (**ELK**), EVI1, **FOS** (**FOSB**, ΔFOSB, **FRA1**, **FRA2**), GLI, HOX-2.4, HOX-7.1, HOX11, IRF-2 [3], **JUN** (**JUNB**, **JUND**), LYL1, **MYB** (**MBM2**), **MYC**, **MYCL**, **MYCN**, **p53**, FKH2/QIN, **RB1**, RBTN1, RBTN2, **REL**, **TAL1**, SKI, TRE, **VAV**, **WT1**

Class 10. DNA repair enzymes
  MLH1, MSH2

Class 11. Mitochondrial membrane factor
  BCL2

Class 12. Function unknown
  AKT, DLK, LBC [4], LCO/LCA, NRL (MAF), MEL, MELF, SCC, TLM

This table lists gene products that have been shown to be tumorigenic or that are specifically expressed in at least one type of tumour cell. Those in bold type are described in individual entries in Section II. Those in brackets are discussed in the preceding bold type entry. Superscripts refer to the reference list below for recently discovered genes. For details of other genes see R. Hesketh, *The Oncogene Handbook*, Academic Press, 1994.

References

[1] Kouhara, H. et al. (1994) Oncogene 9, 455–462.
[2] Chan, A.M.-L. et al. (1994) Oncogene 9, 1057–1063.
[3] Yamamoto, H. et al. (1994) Oncogene 9, 1423–1428.
[4] Toksoz, D. and Williams, D.A. (1994) Oncogene 9, 621–628.

Table 6. *Chromosome locations of human proto-oncogenes and tumour suppressor genes*

1	ECK	3q27	LAZ3
1	EEK	4	FLK1/KDR
1	ERK	4q11–q21	KIT
1	TPR	4q21	MLLT2/AF4
1p13	NRAS	4q26	IL2
1p32	AF-1p	5/17/18 (elements)	TRE
1p32	BLYM	5q	GAP
1p32	MYCL1	5q21	FER
1p32	TAL1	5q21	MCC
1p32–p31	JUN	5q21–q22	APC
1p33	SIL	5q31	IL3
1p33–p34	TIE	5q31.3–q33.2	FGFA
1p34	MPL	5q33	PDGFRB
1p35–p32	LCK	5q33.3–q34	CSF1R
1p36	NB1	5q35	FLT4
1p36.2–p36.1	FGR	5q35	NPM
1q22–q24	SKI	6p21	PIM1
1q23	PBX1	6p23–p22.3	FIM1
1q23–q24	TRK	6q21	FYN
1q23–q31	TRKB	6q21–q22	ROS1
1q23–q31	TRKC	6q22–q23	MYB
1q24–q25	ABL2 (ARG)	6q23	CAN
2p13–p12	REL	6q24–q27	MAS
2p22–p21	MSH2	6q27	AF6
2p23	ALK	7	TIM
2p24.1	MYCN	7p13–p12	EGFR
2p25	ODC1	7p15	MYCLK1
2q14–q21	HIS1	7q31	MET
2q14–q21	LCO	7q31	WNT2
2q33–qter	INHA	7q32–q36	EPHT
3p14	HRCA1	7q33–q36	RAFB1
3p14–p21	LC1	8p12	FLT2
3p21.3	Integrin-α_{RLC}	8q11–q12	MOS
3p24.1–p22	THRB	8q13–qter	LYN
3p25	RAF1	8q22	MYBL1
3p25–p26	VHL	8q22	ETO/MTG8
3q22	RYK	8q24	MYC
3q26	EVI	8q24	PVT1
3q26	EAP	8q24.1	NOV
3q27	BCL6	9p21	MLM

Table 6. *Continued*

9p21	*MTS1/CDK4I, MTS2*	15q21	*PML*
9p34.1	*ABL1*	15q25–q26	*FPS/FES*
9q22	*MLLT3/AF9*	16p13	*BCM*
9q31	*BCNS*	16p13.12–p13.13	*MYH11*
9q34	*DEK*	16p13.3	*TSC2*
9q34	*SET*	16p22–q23	*MAF*
9q34	*TAL2*	16q	*CMAR/CAR*
9q34	*TAN1*	16q22	*CBFB*
9q34	*TSC1*	16q22.1	*UVO*
10p11.2	*EST*	17p13.1	*TP53*
10q11.2	*RET*	17q	*BTR*
10q24	*HOX11*	17q11.2	*EVI2B*
10q24	*NFKB2/LYT10*	17q11.2	*NF1*
11p12–p11.2	*SPI1*	17q11.2–q12	*THRA1*
11p13	*RBTNL1*	17q12–q21	*BRCA1*
11p13	*WT1*	17q21	*PHB*
11p15	*RBTN1*	17q21	*RARA*
11p15.5	*HRAS*	17q21–q22	*HER2*
11p15.5	*BWS*	17q21–q22	*WNT3*
11q13	*BCL1*	17q21.3	*NME1, NME2*
11q13	*EMS1*	17q22	*HLF*
11q13	*INT2*	18q21	*BCL2*
11q13	*MEN1*	18q21	*DCC*
11q13	*SEA*	18q21.3	*YES1*
11q13.3	*HSTF1*	19p13	*E2A*
11q23	*MLL*	19p13.2	*LYL1*
11q23	*PLZF*	19p13.2	*JUNB*
11q23–q24	*ERGB*	19p13.2	*JUND*
11q23.3	*ETS1*	19p13.2	*VAV*
11q23	*RCK*	19p13.3	*MLLT1/ENL/LGT19*
11q23.3–qter	*CBL*	19CEN–p13.2	*MEL*
11q24	*FLI1*	19q13.1	*BCL3*
12p12.1	*KRAS2*	19q13.1	*UFO*
12p13	*TEL*	20q11	*HCK*
12q13	*ATF1*	20q13.3	*SRC*
12p13	*HST2*	21q22	*AML1*
12q13	*HER3*	21q22.3	*ERG*
12q13	*WNT1*	21q22.3	*ETS2*
12q13–q14.3	*GLI1*	22q11.2	*BCR*
12q22	*BTG1*	22q12	*EWS*
13q12	*FLT1*	22q12	*NF2*
13q12	*FLT3/FLK2*	22q12.3–q13.1	*PDGFB*
13q14.2	*RB1*	Xp11.2	*ELK1*
14q13	*FKH2/QIN*	Xp11.2	*RAFA1*
14q24.3	*FOS*	Xp11.3–p11.23	*TIMP*
14q32	*AKT*	Xq13	*MYBL2*
14q32.3	*ELK2*	Xq13	*AFX1*
15	*CSK*	Xq27	*DBL*
15q13–q21	*LTK/TYK1*	Xq28	*c6.1A/c6.1B (MTCP1)*

THE
ONCOGENES

IDENTIFICATION

v-*abl* is the transforming gene of the replication defective Abelson murine leukaemia virus (Ab-MuLV), originally isolated from a mouse infected with Moloney murine leukaemia virus (Mo-MuLV) after chemical thymectomy. v-*abl* is also carried by the ABL-MYC murine retrovirus derived from Ab-MuLV. The Hardy-Zuckerman 2 feline sarcoma virus (HZ2-FeSV) has transduced the (feline) *Abl* gene. ABL (*ABL1*) is the human homologue of *Abl* [1,2].

RELATED GENES

ABL contains regions homologous to the kinase and homology regions 2 and 3 (SH2, SH3) of SRC (see **SRC**). Other related genes: *ABL2/ARG* (*A*belson-*r*elated gene), *EPH*, *NCP94*, *TKR11* and *TKR16*, *Drosophila melanogaster Dash* and *Caenorhabditis elegans Abl*.

	ABL	**v-*abl***
Nucleotides (kb)	225	5.7(Ab-MuLV)
Chromosome	9q34.1	
Mass (kDa): predicted	123	
expressed	145*ABL*	P160, P120,
	(with alternative N-termini)	P90, P100

Cellular location

145*ABL*: Mainly nucleus, some cytoplasm/plasma membrane. v-*abl*: Plasma membrane.

Tissue distribution

ABL expression is widespread but is particularly strong in the spleen, testis and thymus [3]. In germ cells there is a novel transcript, restricted to post-meiotic spermatogenic cells [4].

PROTEIN FUNCTION

ABL has weak tyrosine kinase activity and a sequence-specific DNA binding activity for the EP element present in the enhancers of several viruses (hepatitis B virus, polyomavirus) and in the *Myc* promoter [5].

ABL and v-ABL proteins do not function as receptors and specific targets for their tyrosine kinase activity have not been characterized, although transformation by Ab-MuLV causes phosphorylation of enolase, vinculin and p42 and serine phosphorylation of ribosomal protein S6. The tyrosine kinase activity of v-ABL causes erythroid bursts in fetal liver cells in the absence of erythropoietin, renders the proliferation of mast cells and other types of cell independent of IL3 and in fibroblasts reduces the number of EGFRs and stimulates secretion of an EGF-like growth factor. All myristylated, tyrosine kinase-active forms of ABL associate with PtdIns3-kinase [6].

Activated ABL proteins may thus modulate the normal mechanisms that regulate growth factor-stimulated proliferation, (for example, by activating PtdIns metabolism or the transcription of early genes including *Fos*), an inference strengthened by the finding that ABL is phosphorylated by p34^{CDC2} [7].

Cancer

Over 90% of chronic myeloid leukaemia (CML) cases involve the balanced translocation t(9;22)(q34;q11) of a fragment of the long arm of chromosome 9 to the long arm of chromosome 22, generating a shortened, hybrid chromosome (the Philadelphia chromosome, Ph[1]) containing a *BCR–ABL* chimeric gene (see **BCR**) [8]. The Ph[1] chromosome also occurs in 10–20% of patients with acute lymphoblastic leukaemias (ALL).

Transgenic animals

Haematopoietic stem cells expressing v-*abl* initiate leukaemogenesis in mice. Animals with a homozygous deletion of *Abl* (*Abl*[m1]) have increased perinatal mortality and decreased levels of B and T cell precursors. Plasmacytoma development in *Abl* transgenic mice occurs after a translocation in *Myc* that causes over-expression of MYC protein and is accelerated by crossing with transgenic *Myc* mice [9].

In animals

Mo-MuLV induces lymphocytic leukaemias in mice and the acute transforming virus HZ2-FeSV causes feline sarcomas.

In vitro

Abl does not transform primary fibroblasts but does transform haematopoietic cells, NIH 3T3 fibroblasts and lymphoid cells and is thus unique among murine retroviruses. ABL may be activated to transform fibroblasts by a single point mutation (Phe420 to Val). Phe420 is adjacent to the predicted major site of tyrosine phosphorylation in ABL (Tyr412) and is perfectly conserved among tyrosine kinases with N-terminal SH3 domains [10].

Overexpression of *Myc* acts synergistically with the expression of *Abl* oncogenes in transformation, whereas dominant negative mutations in MYC that leave the dimerization motif intact (see **MYC**) reduce transformation by v-*abl* or by P185$^{BCR-ABL}$ [11].

GENE STRUCTURE

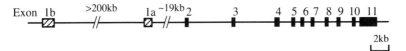

TRANSCRIPTIONAL REGULATION

Two specific promoters utilize exon 1a or 1b: mRNAs 1a and 1b are equivalent to mouse type I and IV mRNAs, respectively [12]. There are four murine *Abl* mRNAs (types I, II, III and IV) that have alternative 5′ sequences encoded by differential splicing of exons 1a and 1b to a common 3′ sequence. Human 1a and 1b *ABL* promoter sequences show high homology [13]. The 1a promoter contains seven SP1 sites and a TTAA sequence that may function as a TATA box. The 1b promoter contains at least 12 protein binding elements, including seven SP1 motifs and four CCAAT boxes but no TATA box.

PROTEIN STRUCTURE

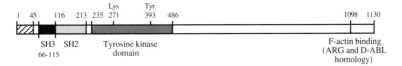

Lys271 (Lys290 in type 1b ABL) is essential for kinase activity. The highly conserved SH2 motif FLVRES is critical for binding to tyrosine phosphorylated proteins and transforming potential [14]. The affinity of ABL for F-actin is enhanced by the BCR sequences present in BCR–ABL (see ***BCR***). All ABL proteins (p150[ABL], p160[v-abl], P210[BCR-ABL]) are phosphorylated at two C-terminal sites by protein kinase C [15], although this region is not required either for ABL kinase activity or for transformation by v-ABL.

The structure of the SH2 domain of ABL in solution has been shown by multidimensional NMR spectroscopy to comprise a compact sphere with a large three-stranded antiparallel β sheet, a second smaller β sheet and a C-terminal α helix enclosing the hydrophobic core [16]. The putative phosphotyrosyl binding site is formed by conserved residues in the large β sheet and in a short amphipathic helix.

Murine *Abl*, from which v-*abl* was acquired, encodes a protein with 85% homology to human ABL. In v-ABL upstream fusion of *gag* provides a myristylated N-terminus that directs membrane localization and activates tyrosine phosphorylation and transformation potential. The two prototype strains of Ab-MuLV encode different v-ABL proteins (P120 and P160). The C-terminal 1010 amino acids of P160 are identical to those of murine ABL. A 263 codon deletion in the centre of P160 gives rise to P120. Variant weakly oncogenic forms (P90, P100) have also been isolated.

ABL ACTIVATION

ABL tyrosine kinase activity and transformation potential may be activated by:

(1) The formation of the fusion BCR–ABL protein in which BCR sequences replace the ABL first exon (see **BCR**).

(2) Deletion of the non-catalytic SH3 (negative regulatory) region [17]. The retention of an N-terminal myristylation site is essential for transforming activity. ABL differs from members of the SRC family of protein tyrosine kinases in that it does not contain a C-terminal regulatory tyrosine (Tyr527 in SRC).

(3) Hyperexpression of ABL (>500-fold more than the normal endogenous concentration). This may reflect the presence of cellular factors that normally inhibit the kinase [18].

(4) N-terminal deletions or an in-frame deletion within the last exon [19].

SEQUENCE OF ABL

```
   1  MLEICLKLVG CKSKKGLSSS SSCYLEEALQ RPVASDFEPQ GLSEAARWNS
  51  KENLLAGPSE NDPNLFVALY DFVASGDNTL SITKGEKLRV LGYNHNGEWC
 101  EAQTKNGQGW VPSNYITPVN SLEKHSWYHG PVSRNAAEYL LSSGINGSFL
 151  VRESESSPGQ RSISLRYEGR VYHYRINTAS DGKLYVSSES RFNTLAELVH
 201  HHSTVADGLI TTLHYPAPKR NKPTVYGVSP NYDKWEMERT DITMKHKLGG
 251  GQYGEVYEGV WKKYSLTVAV KTLKEDTMEV EEFLKEAAVM KEIKHPNLVQ
 301  LLGVCTREPP FYIITEFMTY GNLLDYLREC NRQEVNAVVL LYMATQISSA
 351  MEYLEKKNFI HRDLAARNCL VGENHLVKVA DFGLSRLMTG DTYTAHAGAK
 401  FPIKWTAPES LAYNKFSIKS DVWAFGVLLW EIATYGMSPY PGIDLSQVYE
 451  LLEKDYRMER PEGCPEKVYE LMRACWQWNP SDRPSFAEIH QAFETMFQES
 501  SISDEVEKEL GKQGVRGAVS TLLQAPELPT KTRTSRRAAE HRDTTDVPEM
 551  PHSKGQGESD PLDHEPAVSP LLPRKERGPP EGGLNEDERL LPKDKKTNLF
 601  SALIKKKKKT APTPPKRSSS FREMDGQPER RGAGEEEGRD ISNGALAFTP
 651  LDTADPAKSP KPSNGAGVPN GALRESGGSG FRSPHLWKKS STLTSSRLAT
 701  GEEEGGGSSS KRFLRSCSAS CVPHGAKDTE WRSVTLPRDL QSTGRQFDSS
 751  TFGGHKSEKP ALPRKRAGEN RSDQVTRGTV TPPPRLVKKN EEAADEVFKD
 801  IMESSPGSSP PNLTPKPLRR QVTVAPASGL PHKEEAEKGS ALGTPAAAEP
 851  VTPTSKAGSG APGGTSKGPA EESRVRRHKH SSESPGRDKG KLSRLKPAPP
 901  PPPAASAGKA GGKPSQSPSQ EAAGEAVLGA KTKATSLVDA VNSDAAKPSQ
 951  PGEGLKKPVL PATPKPQSAK PSGTPISPAP VPSTLPSASS ALAGDQPSST
1001  AFIPLISTRV SLRKTRQPPE RIASGAITKG VVLDSTEALC LAISRNSEQM
1051  ASHSAVLEAG KNLYTFCVSY VDSIQQMRNK FAFREAINKL ENNLRELQIC
1101  PATAGSGPAA TQDFSKLLSS VKEISDIVQR (1130)
```

Domain structure

1–26	Type 1a N-terminus (underlined): corresponding N-terminus of type 1b ABL:
	MGQQPGKVLGDQRRPSLPALHFIKGAGKKESSRHGGPHCNVFVEH
26–27	Breakpoint for translocation to form BCR–ABL oncogene
248–256 and 271	ATP binding
363	Active site
393	Autophosphorylation site
61–121	SH3 domain
127–213	SH2 domain (italics)

DATABASE ACCESSION NUMBERS

	PIR	SWISSPROT	EMBL/GENBANK	REFERENCES
Human *ABL1*	A25582	P00519	M14752	11
			X16416	20, 21

References

1 **Rosenberg, N. and Witte, O. (1988) Adv. Virus Res. 35, 39–81.**
2 **Ramakrishnan, L. and Rosenberg, N. (1989) Biochim. Biophys. Acta 989, 209–224.**
3 Van Etten, R.A. et al. (1989) Cell 58, 669–678.
4 Ponzetto, C. and Wolgemuth, D.J. (1985) Mol. Cell. Biol. 5, 1791–1794.
5 Dikstein, R. et al. (1992) Cell 69, 751–757.
6 Varticovski, L. et al. (1991) Mol. Cell. Biol. 11, 1107–1113.
7 Kipreos, E.T. and Wang, J.Y.J. (1992) Science 256, 382–385.
8 Nowell, P.C. and Hungerford, D.A. (1960) Science 132, 1497–1499.
9 Rosenbaum, H. et al. (1992) EMBO J. 9, 897–905.
10 Jackson, P.K. et al. (1993) Oncogene 8, 1943–1956.
11 Sawyers, C.L. et al. (1992) Cell 70, 901-910.
12 Fainstein, E. et al. (1989) Oncogene 4, 1477–1481.
13 Zhu, Q.S. et al. (1990) Oncogene 5, 885–891.
14 Zhu, G. et al. (1993) J. Biol. Chem. 268, 1775–1779.
15 Pendergast, A.M. et al. (1987) Mol. Cell. Biol. 7, 4280–4289.
16 Overduin, M. et al. (1992) Cell 70, 697–704.
17 Shore, S.K. et al. (1990) Proc. Natl Acad. Sci. USA 87, 6502–6506.
18 Pendergast, A.M. et al. (1991) Proc. Natl Acad. Sci. USA 88, 5927–5931.
19 Goga, A. et al. (1993) Mol. Cell. Biol. 13, 4967–4975.
20 Groffen, J. et al. (1983) Nature 304, 167–169.
21 Shtivelman, E. et al. (1986) Cell 47, 277–284.

BCL1

IDENTIFICATION

BCL1 (_B cell leukaemia/lymphoma-1_) was detected with a probe specific for chromosome 11 in DNA isolated from a chronic lymphocytic leukaemia (CLL) cell line.

RELATED GENES

BCL1 is identical to human cyclin D1 and related to other cyclins. The murine homologue is _Cyl-1_.

Nucleotides (kb)		Not fully mapped
Chromosome		11q13
Mass (kDa):	predicted	33.7
	expressed	34

Cellular location

Cytoplasm.

Tissue distribution

Expressed in many cells, including proliferating macrophages, but not in cells of other lymphoid or myeloid lineages. Transcription varies during the cell cycle, being maximal in G_1 [1].

Protein function

Unknown. BCL1 is phosphorylated in G_1 and it directly activates $p34^{CDC2}$ kinase. In human lung fibroblasts D type cyclins associate with many other proteins, including the proliferating cell nuclear antigen (PCNA) [2].

Cancer

The t(11;14)(q13;q32) translocation, in which _BCL1_ becomes juxtaposed to J_H on chromosome 14, leading to overexpression of _BCL1_, occurs in several B cell malignancies (diffuse, small and large cell lymphomas), B cell chronic lymphocytic leukaemia (CLL) and multiple myeloma. Most breakpoints map ~110 kb 5' (centromeric) to the _BCL1_ gene at the major translocation cluster (MTC) although in some cases of intermediately differentiated lymphoma breakpoints lie outside this region [3].

BCL1 is part of an 11q13 region that includes _INT2_ and _HSTF1_ that is amplified in 15–20% of human breast and squamous cell carcinomas [4] and in bladder tumours [5], although in breast tumours _BCL1_ expression is not invariably associated with that of _INT2_ and _HSTF1_ [6]. Anomalous expression of D-type cyclins occurs in variety of tumours [7–13].

In vitro

BCL1/cyclin D1 cooperates with *H-ras* to transform primary rat embryo fibroblasts and these immortalized cells are tumorigenic in nude mice [14]. The transforming action of BCL1 may be mediated by its overcoming the negative regulation normally exerted by RB1 on D-type cyclins [15].

SEQUENCE OF BCL1

```
  1  MEHQLLCCEV ETIRRAYPDA NLLNDRVLRA MLKAEETCAP SVSYFKCVQK
 51  EVLPSMRKIV ATWMLEVCEE QKCEEEVFPL AMNYLDRFLS LEPVKKSRLQ
101  LLGATCMFVA SKMKETIPLT AEKLCIYTDN SIRPEELLQM ELLLVNKLKW
151  NLAAMTPHDF IEHFLSKMPE AEENKQIIRK HAQTFVALCA TDVKFISNPP
201  SMVAAGSVVA AVQGLNLRSP NNFLSYYRLT RFLSRVIKCD PDCLRACQEQ
251  IEALLESSLR QAQQNMDPKA AEEEEEEEE VDLACTPTDV RDVDI (295)
```

Domain structure

56–165   Region of homology with A-type cyclins (underlined)

DATABASE ACCESSION NUMBERS

	PIR	SWISSPROT	EMBL/GENBANK	REFERENCES
Human *BCL1*	A40034, A41523	P24385	M64349, M73554, M74092	16
	B40268, S14794		X59789, X59485, Z23022	17

References

1 Matsushime, H. et al. (1991) Cell 65, 701-713.
2 Xiong, Y. et al. (1992) Cell 71, 505–514.
3 de Boer, C.J. et al. (1993) Cancer Res. 53, 4148–4152.
4 Theillet, C. et al. (1990) Oncogene 5, 147–149.
5 Proctor, A.J. et al. (1991) Oncogene 6, 789–795.
6 Faust, J.B. and Meeker, T.C. (1992) Cancer Res. 52, 2460–2463.
7 Keyomarsi, K. and Pardee, A.B. (1993) Proc. Natl Acad. Sci. USA 90, 1112–1116.
8 Buckley, M.F. et al. (1993) Oncogene 8, 2127–2133.
9 Palmero, I. et al. (1993) Oncogene 8, 1049–1054.
10 Leach, F.S. et al. (1993) Cancer Res. 53, 1986–1989.
11 Williams, R.T. et al. (1993) J. Biol. Chem. 268, 8871–8880.
12 Foulkes, W.D. et al. (1993) Br. J. Cancer 67, 268–273.
13 Rosenberg, C.L. (1993) Oncogene 8, 519–521.
14 Lovec, H. et al. (1994) Oncogene 9, 323–326.
15 Hinds, P.W. et al. (1994) Proc. Natl Acad. Sci. USA 91, 709–713.
16 Withers, D.A. et al. (1991) Mol. Cell. Biol. 11, 4846–4853.
17 Motokura T. et al. (1991) Nature 350, 512–550.

BCL2

IDENTIFICATION

BCL2 (*B cell leukaemia/lymphoma-2*) was detected with a probe specific for chromosome 18 in DNA isolated from a pre-B cell acute lymphocytic leukaemia cell line.

RELATED GENES

BCLX and *BAX*. Two mRNAs are transcribed from human *BCLX* encoding BCLX$_L$ (41% identical to BCL2α) and BCLX$_S$ (identical to BCLX$_L$ save for a 63 amino acid deletion). BCL2 has weak homology to MCL1, murine A1, E1B 19kDa protein, LMW5-HL African swine fever virus gene product, Epstein–Barr virus protein BHRF1 (see **DNA Tumour Viruses, EBV**) and *Caenorhabditis elegans ced-9*.

Nucleotides (kb)		>370
Chromosome		18q21
Mass (kDa):	predicted	26 (BCL2α)/22 (BCL2β)
	expressed	28/30

Cellular location

BCL2α: Inner mitochondrial membrane; some in endoplasmic reticulum and nuclear membranes. BCL2β: cytoplasm.

Tissue distribution

Generally expressed in tissues characterized by apoptotic cell turnover and restricted to long-lived progenitor cells and post-mitotic cells that have an extended lifespan [1]. Restricted within germinal centres to regions implicated in the selection and maintenance of plasma cells and memory B cells, and showing stage-specific expression during B cell development [2]. Expressed in surviving T cells in the thymic medulla and in proliferating precursors, but not in post-mitotic maturation stages, of all haematopoietic lineages. Also expressed in glandular epithelium under hormonal or growth factor control, in complex differentiating epithelium characterized by long-lived stem cells and in some neurons [3].

PROTEIN FUNCTION

Overexpression of BCL2 inhibits apoptosis induced by deprivation of growth factors and BCL2 may be functionally equivalent to the product of the Epstein–Barr virus early gene BHRF1 (see **DNA Tumour Viruses, EBV**) [4,5–8]. BCL2 prevents γ-irradiation-induced apoptosis and functions in an antioxidant pathway to inhibit lipid peroxidation [9]. Glucocorticoid-induced apoptosis of pre-B-lymphocytes is blocked by the expression of high levels of BCL2 by a mechanism that requires the concurrent repression of *MYC* [10] (see *MYC*). In fibroblasts in which the overexpression of MYC is induced, the apoptotic cell death that would normally occur is prevented by the co-expression of BCL2 [11, 12]. Thus the proto-oncogenes *MYC* and *BCL2* can cooperate to prevent apoptosis and cause continuous cell proliferation in the absence of mitogens, although the cells do not appear to be transformed. In human cells BCL2 associates with the RAS-related protein R-RAS p23, indicating that a protein that may be involved in signal transduction is also associated with apoptosis [13].

The BCL2-related protein BCLX$_L$ is as effective as BCL2 in inhibiting cell death following growth factor withdrawal [14]. The truncated form of BCLX$_L$, BCLX$_S$, inhibits the ability of BCL2 to enhance the survival of growth factor-deprived cells.

BCL2 forms dimers with BAX, a conserved homologue that is expressed in a predicted membrane form (α) and in two cytosolic forms (β and γ) [15]. Overexpression of BAX can accelerate apoptosis and BAX thus appears to modulate the death repressor activity of BCL2.

Cancer

The chromosomal translocation t(14;18)(q32;q21) is a specific abnormality of human lymphoid neoplasms that occurs in >85% of follicular small cleaved B cell lymphomas and ~20% diffuse lymphomas [16]. The major breakpoint region (MBR) on chromosome 18, involved in 60% of these cases, is within the 3' untranslated part of *BCL2* exon 3 [17]. This region contains a target sequence, also present in the *Dxp* genes of the immunoglobulin (Ig) diversity (D$_H$) family, to which BCLF proteins bind to mediate chromosomal translocation [18]. The minor cluster region (MCR) (40%) is ~20 kb downstream of *BCL2*. Additional breakpoints occur at the 5' and 3' ends of *BCL2* [19]. These translocations create a *BCL2*/Ig fusion gene. However, although the neoplastic germinal centres in most follicular lymphomas express high levels of BCL2 protein whereas normal germinal centres do not, BCL2 is also present in normal T and B cells and in hairy cell leukaemias and Ki-1 lymphomas that do *not* involve the 14;18 translocation [20].

In ~10% of chronic lymphocytic leukaemias (CLL) *BCL2* is translocated to the Igκ or Igλ light chain gene [21]. The chromosome 18 breakpoints involved are within the 5' end of the *BCL2* gene, the variant cluster region (VCR). The simultaneous presence of MBR (or MCR) translocations and of minor rearrangements involving deletions in VCR occurs in some follicular lymphomas [22].

BCL2 is expressed in normal and malignant plasma cells from myeloma patients [23, 24] and in a number of human lymphoid and myeloid cell lines and tissues [25, 26]. High expression of *BCL2* occurs in some human neuroblastoma and small cell lung carcinoma cell lines and lower levels of the protein occur in a variety of other neural crest-derived tumours and tumour cell lines, including some neuroepitheliomas, Ewing's sarcomas, neurofibromas and melanomas [27,28].

Transgenic animals

In transgenic mice that overexpress *Bcl-2* the lifetime of immunoglobulin secreting cells and memory B cells is extended and the proportion of CD4⁻8⁺ thymocytes is increased [29,30]. The response to immunization is enhanced, consistent with reduced death of activated T cells, and the overproduction of BCL2 substantially alters the V_H gene repertoire in B cells [31,32]. The introduction of *Bcl-2* into *scid* mice (in which the failure to make productive rearrangements of Ig and TCR genes causes early abortion of lymphopoiesis) permits the accumulation of almost normal numbers of Ig⁻ B-lymphoid cells [33]. *TCR/Bcl-2/scid* mice develop normal numbers of CD4⁺8⁺ thymocytes, indicating that expression of the TCR is necessary for T cells to respond to BCL2. Thus *BCL2* sustains immune responsiveness.

Mice transgenic for a *Bcl-2/Ig* fusion gene show an expansion of the lymphoid compartment and mature B cells from these mice show a survival advantage *in vitro* [34]. Mice doubly transgenic for *Bcl-2* and *Myc* under the control of the Ig_H enhancer show hyper-proliferation of pre-B and B cells and develop tumours which appear at earlier times than in Eµ-*Myc* mice and display the phenotype of primitive haematopoietic cells [35]. Thus, by extending cell survival, BCL2 may increase the chance of secondary genetic changes responsible for tumorigenicity.

In vitro

BCL2 expressed from a retroviral vector does not morphologically transform NIH 3T3 cells, render FDCP-1 cells tumorigenic or immortalize normal bone marrow cells, but does immortalize pre-B cells from Eµ-*Myc* transgenic mice, some of which become tumorigenic. In addition, whilst not abolishing the growth factor requirements of some established haematopoietic cell lines, it promotes their extended survival in G_0 in the absence of growth factors [36].

GENE STRUCTURE

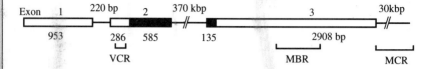

Alternative promoters utilize either exons 2 and 3 or exons 1, 2 and 3 [37]. The untranslated region is GC-rich and contains an SP1 binding site.

TRANSCRIPTIONAL REGULATION

The human *BCL2* 5′ untranslated region contains a unique negative regulatory element (NRE) the activity of which may vary during B cell development[38].

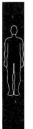

SEQUENCE OF BCL2α

```
  1  MAHAGRTGYD NREIVMKYIH YKLSQRGYEW DAGDVGAAPP GAAPAPGIFS
 51  SQPGHTPHPA ASRDPVARTS PLQTPAAPGA AAGPALSPVP PVVHLTLRQA
101  GDDFSRRYRR DFAEMSSQLH LTPFTARGRF ATVVEELFRD GVNWGRIVAF
151  FEFGGVMCVE SVNREMSPLV DNIALWMTEY LNRHLHTWIQ DNGGWDAFVE
201  LYGPSMRPLF DFSWLSLKTL LSLALVGACI TLGAYLGHK (239)
```

Domain structure

34–85   Domain II (italics): 64% conserved between mouse and human BCL2 but poorly conserved in the chicken protein

136–155   BCL2 homology 1 domain (underlined)

187–202   BCL2 homology 2 domain (underlined)

219–232   Transmembrane domain (underlined, italics)

217–239   Mitochondrial outer membrane targeting signal (underlined, italics)[39].

SEQUENCE OF BCL2β

```
  1  MAHAGRTGYD NREIVMKYIH YKLSQRGYEW DAGDVGAAPP GAAPAPGIFS
 51  SQPGHTPHPA ASRDPVARTS PLQTPAAPGA AAGPALSPVP PVVHLTLRQA
101  GDDFSRRYRR DFAEMSSQLH LTPFTARGRF ATVVEELFRD GVNWGRIVAF
151  FEFGGVMCVE SVNREMSPLV DNIALWMTEY LNRHLHTWIQ DNGGWVGASG
201  DVSLG (205)
```

Domain structure

196–205   Divergence between BCL2β and BCL2α (alternatively spliced versions of the same gene).

DATABASE ACCESSION NUMBERS

	PIR	*SWISSPROT*	*EMBL/GENBANK*	*REFERENCES*
Human *BCL2α*	A24428, A29409	P10415	M13994	*40*
			M14745	*41*
Human *BCL2β*	B29409	P10416	M13995	*40*
Human *BCLX_L*			L20121	*18*
Human *BCLX_S*			L20122	*18*
Human *BAXα*			L22473	*19*
Human *BAXβ*			L22474	*19*
Human *BAXγ*			L22475	*19*

References

1 Villuendas, R. et al. (1991) Am. J. Pathol. 139, 989–993.
2 Merino, R. et al. (1994) EMBO J. 13, 683–691.

3   Hockenbery, D. et al. (1991) Proc. Natl Acad. Sci. USA 88, 6961–6965.
4   Korsmeyer, S.J. (1992) Blood 80, 879–886.
5   Hockenbery, D. et al. (1990) Nature 348, 334–336.
6   Borzillo, G.V. et al. (1992) Oncogene 7, 869–876.
7   Garcia, I. et al. (1992) Science 258, 302–304.
8   Allsopp, T.E. et al. (1993) Cell 73, 295–307.
9   Hockenbery, D. et al. (1993) Cell 75, 241–251.
10 Alnemri, E.S. et al. (1992) Cancer Res. 52, 491–-495.
11 Bissonnette, R.P. et al. (1992) Nature 359, 552–554.
12 Fanidi, A. et al. (1992) Nature 359, 554–556.
13 Fernandez-Sarabia, M.J. and Bischoff, J.R. (1993) Nature 366, 274–275.
14 Boise, L.H. et al. (1993) Cell 74, 597–608.
15 Oltvai, Z.N. et al. (1993) Cell 74, 609–619.
16 Tanaka, S. et al. (1992) Blood 79, 229–237.
17 Limpens, J. et al. (1991) Oncogene 6, 2271–2276.
18 Aoki, K. et al. (1994) Oncogene 9, 1109–1115.
19 Weiss et al. (1987) New Engl. J. Med. 317, 1185–1189.
20 Pezzella, F. et al. (1992) Brit. J. Cancer 65, 87–89.
21 Tashiro, S. et al. (1992) Oncogene 7, 573–-577.
22 Seite, P. et al. (1993) Oncogen, 8, 3073–3080.
23 Hamilton, M.S. et al. (1991) Leukemia 5, 768–771.
24 Pettersson, M. et al. (1992) Blood 79, 495–502.
25 Delia, D. et al. (1992) Blood 79, 1291–1298.
26 Haury, M. et al. (1993) Oncogene 8, 1257–1262.
27 Reed, J.C. et al. (1991) Cancer Res. 51, 6529–6538.
28 Ikegaki, N. et al. (1994) Cancer Res. 54, 6–8.
29 Nunez, G. et al. (1990) Nature 353, 71–73.
30 Sentman, C.L. et al. (1991) Cell 67, 879–888.
31 Yeh, T.M. et al. (1991) Int. Immunol. 3, 1329–1233.
32 Katsumata, M. et al. (1992) Proc. Natl Acad. Sci. USA 89, 11376–11380.
33 Strasser, A. et al. (1994) Nature 368, 457–460.
34 McDonnell, T.J. et al. (1989) Cell 57, 79–88.
35 Strasser, A. et al. (1990) Nature 348, 331–333.
36 Vaux, D.L. et al. (1988) Nature 335, 440–442.
37 Seto, M. et al. (1988) EMBO J. 7, 123–131.
38 Young, R.L. and Korsmeyer, S.J. (1993) Mol. Cell. Biol. 13, 3686–3697.
39 Nguyen, M. et al. (1993) J. Biol. Chem. 268, 25265–25268.
40 Tsujimoto, Y. and Croce, C. (1986) Proc. Natl Acad. Sci. USA 83, 5214–5218.
41 Cleary, M.L. et al. (1986) Cell 47, 19–28.

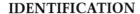
IDENTIFICATION

BCL3 (<u>B c</u>ell <u>l</u>eukaemia/lymphoma-<u>3</u>) was detected by molecular cloning of the breakpoint junction of the 14;19 translocation.

RELATED GENES

BCL3 is a member of the I-κB family. The seven ankyrin repeat regions in BCL3 are homologous to those in the human immediate early response gene product MAD3, the β subunit of the heteromeric DNA binding protein GABP, TAN1, LYT10, *notch* (*Drosophila melanogaster*), *Xnotch* (*Xenopus laevis*), *lin-12* and *glp-1* (*Caenorhabditis elegans*), SW14/SW16 (*Saccharomyces cerevisiae*), *cdc*10 (*S. pombe*).

Nucleotides (kb)		~10–11
Chromosome		19q13.1
Mass (kDa):	**predicted**	46.8
	expressed	28/30

Cellular location

Nucleus.

Tissue distribution

B Lymphocytes. mRNA expression increases seven-fold in normal human T cells between 15 min and 8 h after stimulation by PHA [1] and is abundant in B cell lines just prior to the Ig switch.

PROTEIN FUNCTION

Probable transcription factor. Phosphorylated BCL3 functions as a form of I-κB specific for the p50 subunit of NF-κB, rather than the NF-κB heterodimer (see ***REL***), inhibiting its translocation to the nucleus and binding to DNA [2-5], and increasing κB-dependent *trans* activation in intact cells by acting as an anti-repressor of inhibitory p50/NF-κB homodimers [6]. BCL3 does not inhibit the DNA binding activity of REL protein or its ability to *trans*-activate genes linked to a κB motif [7]. However, BCL3 also associates tightly with homodimers of p50B, a protein closely related to p50 [8]. Formation of the BCL3/p50 ternary complex permits BCL3 directly to *trans*-activate transcription via κB sites.

Cancer

The (14;19)(q32;q13.1) translocation occurs in some cases of B cell chronic lymphocytic leukaemia (B-CLL): *BCL3* is adjacent to the breakpoints involved and recombination occurs between the *BCL3* and Ig$_H$ loci[9]. Rearrangement of a gene designated *BCL3* and *BCL5* (17q22) has been reported in prolymphocytic leukaemia but this gene is unrelated to the chromosome 19 B-CLL-associated gene.

GENE STRUCTURE

BCL3 has not been fully mapped but consists of at least seven exons.

SEQUENCE OF BCL3

```
  1  MDEGPVDLRT RPKAAGLPGA ALPLRKRPLR APSPEPAAPR GAAGLVVPLD
 51  PLRGGCDLPA VPGPPHGLAR PEALYYPGAL LPLYPTRAMG SPFPLVNLPT
101  PLYPMMCPME HPLSADIAMA TRADEDGDTP LHIAVVQGNL PAVHRLVNLF
151  QQGGRELDIY NNLRQTPLHL AVITTLPSVV RLLVTAGASP MALDRHGQTA
201  AHLACEHRSP TCLRALLDSA APGTLDLEAR NYDGLTALHV AVNTECQETV
251  QLLLERGADI DAVDIKSGRS PLIHAVENNS LSMVQLLLQH GANVNAQMYS
301  GSSALHSASG RGLLPLVRTL VRSGADSSLK NCHNDTPLMV ARSRRVIDIL
351  RGKATRPAST SQPDPSPDRS ANTSPESSSR LSSNGLLSAS PSSSPSQSPP
401  RDPPGFPMAP PNFFLPSPSP PAFLPFAGVL RGPGRPVPPS PAPGGS (466)
```

Domain structure

1–112	Proline-rich domain
120–156, 157–189, 190–226, 227–260, 261–293, 294–326, 327–359	Seven repeated ankyrin motifs (underlined)
357–446	Serine/proline-rich domain

DATABASE ACCESSION NUMBERS

	PIR	SWISSPROT	EMBL/GENBANK	REFERENCES
Human *BCL3*	A34794	P20749	M31731, M31732	*1*

References

1 Ohno, H. et al. (1990) Cell 60, 991–997.
2 Nolan, G.P. et al. (1993) Mol. Cell. Biol. 13, 3557–3566.
3 Hatada, E.N. et al. (1992) Proc. Natl Acad. Sci. USA 89, 2489–2493.
4 Naumann, M. et al. (1993) EMBO J. 12, 213–222.
5 Franzoso, G. et al. (1993) EMBO J. 12, 3893–3901.
6 Franzoso, G. et al. (1992) Nature 359, 339–342.
7 Kerr, L.D. et al. (1992) Genes Devel. 6, 2352–2363.
8 Bours, V. et al. (1993) Cell 72, 729–739.
9 Ohno, H. et al. (1993) leukaemia 7, 2057–2063.

BCR

IDENTIFICATION

BCR (*b*reakpoint *c*luster *r*egion) is the first defined member of a small gene family localized on human chromosome 22, detected by screening DNA with a probe specific for the Philadelphia translocation breakpoint [1].

RELATED GENES

Three *BCR* related loci, *BCR2*, *BCR3* and *BCR4*; human *ABR* [2].

Nucleotides (kb)	130
Chromosome	22q11.2
Mass (kDa): predicted	143
expressed	160
	P210$^{BCR-ABL}$/P185$^{BCR-ABL}$

Cellular location

Cytoplasm

Tissue distribution

Widely expressed in many types of human haematopoietic and non-haematopoietic cells and cell lines [3].

PROTEIN FUNCTION

BCR has serine/threonine protein kinase activity [4], contains a central domain with homology to guanine nucleotide exchange proteins and has a C-terminal domain (absent in P210$^{BCR-ABL}$ and P185$^{BCR-ABL}$) that possesses *in vitro* GTPase activating protein activity [5]. BCR has autophosphorylating activity *in vitro* and phosphorylates histones and casein[6].

BCR/ABL exists *in vivo* associated with the GRB2/SOS complex that links tyrosine kinases to the RAS signalling system [7,8]. In myeloid cells expressing P210$^{BCR–ABL}$ the SHC protein that interacts with GRB2 is constitutively phosphorylated [9].

Cancer

The formation of the Philadelphia chromosome (Ph^1) in acute lymphoblastic leukaemia (ALL) and chronic myeloid leukaemia (CML) generates a chimeric *BCR–ABL* gene (see **ABL**). The proliferation *in vitro* of blast cells from CML patients is selectively suppressed by antisense oligodeoxynucleotides directed against the *BCR–ABL* junction [10].

Transgenic animals

Mice transgenic for a P185$^{Bcr-Abl}$ DNA construct develop aggressive leukaemias with early onset and rapid progression, consistent with there being a critical role for the *BCR–ABL* gene product of the Ph[1] chromosome in human leukaemia [11].

In vitro

In general BCR/ABL proteins are non-transforming but P210[BCR-ABL] or P185[BCR-ABL] (or v-ABL) induces both lymphoid and myeloid colonies in bone marrow cells, although only the lymphoid colonies are tumorigenic [12].

GENE STRUCTURE AND THE FORMATION OF THE PHILADELPHIA CHROMOSOME

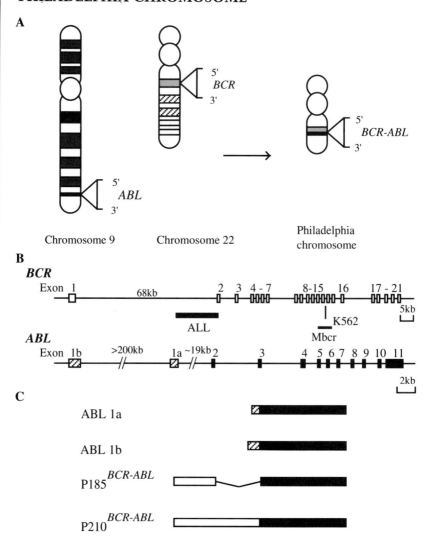

(a) The standard 9:22 reciprocal translocation occurs in about 92% of CML cases with a Ph[1] chromosome, resulting in a *BCR–ABL* chimeric gene on that chromosome. This translocation places *ABL* within the *BCR* gene on chromosome 22. The reciprocal recombination product is 5'-*ABL*/3'-*BCR* on the 9q+ derivative which is also transcriptionally active [13]. Between 5 and 8% of CML cases carry variant translocations which are either (i) Ph[1] negative, in which chromosome 22 is microscopically normal, or (ii) complex variants, in which up to three other chromosomes participate in translocation with chromosomes 9 and 22. The latter includes t(9;22;11)(q34;q11;q13) in which *BCR* 3' of the breakpoint moves to 11q13, the breakpoint occurring 5' of exon 4 [14].

(b) Ph[1] chromosome breakpoints occur between exons 1a and 2 and also between exons 1a and 1b of *ABL*. The fused *BCR–ABL* gene contains the *BCR* exons 5' of the breakpoint and all *ABL* exons except the first alternative exon. Thus in some CML patients the *ABL* gene located on the Ph[1] chromosome retains an intact exon 1a.

In the *BCR* gene Mbcr (major breakpoint cluster region) indicates the region in which breakpoints in CML are located [15]. Twenty-six codons from the 5' end of *ABL* are replaced by 927 codons from the *BCR* gene and fused to 1104 amino acids from ABL, generating P210$^{BCR-ABL}$. Two minor breakpoint cluster regions (mbcr2 and mbcr3) are located within the 3' half of the first *BCR* intron. K562 indicates the breakpoint in the K562 CML-derived cell line.

The breakpoint in the *ABL* sequence is in close proximity to that occurring in the generation of v-*abl*: thus the mechanism of activation of *ABL* in CML and of *Abl* by Ab-MuLV is similar, although the N-terminal deletion in v-*abl* is much larger and internal/frame shift mutations do not occur in the *BCR–ABL* gene.

ALL indicates the 3' region of intron 1 in which Mbcr-negative, Ph[1]-positive ALL breakpoints occur giving rise to a *BCR–ABL* mRNA that is translated into P185$^{BCR-ABL}$ (426 *BCR* encoded amino acids fused to 1104 from *ABL*) [16]. In ALL the breakpoints may also occur within Mbcr [17].

(c) This shows the structures of types 1a and 1b ABL and the chimeric proteins P185$^{BCR-ABL}$ and P210$^{BCR-ABL}$, indicating the coding regions of the genes from which they are derived. Both forms of BCR/ABL retain the SH3 domain and lack a myristylation signal, but tyrosine kinase activity is conferred by the additional N-terminal domain, specifically by sequences encoded by the first *BCR* exon [18]. P210$^{BCR-ABL}$ has a tyrosine kinase activity similar to that of v-ABL, potential substrates being RAS-GAP and its associated proteins p192 and p62 [19]. P185$^{BCR-ABL}$ has a fivefold greater tyrosine kinase activity, is a more potent transforming agent and is more often associated with acute than chronic leukaemia. ABL DNA binding activity is lost in the P210$^{BCR-ABL}$ protein.

TRANSCRIPTIONAL REGULATION

The *BCR* promoter occupies ~1 kb 5' to exon 1 and contains six SP1 consensus sequences, two CCAAT boxes and no TATA-like boxes [20].

PROTEIN STRUCTURE

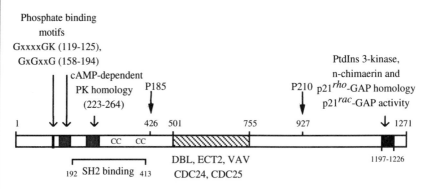

Phosphate binding
motifs
GxxxxGK (119-125),
GxGxxG (158-194)

cAMP-dependent
PK homology
(223-264)

P185

PtdIns 3-kinase,
n-chimaerin and
p21^{rho}-GAP homology
p21^{rac}-GAP activity

P210

1   426 501   755   927   1271

CC   CC

192 SH2 binding 413

DBL, ECT2, VAV
CDC24, CDC25

1197-1226

Cross-hatched box: homology with DBL, VAV, ECT2 [21], *Saccharomyces cerevisiae* CDC24 (regulates cytokinesis in yeast) and CDC25 [22]. Black box: GAP activity for p21^{rac}, homology with a p21^{rho} GAP, PtdIns 3-kinase 85 kDa subunit and *n*-chimaerin (which also has GAP activity for p21^{rac}) [5]. The C-termini of the portions incorporated into P185$^{BCR-ABL}$ and P210$^{BCR-ABL}$ are indicated (P185, P210). The N-terminal 63 amino acids mediate binding to actin [23].

Serine/threonine-rich regions of BCR (192–242 and 298–413) bind to the SH2 domain of ABL in a high affinity, phosphotyrosine-independent interaction [24,25]. This interaction is essential for BCR/ABL-mediated transformation: for the chimeric BCR/ABL proteins the interaction may be inter- or intra-molecular. The effect of the interaction may arise via interference with the binding of a cellular inhibitor to ABL regulatory domains.

SEQUENCE OF BCR

```
   1 MVDPVGFAEA WKAQFPDSEP PRMELRSVGD IEQELERCKA SIRRLEQEVN
  51 QERFRMIYLQ TLLAKEKKSY DRQRWGFRRA AQAPDGASEP RASASRPQPA
 101 PADGADPPPA EEPEARPDGE GSPGKARPGT ARRPGAAASG ERDDRGPPAS
 151 VAALRSNFER IRKGHGQPGA DAEKPFYVNV EFHHERGLVK VNDKEVSDRI
 201 SSLGSQAMQM ERKKSQHGAG SSVGDASRPP YRGRSSESSC GVDGDYEDAE
 251 LNPRFLKDNL IDANGGSRPP WPPLEYQPYQ SIYVGGMMEG EGKGPLLRSQ
 301 STSEQEKRLT WPRRSYSPRS FEDCGGGYTP DCSSNENLTS SEEDFSSGQS
 351 SRVSPSPTTY RMFRDKSRSP SQNSQQSFDS SSPPTPQCHK RHRHCPVVVS
                                  **
 401 EATIVGVRKT GQIWPNDGEG AFHGDADGSF GTPPGYGCAA DRAEEQRRHQ
 451 DGLPYIDDSP SSSPHLSSKG RGSRDALVSG ALESTKASEL DLEKGLEMRK
 501 WVLSGILASE ETYLSHLEAL LLPMKPLKAA ATTSQPVLTS QQIETIFFKV
 551 PELYEIHKEF YDGLFPRVQQ WSHQQRVGDL FQKLASQLGV YRAFVDNYGV
 601 AMEMAEKCCQ ANAQFAEISE NLRARSNKDA KDPTTKNSLE TLLYKPVDRV
 651 TRSTLVLHDL LKHTPASHPD HPLLQDALRI SQNFLSSINE EITPRRQSMT
 701 VKKGEHRQLL KDSFMVELVE GARKLRHVFL FTELLLCTKL KKQSGGKTQQ
 751 YDCKWYIPLT DLSFQMVDEL EAVPNIPLVP DEELDALKIK ISQIKSDIQR
 801 EKRANKGSKA TERLKKKLSE QESLLLLMSP SMAFRVHSRN GKSYTFLISS
 851 DYERAEWREN IREQQKKCFR SFSLTSVELQ MLTNSCVKLQ TVHSIPLTIN
```

```
                              ++
 901 KEDDESPGLY GFLNVIVHSA TGFKQSSNLY CTLEVDSFGY FVNKAKTRVY
 951 RDTAEPNWNE EFEIELEGSQ TLRILCYEKC YNKTKIPKED GESTDRLMGK
1001 GQVQLDPQAL QDRDWQRTVI AMNGIEVKLS VKFNSREFSL KRMPSRKQTG
1051 VFGVKIAVVT KRERSKVPYI VRQCVEEIER RGMEEVGIYR VSGVATDIQA
1101 LKAAFDVNNK DVSVMMSEMD VNAIAGTLKL YFRELPEPLF TDEFYPNFAE
1151 GIALSDPVAK ESCMLNLLLS LPEANLLTFL FLLDHLKRVA EKEAVNKMSL
1201 HNLATVFGPT LLRPSEKESK LPANPSQPIT MTDSWSLEVM SQVQVLLYFL
1251 QLEAIPAPDS KRQSILFSTE V (1271)
```

Domain structure

177   GRB2 SH2 domain binding site (Tyr177) in BCR/ABL. Tyr177 is encoded by exon 1 of *BCR*: mutation blocks BCR/ABL-induced transformation, indicating that GRB2 is involved in oncogenesis as well as in normal development and mitogenesis [7,8]

426–427   Breakpoint for translocation to form P185$^{BCR\text{-}ABL}$ oncogene (**)

927–928   Breakpoint for translocation to form P210$^{BCR\text{-}ABL}$ oncogene (++)

501–755   Homology with DBL, ECT2, VAV, TIM, CDC24 and CDC25 (underlined)

1197–1226   p21^{rac}-GAP activity region (italics)

DATABASE ACCESSION NUMBERS

	PIR	SWISSPROT	EMBL/GENBANK	REFERENCES
Human *BCR*	A26172	P11274	X02596, X52829	20
	A26664		Y00661	26
	A28765		M15025	27
			M24603, M64437	28
				29

References

1   **Konopka, J.B. and Witte, O.N. (1985) Biochim. Biophys. Acta 823, 1–17.**
2   Heisterkamp, N. et al. (1993) J. Biol. Chem. 268, 16903–16906.
3   Collins, S. et al. (1987) Mol. Cell. Biol. 7, 2870–2876.
4   Maru, Y. and Witte, O.N. (1991) Cell 67, 459–468.
5   Diekmann, D. et al. (1991) Nature 351, 400–402.
6   Liu, J. et al. (1993) Oncogene 8, 101–109.
7   Pendergast, A.M. et al. (1993) Cell 75, 175–185.
8   Puil, L. et al. (1994) EMBO J. 13, 764–773.
9   Matsuguchi, T. et al. (1994) J. Biol. Chem. 269, 5016–5021.
10   Szczylik, C. et al. (1991) Science 253, 562–565.
11   Heisterkamp, N. et al. (1990) Nature 344, 251–253.
12   Kelliher, M.A. et al. (1993) Oncogene 8, 1249–1256.
13   Melo, J.V. et al. (1992) Blood 81, 158–165.

14 Koduru, P.R.K. et al. (1993) Oncogene 8, 3239–3247.

15 Sowerby, S.J. et al. (1993) Oncogene 8, 1679–1683.

16 Clark, S.S. et al. (1988) Science 239, 775–777.

17 Hermans, A. et al. (1987) Cell 51, 33–40.

18 Muller, A.J. et al. (1991) Mol. Cell. Biol. 11, 1785–1792.

19 Carlesso, N. et al. 1994) Oncogene 9, 149–156.

20 Shah, N.P. et al. (1991) Mol. Cell. Biol. 11, 1854–1860.

21 Miki, T. et al. (1993) Nature 362, 462–465.

22 Cen, H. et al. (1992) EMBO J. 11, 4007–4015.

23 McWhirter, J.R. and Wang, J.Y.J. (1993) EMBO J. 12, 1533–1546.

24 Pendergast, A.M. et al. (1991) Cell 66, 161–171.

25 Muller, A.J. et al. (1992) Mol. Cell. Biol. 12, 5087–5093.

26 Hariharan, I.K. and Adams, J.M. (1987) EMBO J. 6, 115–119.

27 Heisterkamp, N. et al. (1985) Nature 315, 758–761.

28 Lifshitz, B. et al. (1988) Oncogene 2, 113–117.

29 Mes-Masson, A.M. et al. (1986) Proc. Natl Acad. Sci. USA 83, 9768–9772; Correction: ibid, 84, 2507.

CBL

IDENTIFICATION

v-*cbl* is the oncogene of the acutely transforming Cas NS-1 retrovirus (*C*asitas *B*-lineage *l*ymphoma). CBL was detected by screening human hematopoietic cell lines with a v-*cbl* probe.

RELATED GENES

No homology with other known oncogenes. Sequence homology to the DNA binding and transcriptional activation domains of the yeast regulatory protein GCN4.

		CBL	v-cbl
Nucleotides (bp)		2718	7400 (Cas NS-1 genome)
Chromosome		11q23.3-qter (*CBL2*)	
Mass (kDa):	predicted	100	
	expressed	p135	p100*gag-cbl*

Cellular location

CBL: Cytoplasm. *v-cbl*: Cytoplasm/nucleus.

Tissue distribution

Cbl is expressed in cells of the B, T, erythroid, myeloid and mast cell lineages and is most readily detectable in the thymus and testis [1].

PROTEIN FUNCTION

v-CBL was generated by truncation of 60% of the C-terminus of CBL. This permits the *gag–cbl* fusion protein to enter the nucleus. v-CBL binds to DNA, whereas full-length CBL does not, and thus probably functions as a transcriptional activator [2].

In animals

Cas NS-1 virus is an acutely transforming murine retrovirus that induces pre-B (sIg⁻, Lyb-2⁺, Ly-5 (B220⁺) and pro-B (Mac-1⁺) cell lymphomas and transforms fibroblasts, the *gag–onc* fusion protein appearing to be the responsible agent [3]. v-*cbl* and v-*abl* induce histologically and phenotypically similar tumours although for v-*cbl* there is longer latency and resistance in adult mice.

PROTEIN STRUCTURE

CBL has four potential N-linked glycosylation sites and many Ser/Thr stretches. v-CBL is a truncated form of mouse CBL containing 355 N-terminal amino acids fused behind 32 non-cellular residues[4]. The N-terminus of v-CBL is identical to the first 357 residues of human CBL with four deletions. v-CBL has lost a C-terminal leucine zipper and a 208 residue proline-rich region that occur in CBL and are similar to the activation domains of some transcription factors.

A truncated form of CBL occurs in the cutaneous T cell lymphoma line HUT78 in which 259 C-terminal amino acids are removed: the 72 kDa protein expressed lacks the leucine zipper region and part of the proline-rich domain [5].

SEQUENCE OF CBL

```
  1   MAGNVKKSSG AGGGTGSGGS GSGGLIGLMK DAFQPHHHHH HHLSPHPPGT
 51   VDKKMVEKCW KLMDKVVRLC QNPKLALKNS PPYILDLLPD TYQHLRTILS
101   RYEGKMETLG ENEYFRVFME NLMKKKTKQTI SLFKEGKERM YEENSQPRRN
151   LTKLSLIFSH MLAELKGIFP SGLFQGDTFR ITKADAAEFW RKAFGEKTIV
201   PWKSFRQALH EVHPISSGLE AMALKSTIDL TCNDYISVFE FDIFTRLFQP
251   WSSLLRNWNS LAVTHPGYMA FLTYDEVKAR LQKFIHKPGS YIFRLSCTRL
301   GQWAIGYVTA DGNILQTIPH NKPLFQALID GFREGFYLFP DGRNQNPDLT
351   GLCEPTPQDH IKVTQEQYEL YCEMGSTFQL CKICAENDKD VKIEPCGHLM
401   CTSCLTSWQE SEGQGCPFCR CEIKGTEPIV VDPFDPRGSG SLLRQGAEGA
451   PSPNYDDDDD ERADDTLFMM KELAGAKVER PPSPFSMAPQ ASLPPVPPRL
501   DLLPQRVCVP SSASALGTAS KAASGSLHKD KPLPVPPTLR DLPPPPPPDR
551   PYSVGAESRP QRRPLPCTPG DCPSRDKLPP VPSSRLGDSW LPRPIPKVPV
601   SAPSSSDPWT GRELTNRHSL PFSLPSQMEP RPDVPRLGST FSLDTSMSMN
651   SSPLVGPECD HPKIKPSSSA NAIYSLAARP LPVPKLPPGE QCEGEEDTEY
701   MTPSSRPLRP LDTSQSSRAC DCDQQIDSCT YEAMYNIQSQ APSITESSTF
751   GEGNLAAAHA NTGPEESENE DDGYDVPKPP VPAVLARRTL SDISNASSSF
801   GWLSLDGDPT TNVTEGSQVP ERPPKPFPRR INSERKAGSC QQGSGPAASA
851   ATASPQLSSE IENLMSQGYS YQDIQKALVI AQNNIEMAKN ILREFVSISS
901   PAHVAT (906)
```

Domain structure

124–127	Nuclear localization signal (underlined)
381–419	C_3HC_4-type zinc finger
357–476 and 689–834	Acidic domains
477–688	Proline-rich region
857–892	Leucine zipper (underlined italics)

DATABASE ACCESSION NUMBERS

	PIR	SWISSPROT	EMBL/GENBANK	REFERENCES
Human CBL	A43817	P22681	X57110	4

References

1 Langdon, W.Y. et al. (1989) J. Virol. 63, 5420–5424.
2 Blake, T.J. et al. (1993) EMBO J. 12, 2017–2026.
3 Langdon, W.Y. et al. (1989) Proc. Natl Acad. Sci. USA 86, 1168–1172.
4 Blake, T.J. et al. (1991) Oncogene 6, 653–657.
5 Blake, T.J. and Langdon, W.Y. (1992) Oncogene 7, 757–762.

CRK

IDENTIFICATION

v-*crk* (*C*T10 *r*egulator of *k*inase) is the oncogene of avian sarcoma viruses CT10 and ASV-1. *CRK-I* and *CRK-II* were isolated from embryonic lung cells using the polymerase chain reaction and by screening a human placental cDNA library with a *CRK-I* probe, respectively.

RELATED GENES

CRK proteins contain SH2 and SH3 domains homologous with those present in SRC family proteins, FPS/FES and ABL, RAS-GAP, the PtdIns-specific phospholipase C-Iγ isozymes, α-spectrin, the yeast actin binding protein ABP1p, myosin-I, p85α and p85β (see **SRC**). *CRKL* is 60% homologous to *CRK-II* and maps to chromosome 22q11.

		CRK	v-*crk*
Nucleotides, (bp)		Not fully mapped	2407
Chromosome		17p13	
Mass (kDa):	predicted	39.8	
	expressed	28 (CRK-I)	P47*gag-crk*
		40/42 (CRK-II)	
		36 (CRKL)	

Cellular location

CRK: Cytoplasm. v-*crk*: Cytoplasm.

Tissue distribution

CRK-I (p28) is expressed in human embryonic lung cells. CRK-II (p42) is present in the osteosarcoma cell line 143B, A431 cells and the T cell line H9. CRK-II (p40) is present in a wide variety of cell lines [1].

PROTEIN FUNCTION

P47*gag-crk* causes tyrosine phosphorylation in CT10-infected chick embryo fibroblasts, notably of proteins in the 135–155 kDa range including paxillin [2]. p47 does not itself possess kinase activity and has thus been denoted *C*T10 *r*egulator of *k*inase [3]. P47*gag-crk* immunoprecipitates with a wide range of tyrosine phosphorylated proteins, including the EGF and PDGF receptors and v-SRC, but association with the latter is prevented if autophosphorylation of Tyr416 is blocked [4,5]. Mutational studies indicate that the SH2 domain of P47*gag-crk* binds specifically to tyrosine phosphorylated regions of peptides [6] and shows preferential affinity for binding to phosphotyrosine in the general motif pTyr–hydrophilic–hydrophilic-Ile/Pro [7].

Cancer

The region to which *CRK* maps (17p13) demonstrates frequent deletion or loss of heterozygosity in a wide range of human tumours [8].

In animals

CT10 or ASV-1 cause rapid tumour formation in chickens [9].

In vitro

ASV CT10 transforms chick embryo fibroblasts which are then tumorigenic when injected into chickens [10]. Cell lines expressing CRK-I are tumorigenic in nude mice. CRK-II does not transform cells *in vitro* and is non-tumorigenic [1]. Microinjection of CRK or stable expression of v-CRK causes differentiation of the rat pheochromocytoma cell line PC12 that is abolished by mutations in either the SH2 or SH3 domains [11]. EGF or NGF cause the tyrosyl phosphorylation of v-CRK which associates with the receptors for these ligands.

PROTEIN STRUCTURE

A member of the group of proteins of unrelated function that share homology with non-catalytic regions of SRC, P47$^{gag-crk}$ contains SRC homology regions 2 and 3 (SH2, SH3), transposed with respect to SRC. These regions also occur in phosphatidylinositol-specific phospholipase C-γ [12], where SH2 is duplicated, and P47$^{gag-crk}$ has strong homology with a 180 amino acid region of this protein.

Human CRK-I and CRK-II each contain one SH2 domain together with one and two SH3 domains, respectively [1]. The B and C boxes of SH2, separated by a hinge region, coordinately form the functional phospho-tyrosine binding domain [13]. The binding affinity of v-CRK for tyrosine phosphorylated proteins (e.g. EGFR, PDGF-R, v-SRC) greatly exceeds that of CRK, even though both have identical SH2 domains. This is caused by the presence of a short region N-terminal to the SH2 domain in v-CRK [14].

The P47$^{gag-crk}$ transforming protein comprises 208 *gag*-encoded amino acids fused to 232 novel residues presumed to be from a cellular proto-oncogene. The cellular sequence lacks start and stop codons, so is presumed to be truncated at both ends. The last three amino acids and the stop codon are provided by viral sequences.

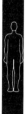

SEQUENCE OF HUMAN CRK-II

```
  1  MAGNFDSEER SSWYWGRLSR QEAVALLQGQ RHGVFLVRDS STSPGDYVLS
 51  VSENSRVSHY IINSSGPRPP VPPSPAQPPP GVSPSRLRIG DQEFDSLPAL
101  LEFYKIHYWD TTTLIEPVSR SRQGSGVILR QEEAEYVRAL FDFNGNDEED
151  LPFKKGDILR IRDKPEEQWW NAEDSEGKRG MIPVPYVEKY RPASASVSAL
201  IGGNQEGSHP QPLGPPEPGP YAQPSVNTPL PNLQNGPIYA RVIQKRVPNA
251  YDKTALALEV GELVKVTKIN VSGQWEGGCN GKRGHFPFTH VRLLDQQNPD
301  EDFS (304)
```

Domain structure

11–104	CRK-II SH2 domain (underlined)
133–184 and 238–290	CRK-II SH3 domains (underlined)

The termination codon for CRK-I (204 amino acids, identical to CRK-II with the substitution of Arg204 for Asn204) is in the same position as that for v-CRK. *CRK-I* lacks a 170 bp sequence present in *CRK-II*: alternative splicing is presumed to remove this region leaving a single SH3 domain in CRK-I. v-CRK is homologous to the N-terminal 203 amino acids of CRK-II with 47 scattered point mutations.

DATABASE ACCESSION NUMBERS

	PIR	SWISSPROT	EMBL/GENBANK	REFERENCE
Human *CRK-I, II*	B45022, A45022		D10656	*1*

References
1 Matsuda, M. et al. (1992) Mol. Cell. Biol. 12, 3482–3489.
2 Birge, R.B. et al. (1993) Mol. Cell. Biol. 13, 4648–4656.
3 Mayer, B.J. et al. (1989) Cold Spring Harbor Symp. Quant. Biol. 53, 907–914.
4 Matsuda, M. et al. (1990) Science 248, 1537–1539.
5 Mayer, B.J. and Hanafusa, H. (1990) Proc. Natl Acad. Sci. USA 87, 2638–2642.
6 Matsuda, M. et al. (1991) Mol. Cell. Biol, 11, 1607–1613.
7 Songyang, Z. et al. (1993) Cell 72, 767–778.
8 Fioretos, T. et al. (1993) Oncogene 8, 2853–2855.
9 Tsuchie, H. et al. (1989) Oncogene 4, 1281–1284.
10 Mayer, B.J. et al. (1988) Nature 332, 272–275.
11 Hempstead, B.L. et al. (1994) Mol. Cell. Biol. 14, 1964–1971.
12 Stahl, M.L. et al. (1988) Nature 332, 269–272.
13 Matsuda, M. et al. (1993) J. Biol. Chem. 268, 4441–4446.
14 Fajardo, J.E. et al. (1993) Mol. Cell. Biol. 13, 7295–7302.

CSF1R/Fms

IDENTIFICATION

v-*fms* is the transforming oncogene of the Susan McDonough (SM-FeSV) and Hardy–Zuckerman (HZ5-FeSV) strains of acutely transforming feline sarcoma virus. *CSF1R/Fms* was detected by screening human placental cDNA with a v-*fms* probe.

RELATED GENES

FMS is closely related to *KIT*, the two receptors for PDGF, human *FRT* (*fms-related tyrosine kinase gene*) and the product of the *FLT3/FLK2* gene (human stem cell tyrosine kinase 1 (STK1)). Each has a distinctive pattern of cysteine spacing in the extracellular domain that includes sequences characteristic of the immunoglobulin (Ig) gene superfamily and in each the kinase domain is interrupted by a hydrophilic spacer of between 64 and 104 amino acids.

FLT1 (*FMS-like tyrosine kinase*, also FLK3) is ~60% homologous to FMS but has a predicted seven Ig-like extracellular domains, compared with five in members of the CSF1R/FMS family. *FLK1* (human *KDR*, murine *Nyk*, rat *TKr-III*) and *FLT4* encode the other members of the class of receptor tyrosine kinases with seven Ig-like loops.

	FMS	v-fms
Nucleotides (kb)	>30	8.2 (SM-FeSV genome)
Chromosome	5q33.3–34	
Mass (kDa): predicted	108	
expressed	gp150	gp140v-*fms* (SM-FeSV)

Cellular location

Transmembrane protein. The ectodomain may be released from cells [1].

Tissue distribution

CSF1R is normally only expressed on monocytes, macrophages and their precursors [2] and at lower levels in normal and malignant B lymphocytes [3] but is also detectable in the human and murine uteroplacental unit [4] and in cell lines derived from human malignant placental trophoblasts. *FMS* is not expressed in normal vascular smooth muscle cells but is activated in intimal smooth muscle cells isolated from an experimental rabbit model of arteriosclerosis [5].

PROTEIN FUNCTION

CSF1R (*FMS*) encodes the receptor for colony stimulating factor-1 (CSF1 or M-CSF) that cooperates with IL2 or IL3 to stimulate bone marrow cells during haematopoiesis [6]. The enhanced expression of *Fms* in pregnant mice indicates a possible role in embryogenesis. *Fms* may also be involved in the induction of macrophage differentiation [7, 8]. Expression of v-*fms* may cause haematopoietic disorders [9].

FMS has intrinsic tyrosine kinase activity and RAF is a substrate *in vitro*. In macrophages CSF1 activates the Na^+/K^+-ATPase, the Na^+/H^+ exchanger and *Fos* and *Myc* transcription. CSF1 also activates the *Src* family kinases SRC, FYN and YES and causes these proteins to associate with the CSF1R [10].

NIH 3T3 fibroblasts are mitogenically stimulated by CSF1 after transfection with the human *FMS* gene, but CSF1 causes barely detectable tyrosine phosphorylation of PLC-γ and no early (5 min) change in $[Ca^{2+}]_i$ [11]. It is possible that CSF1 activates other isoforms of PLC but it seems probable that, despite its structural similarity to the PDGF receptor, activation via FMS does not involve PtdIns(4,5)P_2 hydrolysis.

CSF1 causes weak tyrosine phosphorylation of GAP and strong tyrosine phosphorylation of the GAP associated proteins p62 and p190. Despite the contrast in effects on GAP, CSF1 and PDGF promote equivalent activation of RAS.GTP and stimulate mitogenesis to a similar extent in 3T3 cells [12]. The activated CSF1R associates with the SH2-containing adaptor protein GRB2 and causes the tyrosine phosphorylation of SHC, consistent with the evidence that CSF1 activates a pathway involving RAS [13].

Receptor-mediated endocytosis of FMS and v-FMS follows ligand binding but endocytosis of v-FMS does not require CSF1. The rapid internalization of the FMS receptor does not depend on the tyrosine kinase activity of the receptor or on the presence of the kinase insert region of the cytoplasmic domain although degradation requires both these regions [14]. The kinase insert region is also unnecessary for the growth stimulating activity of the FMS kinase [15, 16].

v-*fms*-mediated transformation appears to be caused by the sustained expression of CSF1-independent tyrosine kinase activity [17]. In SM-FeSV-transformed mink lung epithelial cells PtdIns(4,5)P_2 hydrolysis and PtdIns kinase activities are increased [18].

Cancer

Activating mutations of *FMS* have been detected in patients with primary acute myeloid leukaemia [19].

In animals

Inoculation of SM-FeSV-transformed NIH 3T3 fibroblasts or NRK cells into syngeneic animals or nude mice induces fatal tumours [20].

In vitro

SM-FeSV transforms NIH 3T3, MDCK, NRK, feline embryo fibroblasts and mink lung epithelial cells [21]. This requires tyrosine kinase activity, normal glycosylation and surface membrane expression. The presence of the complete ligand binding domain of CSF1 in v-FMS causes transformed cells to bind CSF1 specifically and CSF1 causes a further two- to threefold increase of phosphotyrosine in gp140$^{v\text{-}fms}$, indicating further increase in the constitutive kinase activity of the transforming protein [11,17]. The expression of a constitutively activated tyrosine phosphatase suppresses transformation by v-*fms* [22].

Expression of a dominant-negative FLK1, the receptor for vascular endothelial growth factor (VEGF-VPF), inhibits glioblastoma cell growth [23].

GENE STRUCTURE

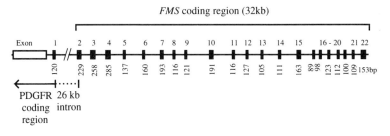

The overall gene structure and encoded amino acid sequence is similar to the PDGF receptor and the two genes may have arisen by duplication. Exon 2 encodes part of the 5′ untranslated sequence of *FMS* mRNA, the initiation codon and the signal peptide [24,25].

In the mouse, integration of Friend MuLV at the 5′ end of *Fms* directly upstream of the region corresponding to exon 2 of the human gene induces transcription as a component of the development of myeloid leukaemia. Proviral insertion is head-to-head with respect to the direction of *Fms* transcription, indicating that the promoter may lie close to exon 2 [26].

PROTEIN STRUCTURE OF FMS AND V-FMS

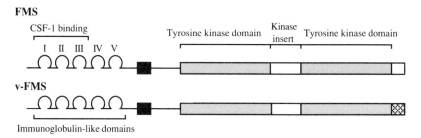

Human and feline FMS proteins share 80.5% identity. v-FMS and FMS differ only by scattered amino acid substitutions except that the 50 C-terminal amino acids of feline FMS are replaced by 14 residues in SM-FeSV v-FMS (cross-hatched box), encoded by a 3′ untranslated region of feline *Fms*, with the elimination of the C-terminal tyrosine of FMS [27]. The mutations that appear critical for the activation of v-FMS are the substitution of two serine residues in the extracellular domain of feline FMS, together with the modification of the C-terminus [28, 29].

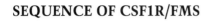

SEQUENCE OF CSF1R/FMS

```
  1  MGPGVLLLLL VATAWHGQGI PVIEPSVPEL VVKPGATVTL RCVGNGSVEW
 51  DGPASPHWTL YSDGSSSILS TNNATFQNTG TYRCTEPGDP LGGSAAIHLY
101  VKDPARPWNV LAQEVVVFED QDALLPCLLT DPVLEAGVSL VRVRGRPLMR
151  HTNYSFSPWH GFTIHRAKFI QSQDYQCSAL MGGRKVMSIS IRLKVQKVIP
201  GPPALTLVPA ELVRIRGEAA QIVCSASSVD VNFDVFLQHN NTKLAIPQQS
251  DFHNNRYQKV LTLNLDQVDF QHAGNYSCVA SNVQGKHSTS MFFRVVESAY
301  LNLSSEQNLI QEVTVGEGLN LKVMVEAYPG LQGFNWTYLG PFSDHQPEPK
351  LANATTKDTY RHTFTLSLPR LKPSEAGRYS FLARNPGGWR ALTFELTLRY
401  PPEVSVIWTF INGSGTLLCA ASGYPQPNVT WLQCSGHTDR CDEAQVLQVW
451  DDPYPEVLSQ EPFHKVTVQS LLTVETLEHN QTYECRAHNS VGSGSWAFIP
501  ISAGAHTHPP DEFLFTPVVV ACMSIMALLL LLLLLLLYKY KQKPKYQVRW
551  KIIESYEGNS YTFIDPTQLP YNEKWEFPRN NLQFGKTLGA GAFGKVVEAT
601  AFGLGKEDAV LKVAVKMLKS TAHADEKEAL MSELKIMSHL GQHENIVNLL
651  GACTHGGPVL VITEYCCYGD LLNFLRRKAE AMLGPSLSPG QDPEGGVDYK
701  NIHLEKKYVR RDSGFSSQGV DTYVEMRPVS TSSNDSFSEQ DLDKEDGRPL
751  ELRDLLHFSS QVAQGMAFLA SKNCIHRDVA ARNVLLTNGH VAKIGDFGLA
801  RDIMNDSNYI VKGNARLPVK WMAPESIFDC VYTVQSDVWS YGILLWEIFS
851  LGLNPYPGIL VNSKFYKLVK DGYQMAQPAF APKNIYSIMQ ACWALEPTHR
901  PTFQQICSFL QEQAQEDRRE RDYTNLPSSS RSGGSGSSSS ELEEESSSEH
951  LTCCEQGDIA QPLLQPNNYQ FC (972)
```

Domain structure

1–23	Signal sequence
24–512	Extracellular domain
513–537	Trans membrane region (underlined)
538–972	Cytoplasmic domain
588–596 and 616	ATP binding domain
683–749	Kinase insert region (underlined)
699, 708, 809	Auto-phosphorylation sites
778	Active site
45, 73, 153, 240, 302, 335, 353, 412, 428 and 480	Potential glycosylation sites
723	Binding site (when phosphorylated) for PtdIns 3-kinase via the two SH2 domains of its p85α subunit [30]
809	Substitution of Tyr809 blocks ligand-dependent mitogenesis but does not inhibit the tyrosine kinase activity of the receptor nor its ability to associate with PtdIns 3-kinase and to induce *Fos* and *Jun* transcription [31] although it does decrease the binding and enzymatic activation of SRC, FYN and YES [10]. Activated Phe809 mutant receptors do not, however, induce *Myc* expression but the co-expression of an exogenous *Myc* gene in cells

expressing only the mutant form of the receptor restores the ability of the cells to proliferate in response to CSF1, implying the existence of an effector interacting with the domain including Tyr809 that is required for *Myc* induction and CSF1-induced mitogenesis

969 Replacement of Tyr969 with Phe enhances transforming potential [17]

DATABASE ACCESSION NUMBERS

	PIR	SWISSPROT	EMBL/GENBANK	REFERENCES
Human *CSF1R*	A24533	P07333	X03663	[32]
Human *FRT*		P16057	D00133	[33]
Human *FLT1*	S09982	P17948	X51602	[34]
Human *FLT4*				[35]

References
1 Downing, J.R. et al. (1991) Mol. Cell. Biol. 9, 2890–2896.
2 **Sherr, C.J. (1988) Biophys. Acta 948, 225–243.**
3 Baker, A.H. et al. (1993) Oncogene 8, 371–378.
4 Pampfer, S. et al. (1992) Biol. Reprod. 46, 48–57.
5 Inaba, T. et al. (1992) J. Biol. Chem. 267, 5693–5699.
6 Stanley, E.R. et al. (1986) Cell 45, 667–674.
7 Rohrschneider, L.R. and Metcalf, D. (1989) Mol. Cell. Biol. 9, 5081–5092.
8 Borzillo, G.V. et al. (1990) Mol. Cell. Biol. 10, 2703–2714.
9 Heard, J.M. et al. (1987) Cell 51, 663–673.
10 Courtneidge, S. et al. (1993) EMBO J. 12, 943–950.
11 Downing, J.R. et al. (1989) EMBO J. 8, 3345–3350.
12 Heidaran, M.A. et al. (1992) Oncogene 7, 147–152.
13 van der Geer, P. and Hunter, T. (1993) EMBO J. 12, 5161–5172.
14 Carlberg, K. et al. (1991) EMBO J. 10, 877–883.
15 Taylor, G.R. et al. (1989) EMBO J. 8, 2029–2037.
16 Shurtleff, S.A. et al. (1990) EMBO J. 9, 2415–2421.
17 Roussel, M.F. et al. (1987) Nature 325, 549–552.
18 Kaplan, D.R. et al. (1987) Cell 50, 1021–1029.
19 Ridge, S.A. et al. (1990) Proc. Natl Acad. Sci. USA 87, 1377–1380.
20 McDonough, S.K. et al. (1971) Cancer Res. 31, 953–956.
21 Donner, L. et al. (1982) J. Virol. 41, 489–500.
22 Zander, N.F. et al. (1993) Oncogene 8, 1175–1182.
23 Millauer, B. et al. (1994) Nature 367, 576–579.
24 Roberts, W.M. et al. (1988) Cell 55, 655–661.
25 Hampe, A. et al. (1989) Oncogene Res. 4, 9–17.
26 Gisselbrecht, S. et al. (1987) Nature 329, 259–261.
27 Woolford, J. et al. (1988) Cell 55, 965–977.
28 Roussel, M.F. et al. (1988) Cell 55, 979–988.
29 **Rohrschneider, L.R. and Woolford, J. (1991) Semin. in Virol. 2, 385–395.**
30 Reedijk, M. et al. (1992) EMBO J. 11, 1365–1372.

31 Roussel, M.F. et al. (1991) Nature 353, 361–363.

32 Coussens, L. et al. (1986) Nature 320, 277–280.

33 Matsushime, H. et al. (1987) Jpn J. Cancer Res. 78, 655–661.

34 Shibuya, M. et al. (1990) Oncogene 5, 519–524.

35 Galland, F. et al. (1993) Oncogene 8, 1233–1240.

DBL

IDENTIFICATION

DBL was identified by NIH 3T3 fibroblast transfection of DNA from a human _d_iffuse _B_ cell _l_ymphoma. *MCF2* and *DBL* represent two activated versions of the same proto-oncogene.

RELATED GENES

The N-terminal region of DBL has homology with vimentin and the central region has homology with human ABR, BCR, ECT2, TIM, VAV and RAS-GRF nucleotide exchange factor.

Nucleotides (kb)	45
Chromosome	Xq27
Mass (kDa): **predicted**	108
expressed	p115 (DBL)
	p66 (oncogenic)

Cellular location

Cytoplasmic: associates with cytoskeletal actin [1].

Tissue distribution

Highly tissue-specific: brain, adrenal glands, gonads.

PROTEIN FUNCTION

Unknown. Microinjection of DBL causes germinal vesicle breakdown and activation of H1 histone kinase in oocytes [2]. *In vitro* it acts as a guanine nucleotide exchange factor for CDC42Hs, the human homologue of the *S. cerevisiae* protein CDC42Sc [3].

Cancer

DBL is expressed in Ewing's sarcoma (tumours of neuroectodermic origin) [4]. Transforming potential is enhanced 50–70-fold on substitution of 5' sequences to form oncogenic *DBL* [5].

Transgenic animals

DBL does not induce neoplasia in transgenic mice but animals that express the DBL protein in their lenses develop cataracts. *DBL* therefore appears capable of interfering with the ability of lens epithelial cells to differentiate into lens fibre cells [6].

In vitro

Transfection of NIH 3T3 cells with DNA from a human nodular poorly differentiated lymphoma (NPDL) generates *NPDL–DBL* that is homologous to oncogenic *DBL* and encodes a 76 kDa protein [7].

PROTEIN STRUCTURE

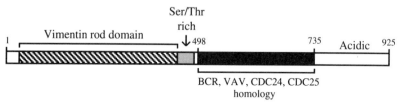

Ser/Thr rich

Vimentin rod domain

↓498

BCR, VAV, CDC24, CDC25 homology

DBL and *MCF2* represent two activated versions of the same proto-oncogene. Activation of the *DBL* oncogene occurs by 5′ fusion of 50 amino acids encoded by an unrelated human gene to 428 amino acids encoded by the 3′ portion of *DBL*, with the loss of the first 497 amino acids of DBL. There is only one (conservative) substitution in the C-terminal 428 amino acids of oncogenic DBL. The loss of the N-terminal 497 amino acids of DBL, rather than the properties of the N-terminus acquired by oncogenic DBL, is responsible for the transforming activity [8]. In MCF2 397 amino acids are removed.

SEQUENCE OF DBL

```
  1   MAEANPRRGK  MRFRRNAASF  PGNLHLVLVL  RPTSFLQRTF  TDIGFWFSQE
 51   DFMPKLPVVM  LSSVSDLLTY  IDDKQLTPEL  GGTLQYCHSE  WIIFRNAIEN
101   FALTVKEMAQ  MLQSFGTELA  ETELPDDIPS  IEEILAIRAE  RYHLLKNDIT
151   AVTKEGKILL  TNLEVPDTEG  AVSSRLECHR  QISGDWQTIN  KLLTQVHDME
201   TAFDGFWEKH  QLKMEQYLQL  WKFEQDFQQL  VTEVEFLLNQ  QAELADVTGT
251   IAQVKQKIKK  LENLDENSQE  LLSKAQFVIL  HGHKLAANHH  YALDLICQRC
301   NELRYLSDIL  VNEIKAKRIQ  LSRTFKMHKL  LQQARQCCDE  GECLLANQEI
351   DKFQSKEDAQ  KALQDIENFL  EMALPFINYE  PETLQYEFDV  ILSPELK VQM
                                                             Δ
401   KTIQLKLENI  RSIFENQQAG  FRNLADKHVR  PIQFVVPTPE  NLVTSGTPFF
451   SSKQGKKTWR  QNQSNLKIEV  VPDCQEKRSS  GPSSSLDNGN  SLDVLKN HVL
                                                             ΔΔ
501   NELIQTERVY  VRELYTVLLG  YRAEMDNPEM  FDLMPPLLRN  KKDILFGNMA
551   EIYEFHNDIF  LSSLENCAHA  PERVGPCFLE  RKDDFQMYAK  YCQNKPRSET
601   IWRKYSECAF  FQECQRKLKH  RLRLDSYLLK  PVQRITKYQL  LLKELLKYSK
651   DCEGSALLKK  ALDAMLDLLK  SVNDSMHQIA  INGYIGNLNE  LGKMIMQGGF
701   SVWIGHKKGA  TKMKDLARFK  PMQRHLFLYE  KAIVFCKRRV  ESGEGSDRYP
751   SYSFKHCWKM  DEVGITEYVK  GDNRKFEIWY  GEKEEVYIVQ  ASNVDVKMTW
801   LKEIRNILLK  QQELLTVKKR  KQQDQLTERD  KFQISLQQND  EKQQGAFIST
851   EETELEHTST  VVEVCEAIAS  VQAEANTVWT  EASQSAEISE  EPAEWSSNYF
901   YPTYDENEEE  NRPLMRPVSE  MALLY (925)
```

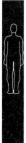

Domain structure

398–925 MCF2 transforming protein (Δ)

498–925 DBL transforming protein (ΔΔ). The DBL breakpoint lies within an *MCF2* exon

498–735 Homology with BCR, VAV, CDC24 and CDC25 (underlined)[9]. Small deletions within this region completely abolish the transforming activity of DBL

343 Putative palmitoylation site

742 Phosphorylation site

DATABASE ACCESSION NUMBERS

	PIR	SWISSPROT	EMBL/GENBANK	REFERENCES
Human *DBL*	A30040	P10911	X12556	10
	A28051	P14919	J03639	11
			X13230	5

References

1 Graziani, G. et al. (1989) Oncogene 4, 823–829.

2 Graziani, G. et al. (1992) Oncogene 7, 229–235.

3 Hart, M.J. et al. (1991) Nature 354, 311–314.

4 Vecchio, G. et al. (1989) Oncogene 4, 897–900.

5 Noguchi, T. et al. (1988) Oncogene 3, 709–715.

6 Eva, A. et al. (1991) New Biol. 3, 158–168.

7 Eva, A. et al. (1987) Oncogene 1, 355–360.

8 Ron, D. et al. (1989) Oncogene 4, 1067–1072.

9 Ron, D. et al. (1991) New Biol. 3, 372–379.

10 Ron, D. et al. (1988) EMBO J. 7, 2465–2473.

11 Eva, A. et al. (1988) Proc. Natl Acad. Sci. USA 85, 2061–2065.

EGFR/ErbB-1

IDENTIFICATION

v-*erbB* is the oncogene of avian <u>e</u>rythro<u>b</u>lastosis virus (AEV), strain AEV-H, detected by hybridizing viral mRNA with cDNA made against the unique sequences of AEV. *EGFR* (*ErbB-1*) encodes the receptor for epidermal growth factor.

RELATED GENES

HER2, HER3, HER4, Drosophila: DER; Xiphophorus maculatus: Xmrk.

		EGFR	*v-erbB*
Nucleotides (kb)		110	7.8 (AEV-H)
Chromosome		7p13–p12	
Mass (kDa):	**predicted**	134	62
	expressed	gp170	68/74

Cellular location

Plasma membrane.

Tissue distribution

Human *EGFR* is widely distributed, except in haematopoietic tissues. Most cells express between 2×10^4 and 2×10^5 receptors.

PROTEIN FUNCTION

EGFR is a receptor for epidermal growth factor (EGF), heparin-binding EGF-like factor (HB-EGF), transforming growth factor α, amphiregulin and vaccinia virus growth factor. EGF binding increases receptor–receptor affinity, activating the cytoplasmic tyrosine kinase domain of EGFR by dimerization and *trans*-phosphorylation: the ligand–receptor complex undergoes receptor-mediated endocytosis [1,2]. In epidermal cells the EGFR is activated by ultraviolet irradiation [3]. EGFR and HER2 heterodimerize and EGF causes the *trans*-phosphorylation of such complexes [4].

EGF acts synergistically with insulin to stimulate DNA synthesis and cell proliferation. Phosphorylated tyrosine residues in the activated EGFR associate with the SH2 domain of growth factor receptor-bound protein 2 (GRB2) which itself is bound to SOS1. This causes the activation of RAS (i.e. increase in GTP.RAS; see *RAS*), leading to the activation of RAF1 and MAP kinase.

The activated EGFR phosphorylates the RAS GTPase-activating protein (GAP), a cytosolic tyrosine kinase [5], EPS8, pp81, lipocortins, pp42 and calmodulin and also stimulates substrate-selective protein tyrosine-phosphatase activity directed towards the EGFR itself and HER2 [6]. In addition to the GRB2/SOS complex, the activated EGFR physically associates with SHC proteins, EPS8, PtdIns 3-kinase and PLCγ [7–9]. EGFR activation increases the intracellular free concentration of Ca^{2+} and causes transient membrane hyperpolarization [10].

In keratinocytes activation of the EGFR specifically stimulates transcription of *K6* and *K16* genes[11].

Cancer

EGFR is amplified by up to 50-fold in some primary tumours, including ~20% of bladder tumours [12], and derived cell lines [13]. Amplification also occurs in ~20% of primary breast tumours where it is strongly associated with early recurrence and death in lymph node-positive patients [14–16].

Three truncated forms of EGFR have been detected in a relatively small proportion of malignancies. Type I lacks the majority of the extracellular domain and does not bind EGF [17]. Type II contains an in-frame deletion of 83 amino acids (520–603) in extracellular domain IV that does not prevent EGF and TGFα binding [18]. Type III has an in-frame deletion of 267 amino acids (29–296) in extracellular domains II and III [19]. Each of these mutations has been detected in glioblastomas and type III has also been detected in 16% of a sample of non-small cell lung carcinomas [20].

In animals

v-*erbB* is the transduced gene in avian retroviruses (e.g. ALV) that causes rapid induction of erythroleukaemia and fibrosarcoma [21].

In vitro

EGFR is a weak transforming agent in NIH 3T3 cells [22] and can induce ligand-independent proliferation of myeloid precursor cells [23].

v-*erbB* transforms chick embryo fibroblasts and stimulates proliferation of erythrocyte progenitor cells although it does not completely block their differentiation.

STRUCTURE OF THE *EGFR* GENE

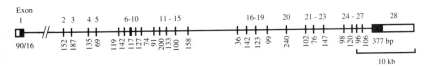

The chicken gene structure (shown above) is highly conserved among vertebrates [24]. The *EGFR* promoter is rich in GC regions and contains overlapping SP1 and T_3 receptor/RXRα binding sites but lacks TATA or CAAT boxes [25]. *EGFR* transcription *in vivo* is positively activated by EGF, cAMP or TPA and is inhibited by T_3R or RAR.

PROTEIN STRUCTURE

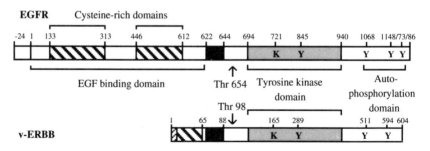

Similar cysteine-rich domains occur in the receptors for insulin, insulin-like growth factor (IGF-I), nerve growth factor (NGF) and low-density lipoprotein (LDL). The 24 amino acid signal sequence (light shading) is proteolytically cleaved from the EGFR. The *gag* encoded (6 amino acids) of v-ERBB (lightly hatched box) also encodes a (putative, cleaved) signal sequence. v-*erbB* is derived from chicken *EGFR*. Chicken and human EGFR share 97% and 65% identity in the tyrosine kinase and C-terminal regions, respectively. In v-ERBB the receptor binding domain and 30 C-terminal residues are deleted and there are eight point mutations, relative to chicken EGFR.

SEQUENCE OF EGFR

```
   1 MRPSGTAGAA LLALLAALCP ASRALEEKKV CQGTSNKLTQ LGTFEDHFLS
  51 LQRMFNNCEV VLGNLEITYV QRNYDLSFLK TIQEVAGYVL IALNTVERIP
 101 LENLQIIRGN MYYENSYALA VLSNYDANKT GLKELPMRNL QEILHGAVRF
 151 SNNPALCNVE SIQWRDIVSS DFLSNMSMDF QNHLGSCQKC DPSCPNGSCW
 201 GAGEENCQKL TKIICAQQCS GRCRGKSPSD CCHNQCAAGC TGPRESDCLV
 251 CRKFRDEATC KDTCPPLMLY NPTTYQMDVN PEGKYSFGAT CVKKCPRNYV
 301 VTDHGSCVRA CGADSYEMEE DGVRKCKKCE GPCRKVCNGI GIGEFKDSLS
 351 INATNIKHFK NCTSISGDLH ILPVAFRGDS FTHTPPLDPQ ELDILKTVKE
 401 ITGFLLIQAW PENRTDLHAF ENLEIIRGRT KQHGQFSLAV VSLNITSLGL
 451 RSLKEISDGD VIISGNKNLC YANTINWKKL FGTSGQKTKI ISNRGENSCK
 501 ATGQVCHALC SPEGCWGPEP RDCVSCRNVS RGRECVDKCK LLEGEPREFV
 551 ENSECIQCHP ECLPQAMNIT CTGRGPDNCI QCAHYIDGPH CVKTCPAGVM
 601 GENNTLVWKY ADAGHVCHLC HPNCTYGCTG PGLEGCPTNG PKIPSIATGM
 651 VGALLLLLVV ALGIGLFMRR RHIVRKRTLR RLLQERELVE PLTPSGEAPN
 701 QALLRILKET EFKKIKVLGS GAFGTVYKGL WIPEGEKVKI PVAIKELREA
 751 TSPKANKEIL DEAYVMASVD NPHVCRLLGI CLTSTVQLIT QLMPFGCLLD
 801 YVREHKDNIG SQYLLNWCVQ IAKGMNYLED RRLVHRDLAA RNVLVKTPQH
 851 VKITDFGLAK LLGAEEKEYH AEGGKVPIKW MALESILHRI YTHQSDVWSY
 901 GVTVWELMTF GSKPYDGIPA SEISSILEKG ERLPQPPICT IDVYMIMVKC
 951 WMIDADSRPK FRELIIEFSK MARDPQRYLV IQGDERMHLP SPTDSNFYRA
1001 LMDEEDMDDV VDADEYLIPQ QGFFSSPSTS RTPLLSSLSA TSNNSTVACI
1051 DRNGLQSCPI KEDSFLQRYS SDPTGALTED SIDDTFLPVP EYINQSVPKR
1101 PAGSVQNPVY HNQPLNPAPS RDPHYQDPHS TAVGNPEYLN TVQPTCVNST
1151 FDSPAHWAQK GSHQISLDNP DYQQDFFPKE AKPNGIFKGS TAENAEYLRV
1201 APQSSEFIGA (1210)
```

Domain structure

1–24	Signal sequence (italics)
25–645	Extracellular domain
646–668	Transmembrane (underlined)
678	Major protein kinase C phosphorylation site (Thr678)
669–1210	Cytoplasmic domain
75–300 and 390–600	Approximate repeats
718–726 and 745	ATP binding
678	Threonine phosphorylation by protein kinase C
693	Threonine phosphorylation by MAP kinase and by EGFR Thr669 (ERT) kinase [26]
1016	Principal binding site for the SH2 domain of PLCγ (Tyr1016)
1172	Principal binding site for the SH2 domain of GAP (Tyr1172)
1016 and 1172	Binding site for protein tyrosine phosphatase 1B [27]
1026, 1070 and 1071	Serine phosphorylation sites [28]
1092, 1110, 1172, 1197	Tyrosine phosphorylation sites (underlined)
128, 175, 196, 352, 361, 413, 444, 528, 568, 603, 623	Putative carbohydrate attachment sites

DATABASE ACCESSION NUMBERS

	PIR	SWISSPROT	EMBL/GENBANK	REFERENCES
Human *EGFR*	A00641	P00533	X00588; X06370	29
	A00642		K01885; K02047	30
	A23062		M38425	31–34

References

1 **Carpenter, G. (1987) Annu. Rev. Biochem. 56, 881–914.**
2 **Laurence, D.J.R. and Gusterson, B.A. (1990) Tumor Biol. 11, 229–261.**
3 Miller, C.C. et al. (1994) J. Biol. Chem. 269, 3529–3533.
4 Qian et al. (1994) Proc. Natl Acad. Sci. USA 91, 1500–1504.
5 Filhol, O. et al. (1994) J. Biol. Chem. 268, 26978–26982.
6 Hernandez-Sotomayor, S.M.T. et al. (1993) Proc. Natl Acad. Sci. USA 90, 7691–7695.
7 Zhu, G. et al. (1992) Proc. Natl Acad. Sci. USA 89, 9559–9563.
8 Segatto, O. et al. (1993) Oncogene 8, 2105–2112.
9 Fazioli, F. et al. (1993) EMBO J. 12, 3799–3808.
10 Peppelenbosch, M.P. et al. (1992) Cell 69, 295–303.
11 Jiang, C.-K. et al. (1993) Proc. Natl Acad. Sci. USA 90, 686–6790.
12 Proctor, A.J. et al. (1991) Oncogene 6, 789–795.
13 **Gullick, W.J. (1991) Br. Med. Bull. 47, 87–98.**
14 Horak, E. et al. (1991) Oncogene 6, 2277–2284.

[15] Borg, A. et al. (1991) Oncogene 6, 137–143.

[16] Paterson, M.C. et al. (1991) Cancer Res. 51, 556–567.

[17] Wong, A.J. et al. (1992) Proc. Natl Acad. Sci. USA 89, 2965–2969.

[18] Humphrey, P.A. et al. (1991) Biophys. Res. Commun. 178, 1413–1420.

[19] Humphrey, P.A. et al. (1990) Proc. Natl Acad. Sci. USA 87, 4207–4211.

[20] Garcia de Palazzo, I.E. et al. (1993) Cancer Res. 53, 3217–3220.

[21] Shu, H.-K.G. et al. (1991) J. Virol. 65, 6177–6180.

[22] Riedel, H. et al. (1988) Proc. Natl Acad. Sci. USA 85, 1477–1481.

[23] Segatto, O. et al. (1991) Mol. Cell. Biol. 11, 3191–3202.

[24] Callaghan, T. et al. (1993) Oncogene 8, 2939–2948.

[25] Xu, J. et al. (1993) J. Biol. Chem. 268, 16065–16073.

[26] Williams, R. et al. (1993) J. Biol. Chem. 268, 18213–18217.

[27] Milarski, K.L. et al. (1993) J. Biol. Chem. 268, 23634–23639.

[28] Kuppuswamy, D. et al. (1993) J. Biol. Chem. 268, 19134–19142.

[29] Ullrich, A. et al. (1984) Nature 309, 418–425.

[30] Lin, C.R. et al. (1984) Science 224, 843–848.

[31] Simmen, F.A. et al. (1984) Biochem. Biophys. Res. Commun. 124, 125–132.

[32] Haley, J. et al. (1987) Oncogene Res. 1, 375–396.

[33] Mroczkowski, B. et al. (1984) Nature 309, 270–273.

[34] Margolis, B.L. et al. (1989) J. Biol. Chem. 264, 10667–10671.

ELK1, ELK2

IDENTIFICATION

ELK1 and *ELK2* were detected by screening a cDNA library with *ETS2* cDNA.

RELATED GENES

Member of the *ETS* family (see **ETS1, ETS2**) with high homology to SAP-1 (see **FOS**).

		ELK1	ELK2
Chromosome		Xp11.2	14q32.3
Mass (kDa):	predicted	45	
	expressed	Not known	

Cellular location

ELK1: Nuclear. *ELK2*: Nuclear.

Tissue distribution

Restricted to lung and testis [1].

PROTEIN FUNCTION

ELK proteins are transcription factors with DNA sequence specificity (CAGGA) similar to ETS1 and ETS2[2]. ELK1 differs from other ETS proteins in having its ETS DNA binding domain located at the N-terminus of the protein. ELK1 (also called p62^{TCF}), is a component of the ternary complex that activates *FOS* transcription via the serum response element (SRE; see **FOS**) [3].

ΔELK1 lacks 11 C-terminal amino acids of the ETS domain and all of the negative regulatory DNA binding domain of ELK1 [4]. The deleted region includes the SRF interaction domain (ESI) and ΔELK1 therefore has the potential to compete with ELK1 in binding to the SRE and thus inhibit transcriptional activation of *FOS* by SRF and ELK1. ELK1 and ΔELK1 are both activators of and substrates for MAP kinases and ELK1 interacts directly with MAP kinases.

Cancer

ELK genes map close to the translocation breakpoint characteristic of synovial sarcoma [t(X;18)(p11.2;q11.2)] and the 14q32 breakpoints seen in ataxia telangiectasia and other T cell malignancies [5,6].

PROTEIN STRUCTURE

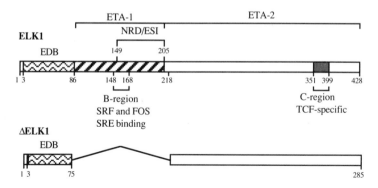

EDB: ETS domain (DNA binding); ETA-1 and ETA-2: ELK1 transcription activation domains; NRD: negative regulatory DNA binding domain; ESI: SRF interaction domain [7]. The efficient formation of a ternary complex at the FOS SRE requires the ELK1 (or SAP-1) ETS domain and the conserved sequence of Box B [8].

SEQUENCE OF ELK1

```
  1  MDPSVTLWQF LLQLLREQGN GHIISWTSRD GGEFKLVDAE EVARLWGLRK
 51  NKTNMNYDKL SRALRYYYDK NIIRKVSGQK FVYKFVSYPE VAGCSTEDCP
101  PQPEVSVTST MPNVAPAAIH AAPGDTVSGK PGTPKGAGMA GPGGLARSSR
151  NEYMRSGLYS TFTIQSLQPQ PPPHPRPAVV LPNAAPAGAA APPSGSRSTS
201  PSPLEACLEA EEAGLPLQVI LTPPEAPNLK SEELNVEPGL GRALPPEVKV
251  EGPKEELEVA GERGFVPETT KAEPEVPPQE GVPARLPAVV MDTAGQAGGH
301  AASSPEISQP QKGRKPRDLE LPLSPSLLGG PGPERTPGSG SGSGLQAPGP
351  ALTPSLLPTH TLTPVLLTPS SLPPSIHFWS TLSPIAPRSP AKLSFQFPSS
401  GSAQVHIPSI SVDGLSTPVV LSPGPQKP (428)
```

Domain structure

3–86   DNA binding ETS domain (EDB: underlined). The truncated protein (residues 1–89) binds autonomously to SRE, unlike the full-length protein, indicating the presence of a negative regulatory domain within ELK1

148–168   B region.

133, 324, 389   Optimal sites for MAP kinase phosphorylation. Other suboptimal sites are 336, 353, 363, 368, 383, 417 and 422

DATABASE ACCESSION NUMBERS

	PIR	SWISSPROT	EMBL/GENBANK	REFERENCES
Human *ELK1*	A41354	P19419	M25269	*1,9*

References

1 Rao, V.N. et al. (1989) Science 244, 66–70.
2 Rao, V.N. and Reddy, E.S.P. (1992) Oncogene 7, 65–70.
3 Hipskind, R.A. et al. (1991) Nature 354, 531–534.
4 Bhattacharya, G. et al. (1993) Oncogene 8, 3459–3464.
5 Kocova, M. et al. (1985) Cancer Genet. Cytogen. 16, 21–30.
6 Rowley, J.D. (1983) Nature 301, 290–291.
7 Janknecht, R. et al. (1994) Oncogene 9, 1273–1278.
8 Treisman, R. et al. (1992) EMBO J. 11, 4631–4640.
9 Janknecht, R. and Nordheim, A. (1992) Nucl. Acids Res. 20, 3317–3324.

EPH

IDENTIFICATION

EPH (*EPHT*) is the prototype of a sub-family of tyrosine kinases, initially isolated from a human genomic library with a v-*fps* probe, that is over-expressed in an <u>e</u>rythropoietin <u>p</u>roducing human <u>h</u>epatocellular (*EPH*) carcinoma cell line.

RELATED GENES

ELK (<u>e</u>ph-<u>l</u>ike <u>k</u>inase); *EEK* (<u>e</u>ph and <u>e</u>lk-related <u>k</u>inase); *ECK* (<u>e</u>pithelial cell <u>k</u>inase); *ERK* (<u>e</u>lk-related <u>k</u>inase). *ERK* is distinct from the *Erk-1, -2* and *-3* family of serine/threonine kinases [1].

Other *EPH*-related genes are: murine *Nuk* (<u>n</u>eural <u>k</u>inase) receptor kinase, murine *Sek*, murine *Mek-4* and chicken *Cek* (<u>c</u>hicken <u>e</u>mbryo <u>k</u>inases 4–10), chicken *Tyro-5*, rat *Ehk-1, Ehk-2* and human *HEK* (<u>h</u>uman <u>e</u>mbryo <u>k</u>inase) and *HEK2*.

Chromosome		7q32–q36
Mass (kDa):	**predicted**	109
	expressed	130

Cellular location

Plasma membrane.

Tissue distribution

EPH is expressed in kidney, testis, liver, lung. *Mek-4, Sek* and *Cek* family genes are expressed during embryonic development.

PROTEIN FUNCTION

EPH is the prototype class IV transmembrane tyrosine kinase receptor. Ligand(s) unknown. Chimeric EGFR–ELK proteins undergo autophos-phorylation of the ELK cytoplasmic domain and stimulate the tyrosine phosphorylation of a set of cellular proteins in response to EGF, indicating that ELK and related proteins function as ligand-dependent receptor tyrosine kinases [2].

Cancer

EPH is overexpressed in several carcinomas [3]. Overexpressed *EPH* renders NIH 3T3 cells tumorigenic [4]. *HEK* is expressed in cell lines derived from human lymphoid tumours [5].

PROTEIN STRUCTURE

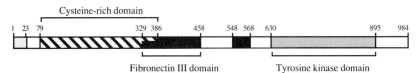

The extracellular domain contains a putative immunoglobulin-like loop at the N-terminus, a single cysteine-rich region and two fibronectin type III repeats [6].

SEQUENCE OF EPH

```
  1  MERRWPLGLG LVLLLCAPLP PGARAKEVTL MDTSKAQGEL GWLLDPPKDG
 51  WSEQQQILNG TPLYMYQDCP MQGRRDTDHW LRSNWIYRGE EASRVHVELQ
101  FTVRDCKSFP GGAGPLGCKE TFNLLYMESD QDVGIQLRRP LFQKVTTVAA
151  DQSFTIRDLA SGSVKLNVER CSLGRLTRRG LYLAFHNPGA CVALVSVRVF
201  YQRCPETLNG LAQFPDTLPG PAGLVEVAGT CLPHARASPR PSGAPRMHCS
251  PDGEWLVPVG RCHCEPGYEE GGSGEACVAC PSGSYRMDMD TPHCLTCPQQ
301  STAESEGATI CTCESGHYRA PGEGPQVACT GPPSAPRNLS FSASGTQLSL
351  RWEPPADTGG RQDVRYSVRC SQCQGTAQDG GPCQPCGVGV HFSPGARGLT
401  TPAVHVNGLE PYANYTFNVE AQNGVSGLGS SGHASTSVSI SMGHAESLSG
451  LSLRLVKKEP RQLELTWAGS RPRSPGANLT YELHVLNQDE ERYQMVLEPR
501  VLLTELQPDT TYIVRVRMLT PLGPGPFSPD HEFRTSPPVS RGLTGGEIVA
551  VIFGLLLGAA LLLGILVFRS RRAQRQRQQR HVTAPPMWIE RTSCAEALCG
601  TSRHTRTLHR EPWTLPGGWS NFPSRELDPA WLMVDTVIGE GEFGEVYRGT
651  LRLPSQDCKT VAIKTLKDTS PGGQWWNFLR EATIMGQFSH PHILHLEGVV
700  TKRKPIMIIT EFMENGALDA FLREREDQLV PGQLVAMLQG IASGMNYLSN
751  HNYVHRDLAA RNILVNQNLC CKVSDFGLTR LLDDFDGTYE TQGGKIPIRW
801  TAPEAIAHRI FTTASDVWSF GIVMWEVLSF GDKPYGEMSN QEVMKSIEDG
851  YRLPPPVDCP APLYELMKNC WAYDRARRPH FQKLQAHLEQ LLANPHSLRT
901  IANFDPRVTL RLPSLSGSDG IPYRTVSEWL ESIRMKRYIL HFHSAGLDTM
951  ECVLELTAED LTQMGITLPG HQKRILCSIQ GFKD (984)
```

Domain structure

1–23	Signal sequence (italics)
24–547	Extracellular domain
79–386	Cysteine-rich domain (cysteines underlined)
548–568	Transmembrane region (underlined)
569–984	Intracellular domain
630–895	Tyrosine kinase domain (underlined)
638–646 and 664	ATP binding region
329–442 and 443–538	Fibronectin type III domains
757	Active site
789	Potential autophosphorylation site
338, 414 and 478	Potential carbohydrate attachment sites

EEK is 57% identical in sequence to EPH. ELK and ECK share >40% and >60% similarity in the extracellular and tyrosine kinase domains, respectively.

DATABASE ACCESSION NUMBERS

	PIR	SWISSPROT	EMBL/GENBANK	REFERENCES
Human *EPH*	A34076	P21709	M18391	7
Human *ECK*			M36395	8
Human *EEK*			X59291	9
Human *ERK*			X59292	9
Human *HEK*			M83941	5

References

1 **Boulton, T.G. et al. (1991) Cell 65, 663–675.**
2 Lhotak, V. and Pawson, T. (1993) Mol. Cell. Biol. 13, 7071–7079.
3 Maru, Y. et al. (1988) Mol. Cell. Biol. 8, 3770–3776.
4 Maru, Y. et al. (1990) Oncogene 5, 445–447.
5 Wicks, I.P. et al. (1992) Proc. Natl Acad. Sci. USA 89, 1611–1615.
6 Pasquale, E.B. et al. (1991) Cell Regul. 2, 523–534.
7 Hirai, H. et al. (1987) Science 238, 1717–1720.
8 Lindberg, R.A. and Hunter, T. (1990) Mol. Cell. Biol. 10, 6316–6324.
9 Chan, J. and Watt, V.M. (1991) Oncogene 6, 1057–1061.

IDENTIFICATION

ERG (*e*ts-*r*elated gene) was detected by screening a cDNA library with *ETS2* cDNA.

RELATED GENES

Member of the *ETS* family (see ***ETS1, ETS2***).

Chromosome	21q22.3
Mass (kDa): predicted	41 (ERG1)
	52 (ERG2)
	54.6 (ERG3)
	38/49/55
expressed	41 (ERG1)/57 (ERG2)/59 (ERG3)

Cellular location

Nuclear.

Tissue distribution

High levels of expression in human tumour-derived cell lines [1,2]. *ERG3* is expressed in a variety of cells [3].

PROTEIN FUNCTION

The *ERG* family encode transcription factors that differ from ETS1 and ETS2 in their sequence specificity, binding weakly to the polyoma virus enhancer PEA3, Mo-MuSV LTR or PU box sequences, but strongly to E74 target sequences, although all of these regions contain a core GGAA motif [4]. In contrast to ETS1, ERG2 is phosphorylated by protein kinase C but not in response to Ca^{2+} ionophore [5].

Cancer

The chromosomal translocation t(22;21)(q12;q22) that occurs in Ewing's sarcoma creates an ERG/EWS fusion protein [6].

PROTEIN STRUCTURE

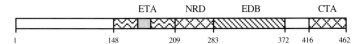

ERG proteins contain a C-terminal DNA binding domain (EDB), two autonomous transcriptional activation domains (ETA, N-terminal and

CTA, C-terminal) and a negative regulatory transcriptional activation domain (NRD) N-terminal to the DNA binding domain [7].

Three ERG2-related isoforms (p38[ERG], p49[ERG] and p55[ERG]) generated by alternative splicing of two exons (A81 and A72) have been detected in human COLO 320 cells[8]. p38[ERG] is colinear with ERG2 but has a truncation of the 5′ coding region that deletes 53 amino acids. The cDNA encoding p55[ERG] contains an additional 72 bp (exon A72) that adds 24 amino acids to the middle of the ORF that are not present in ERG1 or EGR2. The 5′ coding sequence of p55[ERG] also diverges from that of *ERG2*, giving rise to an alternative predicted N-terminus. p49[ERG] has an in-frame deletion of 81 bp (exon A81) and also of exon A72 relative to p55[ERG] [8].

ERG3 is generated by alternative splicing and encodes a 24 amino acid insert with respect to ERG2 [3].

SEQUENCE OF ERG

```
  1  MIQTVPDPAA HIKEALSVVS EDQSLFECAY GTPHLAKTEM TASSSSDYGQ
 51  TSKMSPRVPQ QDWLSQPPAR VTIKMECNPS QVNGSRNSPD ECSVAKGGKM
101  VGSPDTVGMN YGSYMEEKHM PPPNMTTNER RVIVPADPTL WSTDHVRQWL
151  EWAVKEYGLP DVNILLFQNI DGKELCKMTK DDFQRLTPSY NADILLSHLH
201  YLRETPLPHL TSDDVDKALQ NSPRLMHARN TDLPYEPPRR SAWTGHGHPT
251  PQSKAAQPSP STVPKTEDQR PQLDPYQILG PTSSRLANPG SGQIQLWQFL
301  LELLSDSSNS SCITWEGTNG EFKMTDPDEV ARRWGERKSK PNMNYDKLSR
351  ALRYYYDKNI MTKVHGKRYA YKFDFHGIAQ ALQPHPPESS LYKYPSDLPY
401  MGSYHAHPQK MNFVAPHPPA LPVTSSSFFA APNPYWNSPT GGIYPNTRLP
451  TSHMPSHLGT YY (462)
```

Domain structure

1–462   ERG2 generated by alternative splicing of *ERG1* [1,2]
100–462   ERG1
290–374   DNA binding ETS domain (underlined)

N-terminus of ERG2:   MIQTVPDPAAHIKEALS...
N-terminus of p55[ERG]/p49[ERG]:   MASTIKEALS...
Sequence encoded by exon A81:   TPLPHLTSDDVDKALQNSPRLMHARNT
Sequence encoded by exon A72:   GGAAFIFPNTSVYPEATQRITTRP

DATABASE ACCESSION NUMBERS

	PIR	SWISSPROT	EMBL/GENBANK	REFERENCE
Human *ERG2*	A29515	P11308	M17254	2

References
1 Reddy, E.S.P. et al. (1987) Proc. Natl Acad. Sci. USA 84, 6131–6135.
2 Rao, V.N. et al. (1987) Science 237, 635–653.
3 Prasad, D.D.K. et al. (1994) Oncogene 9, 669–673.

4 Reddy, E.S.P. and Rao, V.N. (1991) Oncogene 6, 2285–2289.

5 Murakami, K. et al. (1993) Oncogene 8, 1559–1566.

6 Zucman, J. et al. (1993). EMBO J. 12, 4481–4487.

7 Siddique, H.R. et al. (1993) Oncogene 8, 1751–1755.

8 Duterque-Coquillaud, M. et al. (1993) Oncogene 8, 1865–1873.

ETS1, ETS2

IDENTIFICATION

v-ets (*E t*wenty-six *s*pecific) and v-*myb* are the oncogenes of the acutely transforming avian erythroblastosis virus E26. v-*ets* was detected as a fusion gene with v-*myb* by screening cloned E26 provirus with a v-*myb* probe. *ETS1* and *ETS2* were detected by screening DNA with a v-*ets* probe.

RELATED GENES

ERG, ELK1, ELK2, ELF1, FLI1, SAP-1, TEL, GABPα, PU.1/Spi-1, Spi-1b, Pea-3, Tpl-1, E1A-F, E74A and *E74B* (*Xenopus*, sea urchin and *Drosophila*), ERM, Ets-1 and Ets-2 (*Xenopus*), D-*elg, Elf-1, yan* (*Drosophila*), ERM, ER81 and Er71. Limited homology with the T cell receptor α enhancer binding protein (TCR1α).

		ETS1	*ETS2*	v-*ets*
Nucleotides (kb)		60	20	5.7 (E26)
Chromosome		11q23.3	21q22.3	
Mass (kDa):	**predicted**	50/55	53/54	75
	expressed	51/48/42/39 (alternative splicing)	56	P135*gag-myb-ets*

Cellular location

ETS1: Nuclear. *ETS2*: Nuclear. v-*ets*: Nuclear.

Tissue distribution

ETS1: Expression is high in the thymus, in endothelial cells differentiating or migrating during the development of blood vessels and in migrating neural crest cells [1]. Abundantly expressed in fibroblasts and endothelial cells in invasive tumours.

ETS2: Expression occurs in most tissues and is stimulated in activated T cells.

PROTEIN FUNCTION

The *ETS* family encodes transcription factors that bind to the consensus sequence $^C/_A$GGA$^A/_T$ (ETS binding site (EBS)) [2,3]. The family sequence homology covers ~85 amino acids (the ETS domain), necessary and sufficient for specific binding to EBS *in vitro*. ETS domain proteins interact with *TCRA, TCRB, MB-1, ENDOA*, keratin 18 and MHC class II genes, E74 target sequences, GATA-1, the polyoma virus enhancer and Mo-MuSV LTR [4].

Putative ETS binding sites are present in several T-cell-specific genes including *IL2, IL3, GM-CSF, CD2, CD3, TCRB, TCRG* [5] and in human immunodeficiency virus type 2 (HIV-2) and the HTLV-1LTR [6]. Transcriptional activation of the HTLV-1 LTR requires the synergistic action of ETS1 and SP1 and, in general, ETS proteins appear to function as components of transcription factor complexes to regulate the expression of viral and cellular genes [7].

ETS1 and ETS2 activate the stromelysin 1 and collagenase 1 genes [8] and ETS1 binds to the sequence of the *TCRA* enhancer [9]. ETS1 and ETS2 are phosphorylated in activated T cells, suggesting that they have a role in cell proliferation [10]. *Ets-2* expression is required for germinal vesicle breakdown in *Xenopus* oocytes [11].

Cancer

The *ETS1* and *ETS2/ERG* loci are involved in translocations associated with some leukaemias and with Down's syndrome that may result in activation of these genes[12]. *ETS1* is expressed in tumours of the peripheral nervous system (neuroblastomas and neuroepitheliomas) and in Ewing's sarcoma[13].

In animals

E26 causes erythroblastosis and low-level myeloblastosis in chickens. The potent leukaemogenicity of E26 derives from the fusion of the v-*ets* and v-*myb* genes [14,15]. v-*ets* cooperates with v-*erbA* to cause avian erythro-leukaemia [16].

In vitro

E26 does not transform chick embryo fibroblasts (CEFs) [17] but does transform quail fibroblasts and stimulates the proliferation of CEFs [18], neuroretina cells [19] and NIH 3T3 fibroblasts [20]. v-*ets* can cause weak transformation of erythroid cells [14].

STRUCTURE OF THE *ETS1* AND *ETS2* GENES

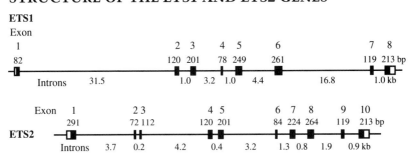

Alternative splicing generates human *ETS1* mRNAs lacking one or both of exons 3 and 5 [21]. The absence of exon 5 causes smaller ETS1 proteins (p39/p42) to be synthesized. The principal proteins have been denoted as ETS1a (~50 kDa: 441 amino acids) and ETS1b (~40 kDa: 354 amino acids) [22]. Scrambled splicing also occurs in which exon 5 or exon 4 splices with exon 2, which normally splices 3' with exon 3 [23].

Regions encoding identical or similar amino acids to ETS2 have retained their genomic organization: the most divergent regions have different organization.

The *ETS1* and *ETS2* promoters lack a TATA or CAAT box and have a high GC content. The *ETS1* promoter has six SP1 sites, AP-1 and AP-2 consensus sequences and binding site motifs for PEA3 and OCT as well as a palindromic region resembling the *FOS* SRE and an ETS1 protein binding site [24,25]. Two negative regulatory elements (NRE1 and NRE2) are present 230 and 350 nucleotides 5' of the promoter, respectively [26]. The human *ETS2* promoter contains a region (–159 to +141) that includes one SP1 site and a GC-rich region and is essential for transcription [27].

PROTEIN STRUCTURE OF CHICKEN p68^{Ets-1}

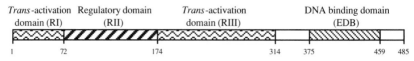

Human ETS1 and chicken p68^{Ets-1} are highly homologous but ETS1 lacks the RI *trans*-activation domain. RII negatively regulates the activity of RI and positively regulates that of RIII.

The exons of human ETS1 are identical in size to those of chicken *Ets-1*, the progenitor of v-*ets* [21]. Human ETS1 and ETS2 are 98% and 95% homologous to v-ETS, respectively. In v-ETS the 13 C-terminal residues of chicken p68^{Ets} have been replaced by 16 C-terminal amino acids and there are two conservative point mutations [28].

SEQUENCE OF ETS1

```
  1  MKAAVDLKPT  LTIIKTEKVD  LELFPSPDME  CADVPLLTPS  SKEMMSQALK
 51  ATFSGFTKEQ  QRLGIPKDPR  QWTETHVRDW  VMWAVNEFSL  KGVDFQKFCM
101  NGAALCALGK  DCFLELAPDF  VGDILWEHLE  ILQKEDVKPY  QVNGVNPAYP
151  ESRYTSDYFI  SYGIEHAQCV  PPSEFSEPSF  ITESYQTLHP  ISSEELLSLK
201  YENDYPSVIL  RDPLQTDTLQ  NDYFAIKQEV  VTPDNMCMGR  TSRGKLGGQD
251  SFESIESYDS  CDRLTQSWSS  QSSFNSLQRV  PSYDSFDSED  YPAALPNHKP
301  KGTFKDYVRD  RADLNKDKPV  IPAAALAGYT  GSGPIQLWQF  LLELLTDKSC
351  QSFISWTGDG  WEFKLSDPDE  VARRWGKRKN  KPKMNYEKLS  RGLRYYYDKN
401  IIHKTAGKRY  VYRFVCDLQS  LLGYTPEELH  AMLDVKPDAD  E  (441)
```

Domain structure

28–130	Homology with chicken p68^{Ets-1} RII domain
97–130	Helix-loop-helix domain (italics)
130–270	Homology with chicken p68^{Ets-1} RIII *trans*-activation domain
331–415	DNA binding ETS domain (underlined)
244–330	Deleted by alternative splicing in ETS1B
251–282	PEST sequence which may target protein cleavage to this region
338	Trp338 is in the centre of a hydrophobic α-helical region essential for the optimal conformation of the ETS binding domain [29].

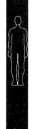

377–383   Nuclear localization signal
337–342   Conserved region I (CRI) conserved in all ETS family proteins
371–379   Conserved region II (CRII) conserved in all ETS family proteins
384–394   Conserved region III (CRIII) conserved in all ETS family proteins

The specific selectivity of ELF1 and E74 for GGAA core-containing sites is conferred on ETS1 by mutation of Lys396 within the conserved region III of ETS1 [30].

An 89 residue region adjacent to the DNA binding domains is conserved with 55% identity in ETS1 and ETS2 but does not occur in other members of the ETS family. This region inhibits DNA binding and activates transcription. The alternatively spliced form of human *ETS1*, lacking exon 7 does not have this inhibitory region and binds to DNA much more efficiently [31].

There is ~65% identity between human ETS1 and ELK1, ETS2, ERG and v-ETS within the 80 amino acid C-terminal DNA binding domains.

SEQUENCE OF ETS2

```
  1  MNDFGIKNMD QVAPVANSYR GTLKRQPAFD TFDGSLFAVF PSLNEEQTLQ
 51  EVPTGLDSIS HDSANCELPL LTPCSKAVMS QALKATFSGF KKEQRRLGIP
101  KNPWLWSEQQ VCQWLLWATN EFSLVNVNLQ RFGMNGQMLC NLGKERFLEL
151  APDFVGDILW EHLEQMIKEN QEKTEDQYEE NSHLTSVPHW INSNTLGFGT
201  EQAPYGMQTQ NYPKGGLLDS MCPASTPSVL SSEQEFQMFP KSRLSSVSVT
251  YCSVSQDFPG SNLNLLTNNS GTPKDHDSPE NGADSFESSD SLLQSWNSQS
301  SLLDVQRVPS FESFEDDCSQ SLCLNKPTMS FKDYIQERSD PVEQGKPVIP
351  AAVLAGFTGS GPIQLWQFLL ELLSDKSCQS FISWTGDGWE FKLADPDEVA
401  RRWGKRKNKP KMNYEKLSRG LRYYYDKNII HKTSGKRYVY RFVCDLQNLL
451  GFTPEELHAI LGVQPDTED (469)
```

Domain structure

359–443   DNA binding ETS domain (underlined)

DATABASE ACCESSION NUMBERS

	PIR	*SWISSPROT*	*EMBL/GENBANK*	*REFERENCES*
Human *ETS1*	A32066	P14921	X14798	[22]
	S10086		J04101	[32]
Human *ETS2*	B32066	P15036	J04102	[33]
			X55181	

References
1 Desbiens, X. et al. (1991) Development 111, 699–713.
2 **Macleod, K. et al. (1993) Trends BioChem. Sci. 17, 251–256.**
3 Karim, F.D. et al. (1990) Genes Devel. 4, 1451–1453.
4 Seth, A. et al. (1994) Oncogene 9, 469–477.

5   Thompson, C.B. et al. (1992) Mol. Cell. Biol. 12, 1043–1053.
6   Gitlin, S.D. et al. (1991) J. Virol. 65, 5513–5523.
7   Gegonne, A. et al. (1993) EMBO J. 12, 1169–1178.
8   Woods, D.B. et al. (1992) Nucl. Acids Res. 20, 699–704.
9   Ho, I.-C. et al. (1990) Science 250, 814–818.
10 Fleischman, L.F. et al. (1993) Oncogene 8, 771–780.
11 Chen, J.H. et al. (1990) Oncogene Res. 5, 277–285.
12 Papas, T.S. et al. (1990) Am. J. Med. Genet. 7 (Suppl), 251–261.
13 Sacchi, N. et al. (1991) Oncogene 6, 2149–2154.
14 Metz, T. and Graf, T. (1991) Genes Devel. 5, 369–380.
15 Metz, T. and Graf, T. (1991) Cell 66, 95–105.
16 Metz, T. and Graf, T. (1992) Oncogene 7, 597–605.
17 Bister, K. et al. (1982) Proc. Natl Acad. Sci. USA 79, 3677–3681.
18 Jurdic, P. et al. (1987) J. Virol. 61, 3058–3065.
19 Amouyel, P. et al. (1989) J. Virol. 63, 3382–3388.
20 Seth, A. and Papas, T.S. (1990) Oncogene 5, 1761–1767.
21 Jorcyk, C.L. et al. (1991) Oncogene 6, 523–532.
22 Reddy, E.S.P. and Rao, V.N. (1988) Oncogene Res. 3, 239–246.
23 Cocquerelle, C. et al. (1992) EMBO J. 11, 1095–1098.
24 Oka, T. et al. (1991) Oncogene 6, 2077–2083.
25 Chen, J.H. and Wright, C.D. (1993) Oncogene 8, 3375–3383.
26 Chen, J.H. et al. (1993) Oncogene 8, 133–139.
27 Mavrothalassitis, G.J. et al. (1990) Oncogene 5, 1337–1342.
28 Lautenberger, J.A. and Papas, T.S. (1993) J. Virol. 67, 610–612.
29 Mavrothalassitis, G.J. et al. (1994) Oncogene 9, 425–435.
30 Bosselut, R. et al. (1993) Nucl. Acids Res. 21, 5184–5191.
31 Wasylyk, C. et al. (1992) Genes Devel. 6, 965–974.
32 Watson, D.K. et al. (1988) Proc. Natl Acad. Sci. USA 85, 7862–7866.
33 Watson, D.K. et al. (1990) Oncogene 5, 1521–1527.

FGR

IDENTIFICATION

v-*fgr* is the oncogene of the acutely transforming Gardner–Rasheed feline sarcoma virus (GR-FeSV). *FGR* was detected by low stringency hybridization screening of human placental DNA with a v-*yes* probe.

RELATED GENES

FGR is a member of the *SRC* tyrosine kinase family (*Blk, FGR, FYN, HCK, LCK/Tkl, LYN, SRC, YES*). GR-FeSV has transduced portions of two distinct cellular genes, γ-actin and *Fgr*.

	FGR	**v-fgr**
Nucleotides (kb)	~15	4.6 (GR-FeSV)
Chromosome	1p36.2–p36.1	
Mass (kDa): predicted	59.5	72
expressed	70	P70$^{gag\text{-}actin\text{-}fgr}$

Cellular location

Cytoplasm: associates with plasma membrane; present in the secondary granules of neutrophils.

Tissue distribution

FGR expression is high in mature peripheral blood monocytes and granulocytes, alveolar and splenic macrophages, human natural killer cells and differentiating myelomonocytic HL60 and U937 cells [1-3]. It is expressed only in the later stages of differentiation of myeloid leukaemia cells, in contrast to *Src* [4].

PROTEIN FUNCTION

FGR is a non-receptor tyrosine kinase. In normal bone marrow-derived monocytic cells *Fgr* mRNA expression is transiently increased by 20-fold by CSF1, GM-CSF or LPS [5] and agents that stimulate the differentiation of HL60 cells also activate transcription and translation [6]. The γ-actin domain inhibits both the kinase activity and oncogenicity of GR-FeSV [7].

Cancer

Fiftyfold amplification of *FGR* occurs in B cells transformed by Epstein–Barr virus [8].

In animals

GR-FeSV is highly infectious to cats, inducing differentiated fibrosarcomas and rhabdosarcomas in young animals [9].

In vitro

FGR does not transform epithelial cells but transforms most mammalian fibroblasts including human [9].

Transgenic animals

Fgr-deficient mice show normal haematopoietic development. Doubly homozygous *Hck⁻/⁻/Fgr⁻/⁻* animals are immunodeficient, having increased susceptibility to infection with *Listeria monocytogenes* [10].

GENE STRUCTURE

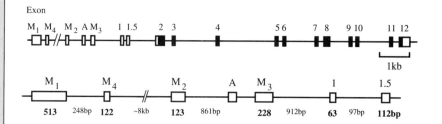

In the expanded diagram of the *FGR* promoter region the sizes of the exons are in bold type. Exons 3–12 closely resemble those of avian *Src* and murine *Lck* [11]. Upstream exons differ and the 5′ untranslated region of *FGR* has an extra intron. In human myelomonocytes differential promoter utilization and alternative splicing gives rise to at least six distinct mRNAs that differ only in their 5′ untranslated regions [12].

   The two predominant RNA species are *FGRA* (EBV-infected B cells) and *FGR4* (myelomonocytic cells). *FGRA* contains exon A linked to exon 1 and downstream exons and in *FGR4* exon M₄ is spliced to exon 1 and downstream exons [13]. Thus in EBV infection a cryptic exon A promoter is activated to regulate the expression of *FGR*, whereas the exon M₄ promoter is used exclusively in myelomonocytic cells. M_1 and M_2 are rarely utilized in mononuclear cells (monocytes, neutrophils and lymphocytes).

TRANSCRIPTIONAL REGULATION

There is a cluster of transcriptional start sites upstream of exon 1a that is rich in GC regions but lacks a TATA box.

PROTEIN STRUCTURE

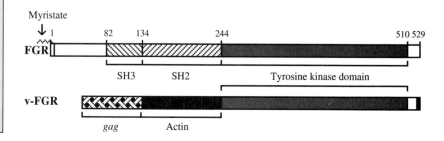

P70*gag-actin-fgr* (663 amino acids) is myristylated in the *gag* N-terminal region (118 amino acids) and includes 151 amino acids of the N-terminus of feline non-muscle actin, 389 of feline FGR and 5 *env* encoded C-terminal amino acids.

SEQUENCE OF FGR

```
  1  MGCVFCKKLE PVATAKEDAG LEGDFRSYGA ADHYGPDPTK ARPASSFAHI
 51  PNYSNFSSQA INPGFLDSGT IRGVSGIGVT LFIALYDYEA RTEDDLTFTK
101  GEKFHILNNT EGDWWEARSL SSGKTGCIPS NYVAPVDSIQ AEEWYFGKIG
151  RKDAERQLLS PGNPQGAFLI RESETTKGAY SLSIRDWDQT RGDHVKHYKI
201  RKLDMGGYYI TTRVQFNSVQ ELVQHYMEVN DGLCNLLIAP CTIMKPQTLG
251  LAKDAWEISR SSITLERRLG TGCFGDVWLG TWNGSTKVAV KTLKPGTMSP
301  KAFLEEAQVM KLLRHDKLVQ LYAVVSEEPI YIVTEFMCHG SLLDFLKNPE
351  GQDLRLPQLV DMAAQVAEGM AYMERMNYIH RDLRAANILV GERLACKIAD
401  FGLARLIKDD EYNPCQGSKF PIKWTAPEAA LFGRFTIKSD VWSFGILLTE
451  LITKGRIPYP GMNKREVLEQ VEQGYHMPCP PGCPASLYEA MEQTWRLDPE
501  ERPTFEYLQS FLEDYFTSAE PQYQPGDQT (529)
```

Domain structure

269–277 and 291	ATP binding region
382	Active site
412	Autophosphorylation site
82–134	SH3 domain (or A box: underlined)

DATABASE ACCESSION NUMBERS

	PIR	*SWISSPROT*	*EMBL/GENBANK*	*REFERENCES*
Human				
FGR (SRC2)	A27676, A28353	P09769	M12719–M12724	*14*
				11
				15

References

1 Ley, T.J. et al. (1989) Mol. Cell. Biol. 9, 92–99.
2 Katagiri, K, et al. (1991) J. Immunol. 146, 701–707.
3 Biondi, A. et al. (1991) Eur. J. Immunol. 21, 843–846.
4 Willman, C.L. et al. (1991) Blood 77, 726–734.
5 Yi, T.L. and Willman, C.L. (1989) Oncogene 4, 1081–1087.
6 Notario, V. et al. (1989) J. Cell Biol. 109, 3129–3136.
7 Sugita, K. et al. (1989) J. Virol. 63, 1715–1720.
8 Cheah, M.S.C., et al. (1986) Nature, 319, 238–240.
9 Rasheed, S. et al. (1982) Virology, 117, 238–244.
10 Lowell, C.A. et al. (1994) Genes Devel. 8, 387–398.
11 Nishizawa, M. et al. (1986) Mol. Cell. Biol. 6, 511–517.

12 Link, D.C. et al. (1992) Oncogene 7, 877–884.

13 Gutkind, J.S. et al. (1991) Mol. Cell. Biol. 11, 1500–1507.

14 Katamine, S. et al. (1988) Mol. Cell. Biol. 8, 259–266.

15 Inoue, K. et al. (1987) Oncogene 1, 301–304.

FLI1

IDENTIFICATION

FLI1 (*Fli-1* (*F*riend *l*eukaemia *i*ntegration-*1*)) was cloned by PCR using partially degenerate *ETS*-domain oligonucleotide primers.

RELATED GENES

FLI1 is a member of the *ETS* family (see **ETS1, ETS2**): it is 80% homologous to ERG2.

Chromosome	11q23–24
Mass (kDa): predicted	51
expressed	55

Cellular location

Nuclear.

Tissue distribution

Human FLI1 is expressed in a subset of erythroleukaemic cell lines. The 5′ untranslated regions of the human and mouse genes are 95% homologous, indicating that expression is post-transcriptionally regulated.

PROTEIN FUNCTION

FLI1 has similar or identical DNA binding properties to ERG2, binding to the ETS2 binding site (GACCGGAAGTG) but not to that of PU.1 [1-3].

Cancer

The chromosomal translocation t(11;22)(q24;q12) that occurs in Ewing's sarcoma creates an EWS/FLI1 fusion protein. FLI1 is expressed in a subset of erythroleukaemic cell lines.

In animals

Mouse *Fli-1* is rearranged or activated by proviral insertion in 75% of Friend murine leukaemia virus-induced erythroleukaemias.

In vitro

EWS/FLI1 has the characteristics of an aberrant transcription factor. It binds to the same *ETS2* consensus sequence as FLI1 but is a more potent *trans*-activator that, in contrast to FLI1, transforms NIH 3T3 cells [4].

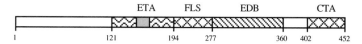

PROTEIN STRUCTURE

```
              ETA      FLS       EDB            CTA
    ┌──────────┬──┬──────────────────────────┬──────┐
    │          │░░│▨▨▨▨▨▨▨▨▨▨▨▨▨▨▨▨▨▨▨▨│  │▨▨▨▨│
    └──────────┴──┴──────────────────────────┴──────┘
    1          121    194   277            360 402  452
```

ERG proteins contain a C-terminal DNA binding domain (EDB) and two autonomous transcriptional activation domains (ETA, N-terminal and CTA, C-terminal) that are 98% homologous to the corresponding region of ERG2. FLI1 also contains an FLS domain (FLI1-specific domain, non-homologous to ERG).

SEQUENCE OF FLI1

```
  1   MDGTIKEALS VVSDDQSLFD SAYGAAAHLP KADMTASGSP DYGQPHKINP
 51   LPPQQEWINQ PVRVNVKREY DHMNGSRESP VDCSVSKCSK LVGGGESNPM
101   NYNSYMDEKN GPPPPNMTTN ERRVIVPADP TLWTQEHVRQ WLEWAIKEYS
151   LMEIDTSFFQ NMDGKELCKM NKEDFLRATT LYNTEVLLSH LSYLRESSLL
201   AYNTTSHTDQ SSRLSVKEDP SYDSVRRGAW GNNMNSGLNK SPPLGGAQTI
251   SKNTEQRPQP DPYQILGPTS SRLANPGSGQ IQLWQFLLEL LSDSANASCI
301   TWEGTNGEFK MTDPDEVARR WGERKSKPNM NYDKLSRALR YYYDKNIMTK
351   VHGKRYAYKF DFHGIAQALQ PHPTESSMYK YPSDISYMPS QHAHQQKVNF
401   VPPHPSSMPV TSSSFFGAAS QYWTSPTGGI YPNPNVPRHP NTHVPSHLGS
451   YY (452)
```

Domain structure

121–194   ETS homology domain (underlined)
277–360   DNA binding ETS domain (underlined)

DATABASE ACCESSION NUMBERS

	PIR	SWISSPROT	EMBL/GENBANK	REFERENCES
Human *ERGB/FLI1*			M98833	5

References

1 Klemsz, M.J. et al. (1993) J. Biol. Chem. 268, 5769–5773.
2 Rao, V.N. et al. (1993) Oncogene 8, 2167–2173.
3 Zhang, L. et al. (1993) Oncogene 8, 1621–1630.
4 May, W.A. et al. (1993) Mol. Cell. Biol. 13, 7393–7398.
5 Watson, D.K. et al. (1992) Cell Growth Differ. 3, 705–713.

FOS

IDENTIFICATION

v-*fos* is the oncogene of the FBJ (Finkel, Biskis and Jinkins, 1966) [1] and FBR (Finkel, Biskis and Reilly) murine osteosarcoma viruses (MuSV) and of the avian transforming virus NK24 [2]. Cellular *FOS* genes were detected by screening DNA with a v-*fos* probe.

RELATED GENES

The *FOS* family are members of the helix–loop–helix/leucine zipper superfamily (see *JUN*). Closely related genes are *FRA1* and *FRA2* ("*FOS*-related *a*ntigens"), *FOSB*, ΔFOSB, r-*fos* (homologous to the third exon of *Fos*) and *Drosophila* dFRA and dJRA. The herpesvirus Marek disease virus (MDV) encodes a gene closely related to the *FOS/JUN* family that is expressed in MDV-transformed lymphoblastoid cells.

	FOS	v-*fos* FBJ-MuSV	v-*fos* FBR-MuSV
Nucleotides (bp)	~3500	4026	3791
Chromosome	14q24.3		
Mass (kDa): predicted	41.6	49.6	60
expressed	55/62	55[v-fos]	P75[gag-fos-fox]

Cellular location

FOS: Nucleus. FBJ-MuSV`: Nucleus. FBR-MuSV: Nucleus.

Tissue distribution

FOS expression is very low in most cell types but there is constitutive high expression in amnion, yolk sac, mid-gestation fetal liver, post-natal bone marrow, normal human skin [3] and in one human pre-B leukaemic cell line but not others of similar origin [4-11]. *FOS* is an immediate early gene, the expression of which is induced rapidly (<5 min) and transiently by growth factors and mitogens. Protein expression is maximal after 90 min [12-15]. In Swiss 3T3 fibroblasts FOS (and FOSB) are mainly required during the G_0 to G_1 transition [16]. However, although in general *FOS* is barely detectable throughout the cell cycle, it may be induced at any stage other than during mitosis [17]. *FOS* is also transiently expressed in IL2- and IL6-dependent mouse myeloma cell lines following withdrawal of growth factor and the onset of apoptosis [18] and in vitamin K_3-induced apoptosis of nasopharyngeal carcinoma cells [19].

PROTEIN FUNCTION

FOS, FOSB, FRA1 and FRA2 form heterodimers with JUN proteins that function as positive or negative transcription factors by binding to specific

DNA sequences (AP-1 sites: consensus sequence $TGA^C/_GTCA$) via basic domains adjacent to the dimerizing helices [20,21]. FOS interacts cooperatively with JUN to inhibit its own transcription. However, for human metallothionein IIA, collagenase, collagen α_1(III), transin, proenkephalin and SV40 genes, FOS/JUN dimers form a potent transcription activating complex. FOS also activates the annexin II and IV, tyrosine hydroxylase, ornithine decarboxylase (*ODC1*), *T1/ST2* and *Fit-1* genes. The stability of dimers increases in the order FOS/FOS<JUN/JUN<FOS/JUN. DNA bends of differing magnitude and orientation are induced by different combinations of FOS and JUN [22] and the ubiquitous DNA-binding protein YY1 may regulate the activity of the *FOS* promoter mainly by affecting its structure [23].

The involvement of members of the *FOS/JUN* family in development is suggested by the observation that *Fos, Fosb* and *Fra-1* and *Jun, Junb* and *Jund* are differentially expressed during development and in adult tissues, consistent with their having distinct functions. In the newborn mouse a large transient (day 1) burst of *Fos* transcription occurs in all major tissues [24].

Cancer

FOS overexpression has been detected in 60% of one sample of human osteosarcomas [25] and in a cell line derived from a pre-B cell acute lymphocytic leukaemia [26].

Transgenic animals

Transgenic mice having a null mutation in *Fos* have low viability at birth (~40%). However, the homozygous mutants that survive have normal growth rates until severe osteopetrosis develops at approximately 11 days [27]. Thus *Fos* is not essential for the growth of most cell types although null mutants show delayed or absent gametogenesis and in most animals there is a reduction of ~75% in the levels of circulating T and B lymphocytes.

In transgenic mice *Fos* expression activated by the FBJ-MuSV LTR causes bone tumours [28]. The expression of FBJ v-*fos* in the epidermis of transgenic mice results in the failure of regulated keratinocyte differentiation and the subsequent development of benign tumours [29].

In animals

The expression of *Fos* by transfection into the highly metastatic murine 3LL cell line induces the expression of the major histocompatibility antigen H-2K^b and reduces the metastatic properties of the cells *in vivo* [30]. FBJ- and FBR-MuSV induce sarcomas in animals [31]. NK24 causes avian nephroblastoma [2].

In vitro

Overexpression of *FOS* does not transform human fibroblasts [32] but does transform rat fibroblasts if (1) an LTR is present to enhance transcription and (2) a 50–100 bp AU-rich element (ARE) 500 bp downstream of the chain terminator and 150 bp upstream of the poly(A) addition signal in the 3′ UTR is removed.

FBJ- and FBR-MuSV both transform cells *in vitro* but FBR-MuSV is more effective. FBR-MuSV immortalizes murine cells in culture: FBJ-MuSV does not. FBR-MuSV v-*fos* transforms human epidermal keratinocyte cells *in vitro* [33]. Internal deletions in the C-terminal half of the FBR-MuSV oncoprotein are responsible for its transforming potential (removing the *trans*-repression domain, preventing binding to the promoter and hence constitutively activating the *Fos* gene).

GENE STRUCTURE

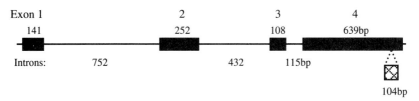

The deletion from murine exon 4 occurring in p55$^{v\text{-}fos}$ (FBJ-MSV) is represented by the crossed box.

TRANSCRIPTIONAL REGULATION OF HUMAN *FOS*

The *FOS* promoter includes a TATA box (–26 to –31 relative to the transcription initiation site), a cAMP response element (–56 to –63), a retinoblastoma control element (–73 to –102), a region *trans*-activated by the hepatitis B virus (HBV) pX (–120 to –220), which also modulates transcription through interactions with the SRE and AP-1 sites [34], two regions of homology with the *HSP70* promoter (–235 to –244 and –252 to –260), an AP-1 site (–291 to –297), a 20 bp dyad symmetry element (DSE: –299 to –318) and a v-*sis*-conditioned medium inducible element (–335 to –347).

The retinoblastoma gene product (p105^{RB}) acts via the retinoblastoma control element to repress *FOS* transcription following stimulation by serum and to lower the concentration of *Fos* mRNA in cells growing in the presence of serum. Deletion of the putative leucine zipper region of p105^{RB} abolishes transcriptional suppression.

The AP-1 site is the target for FOS/JUN heterodimers that inhibit *FOS* transcription. FOS interacts cooperatively with JUN to activate other genes (e.g. human metallothionein IIA, collagenase, collagen α$_1$(III), transin (or stromelysin), SV40) that contain AP-1 sites. FOS interacts with at least one other transcription factor in that it cooperates with NF-κB in activating HIV-1.

The DSE (or serum response element (SRE)) is required for activation by serum, PDGF, TPA or EGF or by pressure in cardiac muscle. Serum responsive factor (p67^{SRF}) in fibroblasts can interact with the DSE via the element CC(A/T)$_6$GG termed the CArG box. p62^{TCF} (ternary complex factor) is an additional protein that interacts directly with the 5' region of the DSE, forms a ternary complex with the DSE and p67^{SRF} and requires both DSE-bound p67^{SRF} and sequences both within and outside the DSE for its interaction with DNA [35,36]. p67^{SRF} is also transcriptionally activated via its C-terminal half by HTLV-1 TAX1 [37]. p67^{SRF} is phosphorylated by casein kinase II but this does not appear to be significant in the growth factor activation of Fos expression [38]. p62^{TCF} is identical to ELK1, the Ets family DNA binding protein (see **ETS1**, **ETS2**) [39]. ELK1/p62^{TCF} is phosphorylated in vitro by MAP kinase and this increases its transcriptional activation capacity [40] and promotes ternary complex formation [41]. This sequence also confers inducibility on a heterologous promoter (the β-globin promoter) but only in response to serum, not PDGF or TPA. This suggests that additional cooperative signals are required for transcriptional activation in response to PDGF or TPA. Sequences closely similar to that of SRE occur in other genes (e.g. actin and Krox-20). An additional SRF accessory protein (SAP) that occurs in two forms (SAP1a and SAP1b) has been isolated: SAP1 is homologous to p62 and has similar DNA binding properties (see **ETS1**, **ETS2**). These accessory proteins contact SRF via a conserved B box sequence (see **ETS1**, **ETS2**) and bind to DNA via an ETS motif ($^C/_A$$^C/_AGGA^A/_T$) that may vary in both its orientation and separation from the SRE [42].

The SRE contains multiple overlapping enhanson elements [43] with which members of both the helix–loop–helix and the CCAAT/enhancer binding protein (C/EBP) transcription factor families [44] and the zinc finger protein SRE-ZBP interact [45]. An additional SRE binding protein (SRE BP) is required for maximal serum induction of Fos [46]. The binding site for SRE BP coincides with that for rNF-IL-6 but the proteins are distinct. The SRE also includes binding sites for DBF/MAPF1 [47–49] and E12 [44].

Fos expression is greatly diminished during muscle cell differentiation and, consistent with this observation, the muscle-specific transcription factor MyoD binds to a region overlapping the SRE to function as a negative regulator of Fos transcription [50].

The v-sis-conditioned medium inducible element, the DSE, the direct repeat region and the cAMP response element can mediate trans-activation by the HTLV-1 TAX protein [51,52].

The Fos gene contains an intragenic regulatory element (FIRE) at the end of exon 1 that can cause premature termination of transcription. Intragenic regulation of transcription also occurs in the Myc and Myb genes [53].

RNA STABILITY

The ARE in many rapidly induced mRNAs is thought to mediate selective degradation. The Fos ARE comprises two domains, (I) within the 5' 49 bp (three AUUUA motifs) that can function as an RNA destabilizer by itself and (II), a 20 bp U-rich sequence in the 3' part of the ARE that enhances the destabilizing capacity of domain I. A second region that regulates mRNA stability is present within the coding sequence. This comprises the

5′ 0.38 kb region which contains multiple destabilizing elements that can function independently to promote both de-adenylation and degradation of mRNA. Within this region two major elements have been defined (CD1 and CD2) that require ribosome assembly and translation to direct mRNA decay. This region also includes a 56 bp purine-rich segment with which at least two protein factors associate to promote rapid degradation [54].

STRUCTURES OF FOS PROTEINS

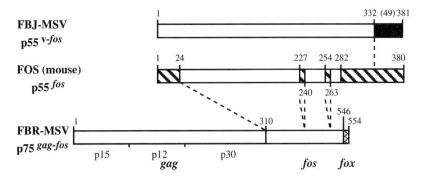

The cross-hatched boxes in FOS represent regions deleted in p75[gag-fos]. The C-terminal 49 amino acids of p55[v-fos] (black box) differ from those of FOS. v-FOS (FBR-MuSV) is myristylated at the N-terminus and this modification, together with its C-terminal mutation, causes loss of *trans*-repression activity [55]. In FBJ-MuSV v-*fos* the central region of the protein alone (Met111 to Ile206) is both necessary and sufficient to transform chick embryo fibroblasts [56].

TRANSCRIPTIONAL AUTOREGULATION BY FOS/JUN DIMERS

The regulatory activity resides in the C-terminal region of the FOS proteins (mutated in the viral proteins of FBJ-MuSV and FBR-MuSV). One of the major post-translational modifications undergone by FOS is serine phospho-esterification in the C-terminus and the negative charge thus conferred on the molecule is crucial for suppression of transcription [57]. Transformation-defective FOS proteins that lack either the leucine zipper region or the N-terminal 110 amino acids inhibit transformation by either v-*fos* or *Ras* [58].

The basic motif KCR (amino acids 153–155 in human FOS) is conserved in FOS, JUN and ATF/CREB family members and redox-regulation of the cysteine residue mediates DNA binding. Nevertheless, the KCR regions of FOS and JUN are not identical in DNA binding and non-basic amino acids (e.g. ISI) in this motif can function efficiently in binding [59]. Reduction of this cysteine by the ubiquitous nuclear redox factor REF-1 stimulates the DNA binding activity of FOS/JUN and JUN/JUN dimers, MYB, NF-κB and ATF/CREB proteins. Replacement of Cys154 by serine enhances the transforming activity of the FOS protein [60].

SEQUENCE HOMOLOGY BETWEEN FOS, FRA1, FRA2 AND FOSB

FOS (chicken)	14-22	60-79	123-208	308-334	344-367
FRA-1 (rat)	11-13	39-58	93-179	217-242	251-275
FRA-2 (chicken)	12-20	46-65	111-197	256-282	300-323
FOSB (mouse)	11-19	54-73	142-227	285-309	315-338

The five homologous regions of the proteins are indicated by shaded regions. The basic and leucine zipper regions occur between FOS residues 123 and 208. The aligned numbers below indicate the amino acids at the extremes of the corresponding regions in the other proteins [61].

SEQUENCE OF FOS

```
  1  MMFSGFNADY EASSSRCSSA SPAGDSLSYY HSPADSFSSM GSPVNAQDFC
 51  TDLAVSSANF IPTVTAISTS PDLQWLVQPA LVSSVAPSQT RAPHPFGVPA
101  PSAGAYSRAG VVKTMTGGRA QSIGRRGKVE QLSPEEEEKR RIRRERNKMA
151  AAKCRNRRRE LTDTLQAETD QLEDEKSALQ TEIANLLKEK EKLEFILAAH
201  RPACKIPDDL GFPEEMSVAS LDLTGGLPEV ATPESEEAFT LPLLNDPEPK
251  PSVEPVKSIS SMELKTEPFD DFLFPASSRP SGSETARSVP DMDLSGSFYA
301  ADWEPLHSGS LGMGPMATEL EPLCTPVVTC TPSCTAYTSS FVFTYPEADS
351  FPSCAAAHRK GSSSNEPSSD SLSSPTLLAL (380)
```

143–160 Basic motif (underlined)
165–193 Leucine zipper (underlined)
139–161 Basic nuclear targeting signal. However, this region is not essential for FOS nuclear localization [62]. Other FOS sequences that resemble known nuclear targeting signals are ineffective in directing pyruvate kinase to the nucleus; FOS may therefore contain a novel nuclear targeting sequence.
362 S6 kinase (RSK) phosphorylation site (Ser362)
374 MAP kinase phosphorylation site (Ser374)

DOMAIN STRUCTURES OF HUMAN FOS, FOSB AND FOSB2

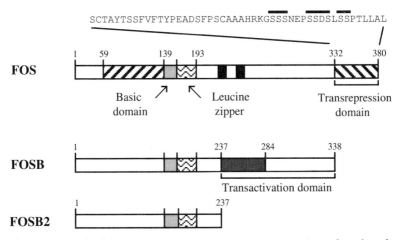

SCTAYTSSFVFTYPEADSFPSCAAAHRKGSSSNEPSSDSLSSPTLLAL

FOS

Basic domain   Leucine zipper   Transrepression domain

FOSB

Transactivation domain

FOSB2

The two hatched boxes represent regions encompassing phosphorylation sites. The bars mark the three groups of C-terminal serine residues in FOS (Ser362–364, Ser368, 369, 371 and Ser373–374). The N-terminal domain (59–139) is phosphorylated *in vitro* by protein kinase C, p34^{CDC2} and a nuclear kinase: the C-terminal region by cAMP-dependent protein kinase, p34^{CDC2} [63], S6 kinase (RSK) and MAP kinase [64].

RELATIONSHIP BETWEEN FOS AND JUN

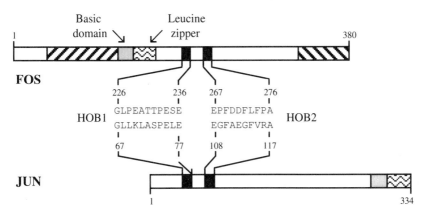

The two homology box regions (HOB1 and HOB2) of FOS lie within a *trans*-activating domain and are conserved in the A1 activation domain of JUN [65]. The FOS sequence is for rat, which is identical to that of human FOS except for the substitution of alanine and threonine by valine and alanine at positions 230 and 231. HOB1 and HOB2 regions also occur in C/EBP and they act cooperatively to stimulate transcription of reporter gene constructs. HOB1 contains a phosphorylation site for MAP kinase.

DATABASE ACCESSION NUMBERS

	PIR	SWISSPROT	EMBL/GENBANK	REFERENCES
FBJ-MuSV v-*fos*	A01344	P01102	V01184	66
			J02084	
FBR-MuSV v-*fos*			KO2712	66
Human *FOS*	A01342	P01100	V01512	67
			K00650 M16287	68, 69

References

1 Finkel, M.P. et al. (1966) Science 151, 698–701.
2 Nishizawa, M. et al. (1987) J. Virol. 61, 3733–3740.
3 Basset-Seguin, N. et al. (1994) Oncogene 9, 765–771.
4 Muller, R. et al. (1983) EMBO J. 2, 679–684.
5 Gonda, T.J. and Metcalf, D. (1984) Nature 310, 249–251.
6 Mason, I. et al. (1985) Differentiation 30, 76–81.
7 Mitchell, R.L. et al. (1985) Cell 40, 209–217.
8 Muller, R. et al. (1985) Nature 314, 546–548.
9 Conscience, J.-F. et al. (1986) EMBO J. 5, 317–323.
10 Kreipe, H. et al. (1986) Differentiation 33, 56–60.
11 Panterne, B. et al. (1992) Oncogene 7, 2341–2344.
12 Muller, R. et al. (1984) Nature 312, 716–720.
13 Bravo, R. et al. (1987) Cell 48, 251–260.
14 Tannenbaum, C.S. et al. (1988) J. Immunol. 140, 3640–3645.
15 Sariban, E. et al. (1985) Nature 316, 64–66.
16 Kovary, K. and Bravo, R. (1991) Mol. Cell. Biol. 11, 4466–4472.
17 Bravo, R. et al. (1986) EMBO J., 5, 695–700.
18 Colotta, F. et al. (1992) J. Biol. Chem. 267, 18278–18283.
19 Wu, F.Y.-H. et al. (1993) Oncogene 8, 2237–2244.
20 **Distel, R.J. and Spiegelman, B. (1990) Adv. Cancer Res. 55, 37–55.**
21 **Ransone, L.J. and Verma, I.M. (1990) Annu. Rev. Cell Biol. 6, 539–557.**
22 Kerppola, T.K. and Curran, T. (1991) Science 254, 1210–1213.
23 Natesan, S. and Gilman, M.Z. (1994) Genes Devel. 7, 2497–2509.
24 Kasik, J.W. et al. (1987) Mol. Cell. Biol. 7, 3349–3352.
25 Wu, J.X. et al. (1990) Oncogene 5, 989–1000.
26 Tsai, L.-H. et al. (1991) Oncogene 6, 81–88.
27 Okada, S. et al. (1994) Mol. Cell. Biol. 14, 382–390.
28 Ruther, U. et al. (1989) Oncogene 4, 861–865.
29 Greenhalgh, D.A. et al. (1993) Oncogene 8, 2145–2157.
30 Kushtai, G. et al. (1990) Int. J. Cancer 45, 1131–1136.
31 Van Beveren, C. et al. (1984) Virology 135, 229–243.
32 Alt, M. and Grassmann, R. (1993) Oncogene 8, 1421–1427.
33 Lee, M.-S. et al. (1993) Oncogene 8, 387–393.
34 Natoli, G. et al. (1993) Mol. Cell. Biol. 14, 989–998.
35 Shaw, P.E. (1992) EMBO J., 11, 3011–3019.
36 Sharrocks, A.D. et al. (1993) Mol. Cell. Biol. 13, 123–132.
37 Fujii, M. et al. (1992) Genes Devel. 6, 2066–2076.
38 Manak, J.R. and Prywes, R. (1993) Oncogene 8, 703–711.
39 Hipskind, R.A. et al. (1991) Nature 354, 531–534.

[40] Marais, R. et al. (1993) Cell 73, 381–393.
[41] Gille, H. et al. (1992) Nature 358, 414–417.
[42] Treisman, R. et al. (1992) EMBO J. 11, 4631–4640.
[43] **Treisman, R. (1992) Trends Biol. Sci. 17, 423–426.**
[44] Metz, R. and Ziff, E. (1991) Oncogene 6, 2165–2178.
[45] Attar, R.M. and Gilman, M.Z. (1992) Mol. Cell. Biol. 12, 2432–2443.
[46] Boulden, A.M. and Sealy, L.J. (1992) Mol. Cell. Biol. 12, 4769–4783.
[47] Ryan, W.A. et al. (1989) EMBO J. 8, 1785–1792.
[48] Walsh, K. (1989) Mol. Cell. Biol. 9, 2191–2201.
[49] Grueneberg, D. et al. (1992) Science 257, 1089–1095.
[50] Trouche, D. et al. (1993) Nature 363, 79–82.
[51] Alexandre, C. and Verrier, B. (1991) Oncogene 6, 543–551.
[52] Wagner, B.J. et al. (1990) EMBO J. 9, 4477–4484.
[53] Lamb, N.J.C. et al. (1990) Cell 61, 485–496.
[54] Schiavi, S.C. et al. (1994) J. Biol. Chem. 269, 3441–3448.
[55] Kamata, N. and Holt, J.T. (1992) Mol. Cell. Biol. 12, 876–882.
[56] Yoshida, T. et al. (1989) Oncogene Res. 5, 79–89.
[57] **Hunter, T. and Karin, M. (1992) Cell 70, 375–387.**
[58] Wick, M. et al. (1992) Oncogene 7, 859–867.
[59] Ng, L. et al. (1994) Nucl. Acids Res. 21, 5831–5837.
[60] Okuno, H. et al. (1993) Oncogene 8, 695–701.
[61] Nishina, H. et al. (1990) Proc. Natl Acad. Sci. USA 87, 3619–3623.
[62] Tratner, I. and Verma, I.M. (1991) Oncogene 6, 2049–2053.
[63] Abate, C. et al. (1991) Oncogene 6, 2179–2185.
[64] Chen, R.-H. et al. (1993) Proc. Natl Acad. Sci. USA 90, 10952–10956.
[65] Sutherland, J.A. et al. (1992) Genes Devel. 6, 1810–1819.
[66] Van Beveren, C. et al. (1983) Cell 32, 1241–1255.
[67] van Straaten, F. et al. (1983) Proc. Natl Acad. Sci. USA 80, 3183–3187.
[68] Treisman, R. (1985) Cell 42, 889–902.
[69] Verma, I.M. et al. (1986) Cold Spring Harb. Symp. Quant. Biol. 51, 949–958.

FOSB

IDENTIFICATION

FOSB was detected by screening cDNA libraries with *FOS* DNA as a probe.

RELATED GENES

FOSB is a member of the helix–loop–helix/leucine zipper superfamily (see *JUN*). Closely related genes are *FOS*, ΔFOSB (*FOSB/SF* or *FOSB2*), *FRA1* and *FRA2* and r-*fos*.

Nucleotides (kb)		~4.6
Mass (kDa):	**predicted**	36
	expressed	52
		37 (FOSB2)

Cellular location

Nucleus.

Tissue distribution

FOSB is an immediate early gene. In stimulated fibroblasts the induction of its transcription is slightly delayed with respect to that of *FOS* [1]. In serum-stimulated Rat-1A cells the expression of ΔFOSB parallels that of FOSB [2].

PROTEIN FUNCTION

FOSB forms heterodimers with JUN proteins that function as positive or negative transcription factors (see **FOS**). FOSB activates transcription of the fibroblast *T1* early response gene [3]. *Fosb* is a more potent *in vitro* transforming agent than *Fos*, having a transforming capacity equivalent to that of v-*fos* [4].

GENE STRUCTURE

The overall structure of the *Fosb* gene is very similar to that of *Fos* [5,6]. The four exons of *Fosb* encode 42, 107, 36 and 153 amino acids, respectively and alternative splicing of exon 4 removes 140 bp to generate a truncated form, ΔFOSB, of 237 amino acids [5].

The murine *Fosb* promoter contains SRE and AP-1 binding sites located in positions that are identical relative to those found in the *Fos* promoter and the activity of the *Fosb* promoter is down-regulated by FOS or FOSB [5].

PROTEIN STRUCTURE

FOS and FOSB are 70% homologous and 42% identical in sequence (see *FOS*). FOSB has a truncated C-terminus relative to FOS but retains the leucine zipper and basic DNA binding regions of FOS. The truncated form of FOS, ΔFOSB (FOSB2), also retains the capacity to form dimers with JUN that bind to AP-1 sites but no longer activate transcription from AP-1-containing promoters or repress the *Fos* promoter [7]. The expression of FOSB2 suppresses transformation by v-*fos*, *Fos* or *Fosb*, presumably by interfering with *trans*-activation events required for transformation [8]. However, overexpression of *Fosb2* does not prevent normal cells from entering the cell cycle in response to serum, indicating that *Fosb2* is not a negative regulator of cell growth [9].

SEQUENCE OF MOUSE FOSB

```
  1  MFQAFPGDYD SGSRCSSSPS AESQYLSSVD SFGSPPTAAA SQECAGLGEM
 51  PGSFVPTVTA ITTSQDLQWL VQPTLISSMA QSQGQPLASQ PPAVDPYDMP
101  GTSYSTPGLS AYSTGGASGS GGPSTSTTTS GPVSARPARA RPRRPREETL
151  TPEEEEKRRV RRERNKLAAA KCRNRRRELT DRLQAETDQL EEEKAELESE
201  IAELQKEKER LEFVLVAHKP GCKIPYEEGP GPGPLAEVRD LPGSTSAKED
251  GFGWLLPPPP PPPLPFQSSR DAPPNLTASL FTHSEVQVLG DPFPVVSPSY
301  TSSFVLTCPE VSAFAGAQRT SGSEQPSDPL NSPSLLAL (338)
```

Domain structure

161–179   Basic, DNA binding motif
183–211   Leucine zipper (underlined)
229–338   *Trans*-activation domain (see *FOS*). All four members of the FOS family that transform established rodent fibroblast cell lines (FBR-v-FOS, FBJ-v-FOS, FOS and FOSB) contain an equivalent C-terminal domain [10,11].

DATABASE ACCESSION NUMBERS

	PIR	SWISSPROT	EMBL/GENBANK	REFERENCES
Mouse *Fosb*	S04108	P13346	X14897	1
			M77748	5

References

1   Zerial, M. et al. (1989) EMBO J., 8, 805–813.
2   Nakabeppu, Y. et al. (1993) Mol. Cell. Biol. 13, 4157–4166.
3   Kalousek, M.B. et al. (1994) J. Biol. Chem. 269, 6866–6873.
4   Schuermann, M. et al. (1991) Oncogene 6, 567–576.
5   Lazo, P.S. et al. (1992) Nucl. Acids Res. 20, 343–350.
6   Nishina, H. et al. (1990) Proc. Natl Acad. Sci. USA 87, 3619–3623.
7   Nakabeppu, Y. and Nathans, D. (1991) Cell 64, 751–759.

8 Yen, J. et al. (1991) Proc. Natl Acad. Sci. USA 88, 5077–5081.

9 Dobrzanski, P. et al. (1991) Mol. Cell. Biol. 11, 5470–5478.

10 Wisdom, R. and Verma, I.M. (1993) Mol. Cell. Biol. 13, 2635–2643.

11 Wisdom, R. and Verma, I.M. (1993) Mol. Cell. Biol. 13, 7429–7438.

FPS/FES

IDENTIFICATION

v-*fps* (*F*ujinami-*P*RCII *s*arcoma) is the oncogene of the acutely transforming Fujinami sarcoma virus (FSV). Four other retroviruses also carry v-*fps*: PRCII and PRCIV (Poultry Research Centre II and IV), UR1 (University of Rochester) and 16L. *fes* (*fe*line *s*arcoma virus) is the cognate gene of *fps* present in three retroviruses (Snyder–Theilen (ST)-FeSV, Gardner–Arnstein (GA)-FeSV and Hardy–Zuckerman 1 (HZ1)-FeSV)[1]. *FPS/FES* was detected by screening human lung carcinoma DNA with a v-*fes* probe.

RELATED GENES

FER, human *FES/FPS*-related tyrosine kinase gene, *Flk* (*f*ps/fes-*l*ike *k*inase, the rat homologue of human *FER*), murine *Fer*T tyrosine kinase and *Drosophila* d*fps*85D. Sequences homologous to *FPS/FES* also occur in the sea urchin genome and vesicular stomatitis virus L polymerase. The FPS/FES family have C-terminal homology with SRC (SH2 and tyrosine kinase domains). FER shares homology with TRK.

	FPS/Fes	v-*fps/fes*
Nucleotides (kb)	13	5.3 (FSV genome)
Chromosome	15q25–q26 (*FES*)	
	5q21 (*FER*)	
Mass (kDa): predicted	94	
expressed	p92^{FES}	P130$^{gag-fps}$, P140$^{gag-fps}$ (FSV)
	p94^{FER}	
	p98^{fps} (chicken)	

Cellular location

FPS/FES: Mainly cytoplasm. v-FPS: Membrane associated. FER: Cytoplasm but also present in the nucleus associated with chromatin.

Tissue distribution

FPS/FES is expressed in immature and differentiated haematopoietic cells of the myeloid lineage and in leukaemic myeloid cells [2–4]. *FER* is ubiquitously expressed [5].

PROTEIN FUNCTION

FPS/FES genes encode cytoplasmic tyrosine kinases that are autophosphorylated. The tissue distribution suggests that its normal role may be in the control of proliferation and differentiation of haematopoietic cells [6] and the introduction of human *FES* into cells can confer the capacity to undergo myeloid differentiation [7]. GM-CSF or IL3 can induce the tyrosine phosphorylation and kinase activity of p92^{fes}.

Expression of v-*fps* causes the phosphorylation of at least nine proteins that are also phosphorylated in response to v-*src*, v-*abl* or v-*fgr* [8] and disrupts gap junctional communication [9]. v-FPS also causes tyrosine phosphorylation of fibronectin receptor proteins and the GAP-associated proteins p62 and p190 [10]. Microinjection of anti-RAS antibody causes reversion of *FPS/FES*-transformed cells [11] and revertant cells derived from *Kras*-transformed cells are resistant to *FPS/FES* transformation.

Cancer

FES/FPS expression is enhanced in some lung cancers and haematopoietic malignancies [12,13]. *FER* is highly expressed in cell lines derived from human kidney carcinomas and glioblastomas [14] and is frequently deleted from chromosome 5 in acute myeloid leukaemia and myelodysplastic syndromes [15].

Transgenic animals

Transgenic mice expressing v-*fps* have severe cardiac or neurological disorders and develop a variety of lymphoid or mesenchymal tumours [16,17]. Lymphoid tumours are monoclonal and appear between 2 and 12 months, indicating a requirement for other genetic changes in addition to the expression of v-*fps*.

In animals

FSV induces fibrosarcomas or myxosarcomas [18,19].

In vitro

Fps/Fes over-expression transforms NIH 3T3 fibroblasts, inducing the expression of *Egr-1*, the *Ras*-related immediate-early gene *RhoB* and the transformation-related 9E3 gene and increasing the concentrations of PtdIns(3)P, PtdIns(3,4)P_2 and PtdIns(3,4,5)P_3 (see **SRC**) [20-24]. FSV transforms erythroid cells, osteoblasts [25,26] and quail myogenic cells [27] and FeSV transforms pre-B cells [28,29]. Rat-2 fibroblasts transfected with v-*fps* are tumorigenic and have metastatic potential [30].

GENE STRUCTURE

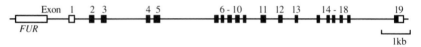

A 9 kb upstream region (*FUR* – *fps/fes* upstream region) encodes a putative 499 amino acid protein of unknown function [31].

PROTEIN STRUCTURE

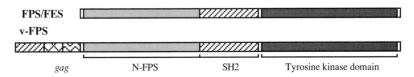

Human and chicken FPS share 70% amino acid identity. In chicken FPS and the derived oncogene P130*gag-fps* the N-terminal domain adjacent to SH2 comprises ~250 amino acids (NFPS) that may determine the subcellular localization. FPS and *gag-fps*-encoded proteins contain an N-terminal potential myristylation site (Gly2), in common with members of the *SRC* family, but, with the exception of the ST-FeSV and GA-FeSV proteins, do not appear to be myristylated or plasma membrane associated [32].

N-terminal *gag* substitution is sufficient to activate the oncogenic potential of *Fps/Fes* although the scattered mutations occurring in most of the forms of v-*fps* can do likewise. However, v-*fps* is linked to N-terminal *gag* sequences in all spontaneously arising, *fps/fes*-containing transforming viruses [33].

SEQUENCE OF FES/FPS

```
  1  MGFSSELCSP QGHGVLQQMQ EAELRLLEGM RKWMAQRVKS DREYAGLLHH
 51  MSLQDSGGQS RAISPDSPIS QSWAEITSQT EGLSRLLRQH AEDLNSGPLS
101  KLSLLIRERQ QLRKTYSEQW QQLQQELTKT HSQDIEKLKS QYRALARDSA
151  QAKRKYQEAS KDKDRDKAKD KYVRSLWKLF AHHNRYVLGV RAAQLHHQHH
201  HQLLLPGLLR SLQDLHEEMA CILKEILQEY LEISSLVQDE VVAIHREMAA
251  AAARIQPEAE YQGFLRQYGS APDVPPCVTF DESLLEEGEP LEPGELQLNE
301  LTVESVQHTL TSVTDELAVA TEMVFRRQEM VTQLQQELRN EEENTHPRER
351  VQLLGKRQVL QEALQGLQVA LCSQAKLQAQ QELLQTKLEH LGPGEPPPVL
401  LLQDDRHSTS SSEQEREGGR TPTLEILKSH ISGIFRPKFS LPPPLQLIPE
451  VQKPLHEQLW YHGAIPRAEV AELLVHSGDF LVRESQGKQE YVLSVLWDGL
501  PRHFIIQSLD NLYRLEGEGF PSIPLLIDHL LSTQQPLTKK SGVVLHRAVP
551  KDKWVLNHED LVLGEQIGRG NFGEVFSGRL RADNTLVAVK SCRETLPPDL
601  KAKFLQEARI LKQYSHPNIV RLIGVCTQKQ PIYIVMELVQ GGDFLTFLRT
651  EGARLRVKTL LQMVGDAAAG MEYLESKCCI HRDLAARNCL VTEKNVLKIS
701  DFGMSREEAD GVYAASGGLR QVPVKWTAPE ALNYGRYSSE SDVWSFGILL
751  WETFSLGASP YPNLSNQQTR EFVEKGGRLP CPELCPDAVF RLMEQCWAYE
801  PGQRPSFSTI YQELQSIRKR HR (822)
```

Domain structure

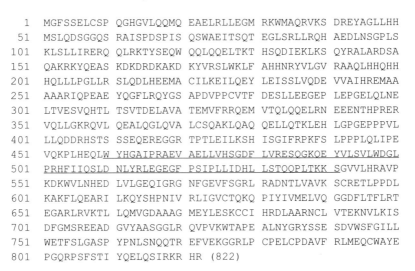

567–575 and 590	ATP binding region (Lys590 is equivalent to SRC Lys295)
683	Active site
713	Autophosphorylation site (equivalent to SRC Tyr416). Lys590 and Tyr713 are essential for kinase and transforming activity [33, 34]

460–541 SH2 domain (underlined). FPS/FES has a group I SH2 domain (Phe or Tyr at the βD5 position) that recognizes phosphopeptides with the general motif P-Tyr-hydrophilic-hydrophilic-hydrophobic [35].

DATABASE ACCESSION NUMBERS

	PIR	SWISSPROT	EMBL/GENBANK	REFERENCES
Human *FES/FPS*	A24673	P07332	X06292	[36]
Human *FER*			J03358	[37]

References
1 Hanafusa, H. (1988) In The Oncogene Handbook, Eds. Curran, T., Reddy, E.P. and Skalka, A., eds, Elsevier, Amsterdam, pp.39–57.
2 Feldman, R.A. et al. (1985) Proc. Natl Acad. Sci. USA 82, 2379–2383.
3 MacDonald, I. et al. (1985) Mol. Cell. Biol. 5, 2543–2551.
4 Samarut, J. et al. (1985) Mol. Cell. Biol. 5, 1067–1072.
5 Feller, S.M. and Wong, T.W. (1992) Biochemistry 31, 3044–3051.
6 Carmier, J.F. and Samarut, J. (1986) Cell 44, 159–165.
7 Yu, G. et al. (1989) J. Biol. Chem. 264, 10276–10281.
8 Kamps, M.P. and Sefton, B.M. (1988) Oncogene 2, 305–315.
9 Kurata, W.E. and Lau, A.F. (1994) Oncogene 9, 329–335.
10 Moran, M.F. et al. (1990) Proc. Natl Acad. Sci. USA 87, 8622–8626.
11 Smith, M.R. et al. (1986) Nature 320, 540–543.
12 Slamon, D.J. et al. (1984) Science 224, 256–262.
13 Jucker, M. et al. (1992) Oncogene 7, 943–952.
14 Hao, Q.L. et al. (1989) Mol. Cell. Biol. 9, 1587–1593.
15 Morris, C. et al. (1990) Cytogenet. Cell Genet. 53, 196–200.
16 Pawson, T. et al. (1989) Mol. Cell. Biol. 9, 5722–5725.
17 Chow, L.H. et al. (1991) Lab. Invest. 64, 457–462.
18 Hanafusa, T. et al. (1980) Proc. Natl Acad. Sci. USA 77, 3009–3013.
19 Sadowski, I. et al. (1988) Oncogene 2, 241–247.
20 Fukui, Y. et al. (1991) Oncogene 6, 407–411.
21 Barker, K. and Hanafusa, H. (1990) Mol. Cell. Biol. 10, 3813–3817.
22 Alexandropoulos et al. (1991) J. Biol. Chem. 266, 15583–15586.
23 Spangler, R. et al. (1989) Proc. Natl Acad. Sci. USA 86, 7017–7021.
24 Feldman, R.A. et al. (1990) Oncogene Res. 5, 187–197.
25 Cogliano, A. et al. (1987) Bone 8, 299–304.
26 Birek, C. et al. (1988) Carcinogenesis 9, 1785–1791.
27 Falcone, G. et al. (1985) Proc. Natl Acad. Sci. USA 82, 426–430.
28 Kahn, P. et al. (1984) Proc. Natl Acad. Sci. USA 81, 7122–7126.
29 Pierce, J.H. and Aaronson, S.A. (1983) J. Virol. 46, 993–1002.
30 Dennis, J.W. et al. (1989) Oncogene 4, 853–860.
31 Roebroek, A.J.M. et al. (1986) Mol. Biol. Rep. 11, 117–125.
32 Beemon, K. and Mattingly, B. (1986) Virology 155, 716–720.
33 Foster, D.A. et al. (1985) Cell 42, 105–115.

34 Weinmaster, G. et al. (1984) Cell 37, 559–568.

35 Songyang, Z. et al. (1994) Mol. Cell. Biol. 14, 2777–2785.

36 Roebroek, A.J.M. et al. (1985) EMBO J., 4, 2897–2903.

37 Hao, Q.L. et al. (1989) Mol. Cell. Biol. 11, 1180–1183.

FRA1, FRA2

IDENTIFICATION

FRA1 and *FRA2* (*FOS*–related antigens) were detected by screening cDNA libraries with *FOS* DNA as a probe.

RELATED GENES

FRA1 and *FRA2* are members of the helix–loop–helix/leucine zipper superfamily (see **JUN**). Closely related genes are *FOS*, *FOSB*, ΔFOSB and r-*fos*.

Mass (kDa): predicted	29 (FRA1); 35 (FRA2)

Cellular location

Nucleus.

Tissue distribution

FRA1 and *FRA2* expression is low in quiescent cells and induced rapidly (*FRA1* detectable after 1 h, *FRA2* after 2 h) and transiently following cell stimulation with a slight lag with respect to FOS [1-4]. After the initial activation period of serum-stimulated quiescent cells when FOS is the principal protein associated with JUN proteins (~3 h), FRA1 and FRA2 are the predominant partners in heterodimers with JUN proteins [5].

PROTEIN FUNCTION

FRA1 and FRA2 form heterodimeric transcription factors with JUN proteins (see **FOS**). In Swiss 3T3 fibroblasts FRA1 and FRA2 are involved in asynchronous growth, rather than being required for the G_0 to G_1 transition [5].

GENE STRUCTURE

The overall structure of the *Fra-1* and *Fra-2* genes is very similar to that of *Fos* (see **FOS**).

PROTEIN STRUCTURE

The structures of FRA1 and FRA2 are closely related to each other and to that of FOS (see **FOS**). Human FRA1 and FRA2 are 45% identical in sequence: FRA1 is 51% identical to FOS.

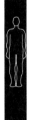

SEQUENCE OF FRA1

```
  1  MFRDFGEPGP SSGNGGGYGG PAQPPAAAQA AQQKFHLVPS INTMSGSQEL
 51  QWMVQPHFLG PSSYPRPLTY PQYSPPQPRP GVIRALGPPP GVRRRPCEQI
101  SPEEEERRRV RRERNKLAAA KCRNRRKELT DFLQAETDKL EDEKSGLQRE
151  IEELQKQKER LELVLEAHRP ICKIPEGAKE GDTGSTSGTS SPPAPCRPVP
201  CISLSPGPVL EPEALHTPTL MTTPSLTPFT PSLVFTYPST PEPCASAHRK
251  SSSSSGDPSS DPLGSPTLLA L (271)
```

Domain structure

111–129 Basic, DNA binding motif
133–161 Leucine zipper (underlined)

SEQUENCE OF FRA2

```
  1  MYQDYPGNFD TSSRGSSGSP AHAESYSSGG GGQQKFRVDM PGSGSAFIPT
 51  INAITTSQDL QWMVQPTVIT SMSNPYPRSH PYSPLPGLAS VPGHMALPRP
101  GVIKTIGTTV GRRRRDEQLS PEEEEKRRIR RERNKLAAAK CRNRRRELTE
151  KLQAETEELE EEKSGLQKEI AELQKEKEKL EFMLVAHGPV CKISPEERRS
201  PPAPGLQPMR SGGGSVGAVV VKQEPLEEDS PSSSSAGLDK AQRSVIKPIS
251  IAGGFYGEEP LHTPIVVTST PAVTPGTSNL VFTYPSVLEQ ESPASPSESC
301  SKAHRRSSSS GDQSSDSLNS PTLLAL (326)
```

Domain structure

130–148 Basic, DNA binding motif
152–180 Leucine zipper (underlined)

DATABASE ACCESSION NUMBERS

	PIR	SWISSPROT	EMBL/GENBANK	REFERENCES
Human *FRA1*	S08010; S15750	P15407	X16707	2
Human *FRA2*	S15749	P15408	X16706	2

References
1 Cohen, D.R. and Curran, T. (1988) Mol. Cell. Biol. 8, 2063–2069.
2 Matsui, M. et al. (1990) Oncogene 5, 249–255.
3 Nishina, H. et al. (1990) Proc. Natl Acad. Sci. USA 87, 3619–3623.
4 Yoshida, T. et al. (1993) Nucl. Acids Res., 21, 2715–2721.
5 Kovary, K. and Bravo, R. (1992) Mol. Cell. Biol. 12, 5015–5023.

FYN

IDENTIFICATION

FYN (formerly *SYN* (src/yes-related novel gene) or *SLK* (src-like kinase)) was originally cloned from a SV40-transformed human fibroblast library. There is no known naturally occurring *fyn*-containing retrovirus.

RELATED GENES

Member of the *SRC* tyrosine kinase family (*Blk, FGR, FYN, HCK, LCK/Tkl, LYN, SRC, YES*).

Nucleotides	Not fully mapped
Chromosome	6q21
Mass (kDa): predicted	60
expressed	$59^{fyn(B)}/p59^{fyn(T)}$

Cellular location

Plasma membrane.

Tissue distribution

$59^{fyn(B)}$ is mainly expressed in the brain and spinal cord but is detectable in most cell types other than epithelial cells [1,2]. $p59^{fyn(T)}$ is mainly expressed in T cells. An additional form, $p72^{fyn}$, has been detected in transformed T cells and in *in vitro* translation systems [3,4]. *FYN* expression is also activated in HL60 cells stimulated to differentiate by TPA [5] and in natural killer cells [6].

PROTEIN FUNCTION

FYN encodes a tyrosine kinase implicated in the control of cell growth. Overexpression of $p59^{fyn(T)}$ enhances IL2 secretion and DNA synthesis in response to anti-CD3 antibody. FYN expression is activated by stimulation of the TCR [7] when it may interact directly with CD3, leading to the phosphorylation and activation of PtdIns-PLCγ₁ and subsequent cellular responses. The CD45 tyrosine phosphatase regulates the tyrosine kinase activity of FYN [8]. In CD45⁻ cells, the TCR is uncoupled from protein tyrosine phosphorylation, PLCγ₁ regulation, accumulation of inositol phosphates $[Ca^{2+}]_i$ responses, diacylglycerol production and protein kinase C activation, suggesting that FYN plays a critical role in coupling the activated TCR to these responses. In T cells, FYN activates the *FOS* and *IL2* promoters: both these activities are inhibited by the tyrosine kinase CSK [9].

   In activated B cells, FYN (and LCK and LYN) all associate with membrane Ig. However, FYN(T) also binds via its SH2 domain to a set of phosphoproteins distinct from those associating with LYN [10]. In pro-B cells IL2 induces activation of FYN and its association with the IL2R β chain [11].

FYN also associates with CD2 and CD5 in T cells, with GAP in thrombin-stimulated platelets, with p125[FAK] in chicken cells and with the PDGF receptor in PDGF-stimulated fibroblasts [12–16].

FYN is expressed in oligodendrocytes and during the initial stages of myelination it is activated by associating with the large myelin-associated glycoprotein (MAG). Its importance for myelination is indicated by impairment of this process in *Fyn*-deficient mice [17].

In polyoma-transformed cells, FYN forms complexes with middle T antigen (as do SRC and YES), an interaction mediated by the C-terminus of FYN [1,18,19].

Cancer

FYN is overexpressed in some human tumour cell lines[1, 20, 21].

Transgenic animals

Mice that do not express FYN show no overt phenotype but increases in thymocyte $[Ca^{2+}]_i$ and proliferation stimulated by activating the TCR or by Thy-1 are markedly reduced, whereas the proliferative response of peripheral T cells remains essentially unaltered [22, 23]. However, disruption of *Fyn* (by the insertion of the β-galactosidase gene) has also been reported to give rise to homozygous *Fyn*-mutant neonates that die from a suckling problem [24].

The overexpression of p59[fyn(T)] in transgenic mice gives rise to T cells that are hyper-stimulatable, showing greatly enhanced phosphotyrosine accumulation and a twofold increase in $[Ca^{2+}]_i$ on activation by Con A or via CD3 or Thy-1[25].

Animals

Chickens inoculated with a recombinant avian retrovirus expressing *fyn* develop fibrosarcomas that may arise from mutations in the kinase or SH2 domains of FYN[26].

In vitro

Overexpression of normal *Fyn* transforms NIH 3T3 cells [20]. Substitution of the N-terminal two-thirds of FYN by the corresponding v-FGR region activates the FYN tyrosine kinase and transforming potential [27].

GENE STRUCTURE

FYN shares the common 12 exon organization of the *SRC* family.

PROTEIN STRUCTURE

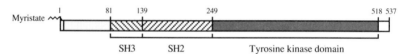

The two *Fyn* mRNAs (brain and thymus forms) arise by mutually exclusive splicing of alternative seventh exons: their products differ by 27 of the 55 amino acids encoded by the exon which is positioned at the beginning of the kinase domain and includes the presumptive nucleotide binding site [28].

SEQUENCE OF FYN

```
  1  MGCVQCKDKE ATKLTEERDG SLNQSSGYRY GTDPTPQHYP SFGVTSIPNY
 51  NNFHAAGGQG LTVFGGVNSS SHTGTLRTRG GTGVTLFVAL YDYEARTEDD
101  LSFHKGEKFQ ILNSSEGDWW EARSLTTGET GYIPSNYVAP VDSIQAEEWY
151  FGKLGRKDAE RQLLSFGNPR GTFLIRESET TKGAYSLSIR DWDDMKGDHV
201  KHYKIRKLDN GGYYITTRAQ FETLQQLVQH YSERAAGLCC RLVVPCHKGM
251  PRLTDLSVKT KDVWEIPRES LQLIKRLGNG QFGEVWMGTW NGNTKVAIKT
301  LKPGTMSPES FLEEAQIMKK LKHDKLVQLY AVVSEEPIYI VTEYMNKGSL
351  LDFLKDGEGR ALKLPNLVDM AAQVAAGMAY IERMNYIHRD LRSANILVGN
401  GLICKIADFG LARLIEDNEY TARQGAKFPI KWTAPEAALY GRFTIKSDVW
451  SFGILLTELV TKGRVPYPGM NNREVLEQVE RGYRMPCPQD CPISLHELMI
501  HCWKKDPEER PTFEYLQSFL EDYFTATEPQ YQPGENL (537)
```

Domain structure

2	Myristate attachment site
12	Protein kinase C phosphorylation site
233–287	Region corresponding to exon 7 (italics): corresponding sequence of FYN(T): EKADGLCFNL TVVSSSCTPQ TSGLAKDAWE VARDSLFLEK KLGQGCFAEV WL
277–285 and 299	ATP binding site
390	Active site
420	Tyrosine autophosphorylation site
531	Phosphorylation site. Mutation of Tyr531 to Phe does not activate the transforming capacity, in contrast to the effect of the equivalent mutation in SRC
87–139	SH3 domain (or A box: underlined). The crystal structure of this domain has been determined at 1.9 Å resolution [29].

Amino acids 83–537 are 80% homologous to YES and 77% to SRC and FGR. The C-terminal 191 amino acids are 86% homologous to SRC; the N-terminal 82 residues are 6% homologous.

DATABASE ACCESSION NUMBERS

	PIR	*SWISSPROT*	*EMBL/GENBANK*	*REFERENCES*
Human *FYN*	A24314, A25389	P06241	M14333	[24]
			M14676	[28, 30]

References
1 Kypta, R.M. et al. (1988) EMBO J. 7, 3837–3844.
2 Yagi, T. et al. (1993) Oncogene 8, 3343–3351.
3 Espino, P.C. et al. (1992) Oncogene 7, 317–322.
4 Da Silva, A.J. and Rudd, C.E. (1993) J. Biol. Chem. 268, 16537–16543.
5 Katagiri, K. et al. (1991) J. Immunol. 146, 701–707.
6 Biondi, A. et al. (1991) Eur. J. Immunol. 21, 843–846.
7 Katagiri, K. et al. (1989) Proc. Natl Acad. Sci. USA 86, 10064–10068.
8 Shiroo, M. et al. (1992) EMBO J. 11, 4887–4897.
9 Takeuchi, M. et al. (1994) J. Biol. Chem. 268, 27413–27419.
10 Malek, S.N. and Desiderio, S. (1993) J. Biol. Chem. 268, 22557–22565.
11 Kobayashi, N. et al. (1993) Proc. Natl Acad. Sci. USA 90, 4201–4205.
12 Bell, G.M. et al. (1992) Mol. Cell. Biol. 12, 5548–5554.
13 Burgess, K.E. et al. (1992) Proc. Natl Acad. Sci. USA 89, 9311–9315.
14 Cichowski, K. et al. (1992) J. Biol. Chem. 267, 5025–5028.
15 Cobb, B.S. et al. (1994) Mol. Cell. Biol. 14, 147–155.
16 Twamley, G.M. et al. (1992) Oncogene 7, 1893–1901.
17 Umemori, H. et al. (1994) Nature 367, 572–576.
18 Cheng, S.H. et al. (1991) J. Virol. 65, 170–179.
19 Pleiman, C.M. et al. (1993) Mol. Cell. Biol. 13, 5877–5887.
20 Kawakami, T. et al. (1986) Mol. Cell. Biol. 6, 4195–4201.
21 Semba, K. et al. (1986) Proc. Natl Acad. Sci. USA 83, 5459–5463.
22 Appleby, M.W. et al. (1992) Cell 70, 751–763.
23 Stein, P.L. et al. (1992) Cell 70, 741–750.
24 Yagi, T. et al. (1993) Nature 366, 742–745.
25 Cooke, M.P. et al. (1991) Cell 65, 281–291.
26 Semba, K. et al. (1990) Mol. Cell. Biol. 10, 3095–3104.
27 Kawakami, T. et al. (1988) Proc. Natl Acad. Sci. USA 85, 3870–3874.
28 Cooke, M.P. and Perlmutter, R.M. (1989) New Biol. 1, 66–74.
29 Noble, M.E.M. et al. (1993) EMBO J. 12, 2617–2624.
30 Peters, D.J. et al. (1990) Oncogene 5, 1313–1319.

HCK

IDENTIFICATION

HCK (*h*aematopoietic *c*ell *k*inase) encodes a *SRC*-family protein tyrosine kinase detected in human cells with v-*src* and murine *Lck* probes.

RELATED GENES

HCK is a member of the *SRC* tyrosine kinase family (*Blk*, *FGR*, *FYN*, *HCK*, *LCK/Tkl*, *LYN*, *SRC*, *YES*). *Hck-2* and *Hck-3* are the murine homologues of *LYN* and *LCK*, respectively.

Nucleotides (kb)	>30
Chromosome	20q11
Mass (kDa): predicted	57
expressed	56/59

Cellular location

Membrane-associated: p56 and p59. Cytoplasm: p59 alone.

Tissue distribution

Expression restricted to haematopoietic cells, predominantly of the myeloid and B lymphoid lineages [1,2]. *HCK* is expressed when acute myeloid leukaemic cells are induced to differentiate *in vitro* to cells with monocytic characteristics [3].

PROTEIN FUNCTION

The expression pattern suggests that HCK, in common with other members of the SRC family, has distinct cell lineage-specific functions and in particular may be involved in the differentiation of monocytes and granulocytes.

Cancer

HCK expression is detectable in several human leukaemia cell lines [1,2,4].

Transgenic animals

Transgenic male mice that are hemizygous for the *Hck* transgene are sterile, indicating that the gene may be important in spermatogenesis[5]. *Hck*-deficient mice show normal haematopoietic development but impaired phagocytosis. The specific activity of LYN is increased in *Hck*[-/-] macrophages, indicating that LYN may compensate for the absence of HCK[6].

STRUCTURE OF THE HUMAN AND MURINE *HCK* GENES

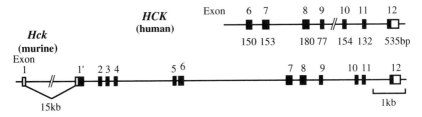

Human *HCK* exons 6–12 are almost identical in size to the corresponding exons of *FGR*, *LCK* and *SRC* [7].

TRANSCRIPTIONAL REGULATION

The murine *Hck* promoter has no TATA or CAAT elements but contains GC-rich regions, three SP1 and two AP-2 consensus binding sites and an LPS-responsive element [8,9]. p59 is generated by translation from a CTG codon 5′ of the ATG used to generate p56 [10].

PROTEIN STRUCTURE

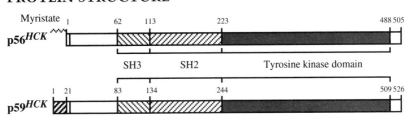

SEQUENCE OF HCK

```
  1  MGSMKSKFLQ VGGNTFSKTE TSASPHCPVY VPDPTSTIKP GPNSHNSNTP
 51  GIREAGSEDI IVVALYDYEA IHHEDLSFQK GDQMVVLEES GEWWKARSLA
101  TRKEGYIPSN YVARVDSLET EEWFFKGISR KDAERQLLAP GNMLGSFMIR
151  DSETTKGSYS LSVRDYDPRQ GDTVKHYKIR TLDNGGFYIS PRSTFSTLQE
201  LVDHYKKGND GLCQKLSVPC MSSKPQKPWE KDAWEIPRES LKLEKKLGAG
251  QFGEVWMATY NKHTKVAVKT MKPGSMSVEA FLAEANVMKT LQHDKLVKLH
301  AVVTKEPIYI ITEFMAKGSL LDFLKSDEGS KQPLPKLIDF SAQIAEGMAF
351  IEQRNYIHRD LRAANILVSA SLVCKIADFG LARVIEDNEY TAREGAKFPI
401  KWTAPEAINF GSFTIKSDVW SFGILLMEIV TYGRIPYPGM SNPEVIRALE
451  RGYRMPRPEN CPEELYNIMM RCWKNRPEER PTFEYIQSVL DDFYTATESQ
501  YQQQP (505)
```

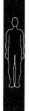

Domain structure

–21–1	21 amino acid N-terminal extension present in the p59 isoform (MGGRSSCEDPGCPRDEERAPR)
247–255 and 269	ATP binding site
360	Active site
390	Auto-phosphorylation site
62–113	SH3 domain (A box: underlined)
114–223	SH2 domain (italics)
224–488	Catalytic domain

Database accession numbers

	PIR	SWISSPROT	EMBL/GENBANK	REFERENCES
Human *HCK*	A27812	P08631	M16591, M16592	*1,2*
Human *HCK*			X59741, X59742, X59743	7

References

1 Ziegler, S.F. et al. (1987) Mol. Cell. Biol. 7, 2276–2285.
2 Quintrell, N. et al. (1987) Mol. Cell. Biol. 7, 2267–2275.
3 Willman, C.L. et al. (1991) Blood 77, 726–734.
4 Perlmutter, R.M. et al. (1988) Biochim. Biophys. Acta 948, 245–262.
5 Magram, J. and Bishop, J.M. (1991) Proc. Natl Acad. Sci. USA 88, 10327–10331.
6 Lowell, C.A. et al. (1994) Genes Devel. 8, 387–398.
7 Hradetzky, D. et al. (1992) Gene, 113, 275–280.
8 Ziegler, S.F. et al. (1991) Oncogene 6, 283–288.
9 Lichtenberg, U. et al. (1992) Oncogene 7, 849–858.
10 Lock, P. et al. (1991) Mol. Cell. Biol. 11, 4363–4370.

HER2/ErbB-2/Neu

IDENTIFICATION

Neu was first identified by transfection with DNA from *neu*roglioblastomas that had arisen in rats exposed *in utero* to ethylnitrosourea. *HER2* was identified by screening genomic and cDNA libraries.

RELATED GENES

HER2/ErbB-2 are members of the *EGFR* family (*EGFR, HER3* and *HER4*). HER2 is ~80% homologous to EGFR and 80% identical to rat NEU.

Nucleotides	Not fully mapped
Chromosome	17q21–q22
Mass (kDa): predicted	138
expressed	gp185
	100 (HER2 ECD)

Cellular location

Plasma membrane. HER2 ECD is a perinuclear cytoplasmic protein.

Tissue distribution

Widely distributed. The pattern of expression is closely similar to that of *EGFR* [1,2], although high levels of *HER2* mRNA occur in melanocytes in which *EGFR* is undetectable. *HER2 ECD* is an alternatively processed form of *HER2* produced in some human breast carcinoma cell lines [3].

PROTEIN FUNCTION

Receptor-like tyrosine kinase activated by NEU differentiation factor (NDF or heregulin (HRG)) or glial growth factors [4] or by NEU protein-specific activating factor (NAF) [5]. Activation by heregulin requires the co-expression of HER4. A 30 kDa glycoprotein secreted from human breast cancer cells and a 25 kDa peptide secreted by activated macrophages also bind to HER2 [6]. NDF stimulates tyrosine phosphorylation of HER2 and the differentiation of human breast cancer cells *in vitro* [7]. Activated HER2 phosphorylates and binds to SHC proteins, as does activated EGFR [8]. The expression of *Neu* causes accumulation of GTP.RAS [9].

TPA stimulates serine/threonine phosphorylation of normal and oncogenic NEU and inhibits the tyrosine kinase activity of oncogenic NEU: thus, like the EGFR oncogenic NEU may be negatively regulated by protein kinase C [10].

Oncogenic activation of *Neu* (by point mutation, overexpression or by truncation of non-catalytic sequences) results in its constitutive phosphorylation and in the tyrosine phosphorylation of PtdInsP_2-specific phospholipase Cγ, which is permanently associated with activated NEU [11].

The truncated version of HER2, HER2 ECD, suppresses the growth-inhibitory effects of antibodies directed against HER2 [3].

Cancer

Unlike the rat *Neu* oncogene *HER2* does not have an activated mutant form. However, *HER2* is overexpressed with high frequency in breast, stomach, ovarian and bladder cancers [12,13] and its over-expression or amplification has been detected in a variety of other cancers [14–16]. In lymph node positive breast cancer patients there is a strong correlation between *HER2* amplification and poor prognosis, although the expression of *HER2* does not appear to promote metastasis. The extracellular region is proteolytically released from COS-7 cells in a form that activates p185[neu] and is similarly released as a 110 kDa protein into the sera of advanced-stage breast carcinoma patients [17]. The SH2 domain protein GRB-7 is concomitantly overexpressed with HER2 in some breast cancers and binds tightly to tyrosine phosphorylated HER2 [18].

Transgenic animals

Transgenic mice carrying an activated *Neu* oncogene develop mammary adenocarcinomas and, occasionally, other tumours [19,20].

In animals

The expression of oncogenic NEU in mouse mammary epithelium can cause ductal carcinoma but may also induce epithelial abnormalities resembling those of human sclerosing adenosis and atypical hyperplasia that may be precursors of ductal carcinoma [21].

In vitro

Overexpression of either human *HER2* or rat *Neu* transforms NIH 3T3 fibroblasts and *Neu*-induced transformation can occur independently of the EGF receptor [22]. Transformation of NIH 3T3 fibroblasts by oncogenic *Neu* causes the cells to exhibit metastatic properties both *in vitro* and *in vivo* [23]. MYC or p105[RB1] can suppress *Neu* transformation and adenovirus E1A protein suppresses *Neu*-induced metastasis of NIH 3T3 cells, although mechanisms additional to the suppression of *Neu* transcription are involved [24]. Monoclonal antibodies directed against p185[HER2] specifically inhibit the proliferation of human breast carcinoma cells [25].

GENE STRUCTURE

There is strict conservation of exon-intron boundaries in the regions encoding the catalytic domains of HER2 and EGFR (see ***EGFR/ErbB-1***). The *HER2* promoter is similar to that of EGFR, having a high GC content, an SP1 binding site and multiple transcription initiation sites but also including both TATA and CAAT boxes [26]. In cells overexpressing HER2, promoter activity is enhanced as a result of the increased abundance of the transcription factor OB2-1 [27].

PROTEIN STRUCTURE

The dominant transforming *Neu* oncogene isolated from rat neuroblastoma

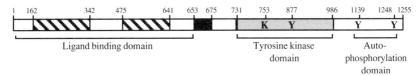

DNA was oncogenically activated by a single point mutation (Val664 to Glu) in the transmembrane domain [28]. The Glu664 mutation confers high-affinity ligand binding on the receptor [29] and enhances tyrosine kinase activity and autophosphorylation of Tyr1248 (the major auto-phosphorylation site). Mutation of Tyr1248 to Phe lowers tyrosine kinase and transforming activities. Thus Tyr1248 negatively regulates transformation, the effect being blocked by phosphorylation [30].

SEQUENCE HOMOLOGY BETWEEN THE PROTEIN KINASE DOMAINS OF HER2 AND SOME VIRAL ONCOGENES

Viral oncogene:	erbB	src	abl	yes	fgr	ros	fps	mil	fms	mos/rel
% homology:	82	43	42	42	41	38	37	28	27	<25

SEQUENCE OF HER2

```
   1 MELAALCRWG LLLALLPPGA ASTQVCTGTD MKLRLPASPE THLDMLRHLY
  51 QGCQVVQGNL ELTYLPTNAS LSFLQDIQEV QGYVLIAHNQ VRQVPLQRLR
 101 IVRGTQLFED NYALAVLDNG DPLNNTTPVT GASPGGLREL QLRSLTEILK
 151 GGVLIQRNPQ LCYQDTILWK DIFHKNNQLA LTLIDTNRSR ACHPCSPMCK
 201 GSRCWGESSE DCQSLTRTVC AGGCARCKGP LPTDCCHEQC AAGCTGPKHS
 251 DCLACLHFNH SGICELHCPA LVTYNTDTFE SMPNPEGRYT FGASCVTACP
 301 YNYLSTDVGS CTLVCPLHNQ EVTAEDGTQR CEKCSKPCAR VCYGLGMEHL
 351 REVRAVTSAN IQEFAGCKKI FGSLAFLPES FDGDPASNTA PLQPEQLQVF
 401 ETLEEITGYL YISAWPDSLP DLSVFQNLQV IRGRILHNGA YSLTLQGLGI
 451 SWLGLRSLRE LGSGLALIHH NTHLCFVHTV PWDQLFRNPH QALLHTANRP
 501 EDECVGEGLA CHQLCARGHC WGPGPTQCVN CSQFLRGQEC VEECRVLQGL
 551 PREYVNARHC LPCHPECQPQ NGSVTCFGPE ADQCVACAHY KDPPFCVARC
 601 PSGVKPDLSY MPIWKFPDEE GACQPCPINC THSCVDLDDK GCPAEQRASP
 651 LTSIISAVVG ILLVVVLGVV FGILIKRRQQ KIRKYTMRRL LQETELVEPL
 701 TPSGAMPNQA QMRILKETEL RKVKVLGSGA FGTVYKGIWI PDGENVKIPV
 751 AIKVLRENTS PKANKEILDE AYVMAGVGSP YVSRLLGICL TSTVQLVTQL
 801 MPYGCLLDHV RENRGRLGSQ DLLNWCMQIA KGMSYLEDVR LVHRDLAARN
 851 VLVKSPNHVK ITDFGLARLL DIDETEYHAD GGKVPIKWMA LESILRRRFT
 901 HQSDVWSYGV TVWELMTFGA KPYDGIPARE IPDLLEKGER LPQPPICTID
 951 VYMIMVKCWM IDSECRPRFR ELVSEFSRMA RDPQRFVVIQ NEDLGPASPL
1001 DSTFYRSLLE DDDMGDLVDA EEYLVPQQGF FCPDPAPGAG GMVHHRHRSS
1051 STRSGGGDLT LGLEPSEEEA PRSPLAPSEG AGSDVFDGDL GMGAAKGLQS
1101 LPTHDPSPLQ RYSEDPTVPL PSETDGYVAP LTCSPQPEYV NQPDVRPQPP
1151 SPREGPLPAA RPAGATLERP KTLSPGKNGV VKDVFAFGGA VENPEYLTPQ
1201 GGAAPQPHPP PAFSPAFDNL YYWDQDPPER GAPPSTFKGT PTAENPEYLG
1251 LDVPV (1255)
```

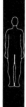

Domain structure

1–21	Signal sequence (italics)
22–652	Extracellular domain
653–675	Transmembrane domain (underlined)
676–1255	Cytoplasmic domain
726–734 and 753	ATP binding site
1139, 1221, 1222, 1248	Phosphorylation sites (underlined)
68, 124, 187, 259, 530, 571, 629	Putative carbohydrate attachment sites

DATABASE ACCESSION NUMBERS

	PIR	SWISSPROT	EMBL/GENBANK	REFERENCES
Human *HER2*	A25491	P04626	X03363	*2,31*

References

1 Coussens, L. et al. (1985) Science 230, 1132–1139.
2 Semba, K. et al. (1985) Proc. Natl Acad. Sci. USA 82, 6497–6501.
3 Scott, G.K. et al. (1993) Mol. Cell. Biol. 13, 2247–2257.
4 Marchionni, M.A. et al. (1993) Nature 362, 312–318.
5 Dobashi, K. et al. (1991) Proc. Natl Acad. Sci. USA 88, 8582–8586.
6 Tarakhovsky, A. et al. (1991) Oncogene 6, 2187–2196.
7 Peles, E. et al. (1992) Cell 69, 205–216.
8 Segatto, O. et al. (1993) Oncogene 8, 2105–2112.
9 Satoh, T. et al. (1990) Proc. Natl Acad. Sci. USA 87, 7926–7929.
10 Cao, H. et al. (1991) Oncogene 6, 705–711.
11 Peles, E. et al. (1991) EMBO J. 10, 2077–2086.
12 Slamon, D.J. et al. (1989) Science 244, 707–712.
13 Wright, C. et al. (1990) Brit. J. Cancer 62, 764–765.
14 Berchuck, A. et al. (1991) Am. J. Obstet. Gynecol. 164, 15–21.
15 Yonemura, Y. et al. (1991) Cancer Res. 51, 1034–1038.
16 Riviere, A. et al. (1991) Cancer 67, 2142–2149.
17 Pupa, S.M. et al. (1993) Oncogene 8, 2917–2923.
18 Stein, D. et al. (1994) EMBO J. 13, 1331–1340.
19 Muller, W.J. et al. (1988) Cell 54, 105–115.
20 Bouchard, L. et al. (1989) Cell 57, 931–936.
21 Bradbury, J.M. et al. (1993) Oncogene 8, 1551–1558.
22 Chazin, V.R. et al. (1992) Oncogene 7, 1859–1866.
23 Yu, D. and Hung, M.-C. (1991) Oncogene 6, 1991–1996.
24 Yu, D. et al. (1993) Cancer Res. 53, 5784–5790.
25 Carter, P. et al. (1992) Proc. Natl Acad. Sci. USA 89, 4285–4289.
26 Chen, Y. and Gill, G.N. (1994) Oncogene 9, 2269–2276.
27 Skinner, A. and Hurst, H.C. (1993) Oncogene 8, 3393–3401.
28 Cao, H. et al. (1992) EMBO J. 11, 923–932.
29 Ben-Levy, R. et al. (1992) J. Biol. Chem. 267, 17304–17313.
30 Akiyama, T. et al. (1991) Mol. Cell. Biol. 11, 833–842.
31 Yamamoto, T. et al. (1986) Nature 319, 230–234.

IDENTIFICATION

HER3/ErbB-3 was detected by screening genomic DNA using v-erbB as a probe and by PCR amplification of genomic DNA using degenerate oligonucleotide primers based on sequences encoding regions of the EGFR family catalytic domains.

RELATED GENES

HER3 is a member of the EGFR family, distinct from EGFR, HER2 and HER4.

Nucleotides	Not fully mapped
Chromosome	12q13
Mass (kDa): predicted	146
expressed	gp160

Cellular location

HER3: Plasma membrane.

Tissue distribution

Widely expressed. Pattern of expression closely similar to that of EGFR and HER2 although HER3 is undetectable in fetal or adult skin fibroblasts. Transcribed in term placenta, the respiratory and urinary tracts, stomach, lung, kidney and brain but not in skeletal muscle or lymphoid cells [1]. Expressed in normal fetal liver, kidney and brain but not in the heart.

PROTEIN FUNCTION

Receptor-like tyrosine kinase. Ligand unknown. Although HER3 has a tyrosine kinase domain that is highly homologous to those of EGFR and HER2, the C-terminal domain and a 29 amino acid region C-terminal to the ATP binding domain diverge markedly. Activated receptors associate with PtdIns 3-kinase, SHC and GRB2 but not with PLCγ or GAP [2].

Cancer

HER3 is expressed in some carcinomas and, with low frequency, in sarcomas. Not detectable in cell lines derived from haematopoietic tumours but overexpressed in a subset of mammary tumour-derived cell lines [3].

GENE STRUCTURE

There is strict conservation of exon–intron boundaries in the regions encoding the catalytic domains of HER3 and EGFR (see **EGFR/ErbB-1**). The

HER3 promoter is similar to that of EGFR, having a high GC content, no TATA box and multiple transcription initiation sites [4]. In cells overexpressing HER3, promoter activity is enhanced as a result of the increased abundance of the transcription factor OB2-1 [5].

PROTEIN STRUCTURE

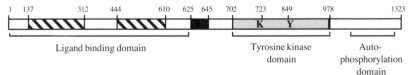

HER3 is ~44% identical in amino acid sequence to EGFR and HER2 in the extracellular domain and ~60% identical in the tyrosine kinase domain (see **EGFR/ErbB-1**). The tyrosine kinase domain homology with EPH, MET, FMS and the insulin receptor is ~30%. There is no significant homology between the C-terminal 353 amino acids of HER3 and the corresponding regions of EGFR, HER2 and HER4 that contain the major tyrosine autophosphorylation sites.

SEQUENCE OF HER3

```
   1 MRANDALQVL GLLFSLARGS EVGNSQAVCP GTLNGLSVTG DAENQYQTLY
  51 KLYERCEVVM GNLEIVLTGH NADLSFLQWI REVTGYVLVA MNEFSTLPLP
 101 NLRVVRGTQV YDGKFAIFVM LNYNTNSSHA LRQLRLTQLT EILSGGVYIE
 151 KNDKLCHMDT IDWRDIVRDR DAEIVVKDNG RSCPPCHEVC KGRCWGPGSE
 201 DCQTLTKTIC APQCNGHCFG PNPNQCCHDE CAGGCSGPQD TDCFACRHFN
 251 DSGACVPRCP QPLVYNKLTF QLEPNPHTKY QYGGVCVASC PHNFVVDQTS
 301 CVRACPPDKM EVDKNGLKMC EPCGGLCPKA CEGTGSGSRF QTVDSSNIDG
 351 FVNCTKILGN LDFLITGLNG DPWHKIPALD PEKLNVFRTV REITGYLNIQ
 401 SWPPHMHNFS VFSNLTTIGG RSLYNRGFSL LIMKNLNVTS LGFRSLKEIS
 451 AGRIYISANR QLCYHHSLNW TKVLRGPTEE RLDIKHNRPR RDCVAEGKVC
 501 DPLCSSGGCW GPGPGQCLSC RNYSRGGVCV THCNFLNGEP REFAHEAECF
 551 SCHPECQPME GTATCNGSGS DTCAQCAHFR DGPHCVSSCP HGVLGAKGPI
 601 YKYPDVQNEC RPCHENCTQG CKGPELQDCL GQTLVLIGKT HLTMALTVIA
 651 GLVVIFMMLG GTFLYWRGRR IQNKRAMRRY LERGESIEPL DPSEKANKVL
 701 ARIFKETELR KLKVLGSGVF GTVHKGVWIP EGESIKIPVC IKVIEDKSGR
 751 QSFQAVTDHM LAIGSLDHAH IVRLLGLCPG SSLQLVTQYL PLGSLLDHVR
 801 QHRGALGPQL LLNWGVQIAK GMYYLEEHGM VHRNLAARNV LLKSPSQVQV
 851 ADFGVADLLP PDDKQLLYSE AKTPIKWMAL ESIHFGKYTH QSDVWSYGVT
 901 VWELMTFGAE PYAGLRLAEV PDLLEKGERL AQPQICTIDV YMVMVKCWMI
 951 DENIRPTFKE LANEFTRMAR DPPRYLVIKR ESGPGIAPGP EPHGLTNKKL
1001 EEVELEPELD LDLDLEAEED NLATTTLGSA LSLPVGTLNR PRGSQSLLSP
1051 SSGYMPMNQG NLGESCQESA VSGSSERCPR PVSLHPMPRG CLASESSEGH
1101 VTGSEAELQE KVSMCRSRSR SRSPRPRGDS AYHSQRHSLL TPVTPLSPPG
1151 LEEEDVNGYV MPDTHLKGTP SSREGTLSSV GLSSVLGTEE EDEDEEYEYM
1201 NRRRRHSPPH PPRPSSLEEL GYEYMDVGSD LSASLGSTQS CPLHPVPIMP
1251 TAGTTPDEDY EYMNRQRDGG GPGGDYAAMG ACPASEQGYE EMRAFQGPGH
1301 QAPHVHYARL KTLRSLEATD SAFDNPDYWH SRLFPKANAQ RT (1342)
```

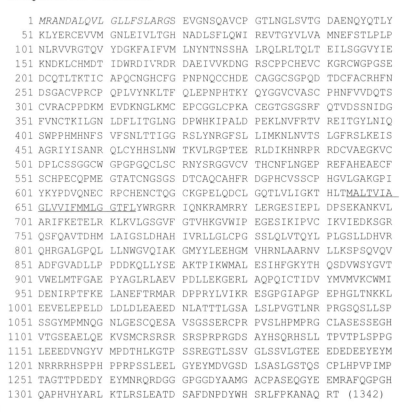

Domain structure

1–19	Signal sequence (italics)
20–643	Extracellular domain
644–664	Transmembrane domain (underlined)
665–1342	Cytoplasmic domain
715–723 and 742	ATP binding site
126, 250, 353, 408, 414, 437, 469, 522, 566, 616	Putative carbohydrate attachment sites

DATABASE ACCESSION NUMBERS

	PIR	SWISSPROT	EMBL/GENBANK	REFERENCES
Human *HER3*	A36223	P21860	M29366	2
			M34309	6

References

1 Prigent, S.A. et al. (1992) Oncogene 7, 1273–1278.
2 Fedi, P. et al. (1994) Mol. Cell. Biol. 14, 492–500.
3 Kraus, M.H. et al. (1989) Proc. Natl Acad. Sci. USA 86, 9193–9197.
4 Suen, T.-C. and Hung, M.-C. et al. (1990) Mol. Cell Biol. 10, 6306–6315.
5 Skinner, A. and Hurst, H.C. (1993) Oncogene 8, 3393–3401.
6 Plowman, G.D. et al. (1990) Proc. Natl Acad. Sci. USA 87, 4905–4909.

HER4/ErbB-4

IDENTIFICATION

HER4 /ErbB-4 was detected by PCR amplification of genomic DNA using degenerate oligonucleotide primers based on sequences encoding regions of the EGFR family catalytic domains.

RELATED GENES

HER4 is a member of the *EGFR* family, distinct from *EGFR*, *HER2* and *HER3*.

Nucleotides (kb)	Not fully mapped
Mass (kDa): predicted	144
expressed	gp180

Cellular location

Plasma membrane.

Tissue distribution

Maximum expression in brain, heart and kidney but also expressed in parathyroid, cerebellum, pituitary, spleen, testis and breast with lower levels detectable in thymus, lung, salivary gland and pancreas.

PROTEIN FUNCTION

The intrinsic tyrosine kinase activity of HER4 is specifically stimulated by a heparin-binding growth factor related to heregulin that has no direct effect on EGFR, HER2 or HER3 [1] and also by heregulin [2]. This growth factor causes phenotypic differentiation of a human mammary tumour cell line.

Cancer

Expressed in a variety of mammary adenocarcinoma and neuroblastoma cell lines [1].

PROTEIN STRUCTURE

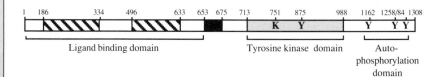

138

The extracellular domains are between 56% and 67% identical to the corresponding regions of HER3 and 43–51% and 34–46% identical to EGFR and HER2. The 50 conserved extracellular cysteines of EGFR, HER2 and HER3 are also conserved in HER4 except for the fourth cysteine in domain IV. The transmembrane 37 amino acids are 73% identical with those of EGFR and the 276 residue catalytic domain is 79%, 77% and 63% identical to those of EGFR, HER2 and HER3, respectively. In the C-terminus homology is much lower (19% (EGFR), 27% (HER2), respectively) but the major tyrosine autophosphorylation sites of EGFR are conserved.

SEQUENCE OF HER4

```
   1 MKPATGLWVW VSLLVAAGTV QPSDSQSVCA GTENKLSSLS DLEQQYRALR
  51 KYYENCEVVM GNLEITSIEH NRDLSFLRSV REVTGYVLVA LNQFRYLPLE
 101 NLRIIRGTKL YEDRYALAIF LNYRKDGNFG LQELGLKNLT EILNGGVYVD
 151 QNKFLCYADT IHWQDIVRNP WPSNLTLVST NGSSGCGRCH KSCTGRCWGP
 201 TENHCQTLTR TVCAEQCDGR CYGPYVSDCC HRECAGGCSG PKDTDCFACM
 251 NFNDSGACVT QCPQTFVYNP TTFQLEHNFN AKYTYGAFCV KKCPHNFVVD
 301 SSSCVRACPS SKMEVEENGI KMCKPCTDIC PKACDGIGTG SLMSAQTVDS
 351 SNIDKFINCT KINGNLIFLV TGIHGDPYNA IEAIDPEKLN VFRTVREITG
 401 FLNIQSWPPN MTDFSVFSNL VTIGGRVLYS GLSLLILKQQ GITSLQFQSL
 451 KEISAGNIYI TDNSNLCYYH TINWTTLFST INQRIVIRDN RKAENCTAEG
 501 MVCNHLCSSD GCWGPGPDQC LSCRRFSRGR ICIESCNLYD GEFREFENGS
 551 ICVECDPQCE KMEDGLLTCH GPGPDNCTKC SHFKDGPNCV EKCPDGLQGA
 601 NSFIFKYADP DRECHPCHPN CTQGCNGPTS HDCIYYPWTG HSTLPQHART
 651 PLIAAGVIGG LFILVIVGLT FAVYVRRKSI KKKRALRRFL ETELVEPLTP
 701 SGTAPNQAQL RILKETELKR VKVLGSGAFG TVYKGIWVPE GETVKIPVAI
 751 KILNETTGPK ANVEFMDEAL IMASMDHPHL VRLLGVCLSP TIQLVTQLMP
 801 HGCLLEYVHE HKDNIGSQLL LNWCVQIAKG MMYLEERRLV HRDLAARNVL
 851 VKSPNHVKIT DFGLARLLEG DEKEYNADGG KMPIKWMALE CIHYRKFTHQ
 901 SDVWSYGVTI WELMTFGGKP YDGIPTREIP DLLEKGERLP QPPICTIDVY
 951 MVMVKCWMID ADSRPKFKEL AAEFSRMARD PQRYLVIQGD DRMKLPSPND
1001 SKFFQNLLDE EDLEDMMDAE EYLVPQAFNI PPPIYTSRAR IDSNRSEIGH
1051 SPPPAYTPMS GNQFVYRDGG FAAEQGVSVP YRAPTSTIPE APVAQGATAE
1101 IFDDSCCNGT LRKPVAPHVQ EDSSTQRYSA DPTVFAPERS PRGELDEEGY
1151 MTPMRDKPKQ EYLNPVEENP FVSRRKNGDL QALDNPEYHN ASNGPPKAED
1201 EYVNEPLYLN TFANTLGKAE YLKNNILSMP EKAKKAFDNP DYWNHSLPPR
1251 STLQHPDYLQ EYSTKYFYKQ NGRIRPIVAE NPEYLSEFSL KPGTVLPPPP
1301 YRHRNTVV (1308)
```

DOMAIN STRUCTURE

1–25	Signal sequence (italics)
26–649	Extracellular domain
650–675	Transmembrane domain (underlined)
676–1308	Cytoplasmic domain

679	Potential protein kinase C phosphorylation site (Ser679)
699	Potential MAP kinase phosphorylation site (Thr699)
713–988	Catalytic domain
725–730 and 751	ATP binding site (underlined)
1162, 1258, 1188, 1284	Phosphorylation sites (underlined)
138, 174, 181, 253, 358, 410, 473, 495, 576, 620	Putative carbohydrate attachment sites

DATABASE ACCESSION NUMBERS

	PIR	*SWISSPROT*	*EMBL/GENBANK*	*REFERENCE*
Human *HER4*			L07868	*1*

References
1 Plowman, G.D. et al. (1993) Proc. Natl Acad. Sci. USA 90, 1746–1750.
2 Plowman, G.D. et al. (1993) Nature 366, 473–475.

HSTF1/Hst

IDENTIFICATION

HSTF1 (*h*eparan *s*ecretory *t*rans*f*orming protein *1*) is a human transforming gene originally detected by NIH 3T3 fibroblast transfection with DNA from *h*uman *s*tomach *t*umours that has no homology with known viral oncogenes. *HST2* is a close homologue of *HSTF1* that was cloned by cross-hybridization with *HSTF1* probes.

The *HSTF1/Hst-1* and *INT2/Int-2* oncogenes are members of the fibroblast growth factor (FGF) family [1-3].

RELATED GENES

The FGF family includes seven proteins: acidic fibroblast growth factor (*FGFA*, aFGF, HBGF-1 or FGF1), basic FGF (*FGFB*, bFGF, HBGF-2 or FGF2), *INT2* (FGF3), *HSTF1* (*Hst-1*/Kaposi-FGF/K-FGF or FGF4), *FGF5*, *HST2*/*Hst-2* (*FGF6*) and keratinocyte growth factor, KGF (FGF7).

	HSTF1	HST2
Nucleotides (kb)	11	8
Chromosome	11q13.3	12p13
Mass (kDa): predicted	22	14
expressed	22	

Cellular location

HSTF1 is glycosylated and secreted, the secreted protein being stabilized by heparin [4]. HST2 also has the characteristics of a heparin-binding growth factor.

Tissue distribution

HSTF1/Hst-1 is expressed at a limited stage of embryonal development [5]. *HST2* is only detectable in leukaemic cell lines [6].

PROTEIN FUNCTION

The members of the FGF family appear to act as paracrine or autocrine growth factors. FGFA and FGFB may function in both cell growth and in differentiation and have been implicated in cell transformation, angiogenesis and embryonic development. HST1 and INT2 induce mesoderm formation in *Xenopus laevis* animal pole cells [7].

Cancer

FGFs have oncogenic potential: they can induce blood vessel formation and are synthesized by many tumour cells [1-3].

HSTF1, together with *INT2* and *BCL1*, is amplified in up to 22% of human breast carcinomas [8,9]. *HSTF1*, *INT2* and anionic glutathione-S-transferase are co-amplified in ~30% of breast carcinomas [10] However, there is no evidence that the HSTF1 or INT2 proteins are expressed in breast tumours. Co-amplification of *HSTF1/INT2* occurs in up to 47% of oesophageal carcinomas [11-13] and *HSTF1* is expressed together with *KIT* in some testicular germ cell tumours [14]. *HSTF1* has also been identified in human DNA from gastric cancers, hepatomas, colon carcinomas[15], melanoma [16], osteosarcoma [17] and in Kaposi's sarcoma [18].

The human FGF receptors *BEK* (*b*acterial *e*xpressed *k*inase) and *FLG* (*F*ms-*l*ike gene, also *FLT2*) are amplified in ~10% of human breast tumours. BEK expression may correlate with that of *MYC* and expression of *FGFR1/FLG* with *HSTF1/INT2/BCL1* [19].

In animals

Hst-1 may be activated by MMTV proviral insertion on either side of the gene: some insertions activate both *Hst-1* and the 17 kb distant *Int-2* gene [20]. *Hst-1* may be involved in tumour progression from a non-metastatic to a metastatic phenotype in the mouse mammary tumour system [21].

In vitro

HSTF1 or *FGF5* genomic and cDNA sequences transfected into NIH 3T3 cells induce morphological transformation, anchorage-independent growth and tumorigenicity [18,22-26].
HST2 transforms NIH 3T3 fibroblasts into cells that are tumorigenic in nude mice [6].

GENE STRUCTURE

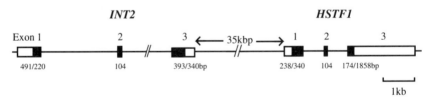

The FGF family has a common genomic organization and each member has a conserved 104 bp exon encoding the central 35 amino acids. *INT2/Int-2* and *HSTF1/Hst-2* are in the same transcriptional orientation.

TRANSCRIPTIONAL REGULATION

The *HSTF1* promoter contains a TATA box and three putative SP-1 binding sites. The 5′ non-coding region and exon 1 are GC-rich regions, a characteristic of house-keeping genes [27]. Expression of *HSTF1* may be regulated by protein factor(s) binding to an enhancer located in the third exon of the gene [28].

PROTEIN STRUCTURE

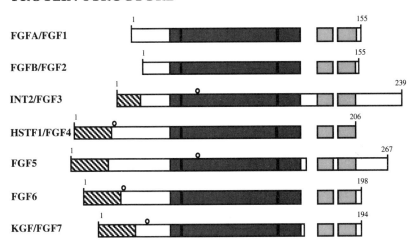

FGF family proteins contain two major regions of homology (heavy and light shading) and there are two absolutely conserved cysteine residues indicated by the vertical bars (see below). The cross-hatched boxes indicate N-terminal signal sequences, circles potential N-glycosylation sites. The human proteins are represented, with the exception of FGF6 for which the structure of the mouse protein is shown.

HSTF1 is homologous to FGFA (38%), FGFB (43%) and mouse INT2 (40%). Murine FGF6 is 66% identical to murine HST1/K-FGF and 39% identical to INT2.

SEQUENCE OF HSTF1 (FGF4)

```
  1  MSGPGTAAVA LLPAVLLALL APWAGRGGAA APTAPNGTLE AELERRWESL
 51  VALSLARLPV AAQPKEAAVQ SGAGDYLLGI KRLRRLYCNV GIGFHLQALP
101  DGRIGGAHAD TRDSLLELSP VERGVVSIFG VASRFFVAMS SKGKLYGSPF
151  FTDECTFKEI LLPNNYNAYE SYKYPGMFIA LSKNGKTKKG NRVSPTMKVT
201  HFLPRL (206)
```

Domain structure

9–20	Potential signal sequence (italics)
88, 155	Conserved cysteine residues (underlined)

SEQUENCE OF HST2 (FGF6)

```
  1  MSRGAGRLQG TLWALVFLGI LVGMVVPSPA GTRANNTLLD SRGWGTLLSR
 51  SRAGLAGEIA GVNWESGYLV GIKRQRRLYC NVGIGFHLQV LPDGRISGTH
101  EENPYSLLEI STVERGVVSL FGVRSALFVA MNSKGRLYAT PSFQEECKFR
151  ETLLPNNYNA YESDLYQGTY IALSKYGRVK RGSKVSPIMT VTHFLPRI (198)
```

Domain structure

12–26	Potential signal sequence (italics)
80, 147	Conserved cysteine residues (underlined)

DATABASE ACCESSION NUMBERS

	PIR	SWISSPROT	EMBL/GENBANK	REFERENCES
Human *HSTF1* (FGF4)	A28417	P08620	J02986	27
(or *HST* or *KS3*)			M17446	18, 22
Human *HST2*	S04204	P10767	X14071, X14072,	29
(*FGF6*)			X14073	

References

1 Burgess, W.H. and Maciag, T. (1989) Ann. Rev. Biochem. 58, 575–606.
2 Goldfarb, M. (1990) Cell Growth Differen. 1, 439–445.
3 Johnson, D.E. and Williams, L.T. (1993) Adv. Cancer Res. 60, 1–41.
4 Delli-Bovi, P. et al. (1988) Mol. Cell. Biol. 8, 2933–2941.
5 Suzuki, H.R. et al. (1992) Devel. Biol. 150, 219–222.
6 Iida, S. et al. (1992) Oncogene 7, 303–310.
7 Paterno, G.D. et al. (1989) Development 106, 79–83.
8 Tsuda, H. et al. (1989) Cancer Res. 49, 3104–3108.
9 Theillet, C. et al. (1990) Oncogene 5, 147–149.
10 Saint–Ruf, C. et al. (1991) Oncogene 6, 403–406.
11 Tsuda, T. et al. (1989) Cancer Res. 49, 5505–5508.
12 Kitagawa, Y. et al. (1991) Cancer Res. 51, 1504–1508.
13 Wagata, T. et al. (1991) Cancer Res. 51, 2113–2117.
14 Strohmeyer, T. et al. (1991) Cancer Res., 51, 1811–1816.
15 Yoshida, T. et al. (1991) Methods Enzymol. 198, 124–138.
16 Adelaide, J., et al. (1988) Oncogene 2, 413–416.
17 Zhan, X. et al. (1987) Oncogene, 1, 369–376.
18 Delli-Bovi, P. et al. (1987) Cell 50, 729–737.
19 Adnane, J. et al. (1991) Oncogene 6, 659–663.
20 Peters, G. et al. (1989) Proc. Natl Acad. Sci. USA 86, 5678–5682.
21 Murakami, A. et al. (1990) Cell Growth Differ. 1, 225–231.
22 Taira, M. et al. (1987) Proc. Natl Acad. Sci. USA 84, 2980–2984.
23 Sakamoto, H. et al. (1988) Biochem. Biophys. Res. Commun. 151, 965–972.
24 Wellstein, A. et al. (1990) Cell Growth Differ. 1, 63–71.
25 Fuller-Pace, F. et al. (1991) J. Cell. Biol, 115, 547–555.

26 Talarico, D. and Basilico, C. (1991) Mol. Cell. Biol. 11, 1138–1145.

27 Yoshida, T. et al. (1987) Proc. Natl Acad. Sci. USA 84, 7305–7309 (erratum ibid, 85, 1967)

28 Sasaki, A. et al. (1991) Jpn. J. Cancer Res. 82, 1191–1195.

29 Marics, I. et al. (1989) Oncogene 4, 335–340.

INT2

IDENTIFICATION

Murine *Int-2* was initially identified as a frequent target for activation by proviral insertion of mouse mammary tumour virus [1]. Human *INT2* was detected by cross-hybridization with mouse *Int-2* probes.

RELATED GENES

INT2/Int-2 and *HSTF1/Hst-1* are members of the fibroblast growth factor (FGF) family (see **HSTF1/Hst**).

Nucleotides (kb)	10
Chromosome	11q13
Mass (kDa): predicted	27
expressed	27.5–31.5

Cellular location

NIH 3T3 cells transformed by mouse *Int-2* cDNA express a series of INT-2-related proteins. The use of different initiation codons gives rise to proteins located in the endoplasmic reticulum, the Golgi apparatus or the nucleus [2]. In highly transformed clonal lines INT-2 proteins undergo further post-translational processing and are secreted, becoming associated with the cell surface and the extracellular matrix [3,4].

Tissue distribution

In addition to its activation in MMTV-induced tumours in mice, *Int-2* is expressed in embryos and in some teratocarcinomas [5]. Murine mRNA expression occurs in specific tissues during development and is rarely detected in adult tissues [6].

PROTEIN FUNCTION

INT2 (and HST1) induces mesoderm formation in *Xenopus laevis* animal pole cells [7]. The complex pattern of murine expression suggests multiple roles for INT2 during fetal development. INT2 secreted by highly transformed cells can be displaced from the cell surface by glycosaminoglycans and the addition of excess heparin causes the cells to revert to normal morphology [3, 4].

Cancer

INT2, together with *HSTF1* and *BCL1*, is amplified in up to 22% of human breast carcinomas [8,9] and one study has detected polymorphism of *INT2* in 61% of lymph-node positive patients [10]. However, there is no evidence that INT2 (or HSTF1) proteins are expressed in breast tumours. Co-amplification of *HSTF1/INT2* occurs in up to 47% of oesophageal carcinomas [11–13]. *INT2* is frequently amplified in squamous cell carcinomas (SCC) of the head and neck. Co-amplification of *INT2* and *EGFR* has been detected in a laryngeal SCC and an SCC metastatic to the neck [14].

Transgenic animals

In mice the *Int-2* transgene causes mammary hyperplasia and in some males prostatic hyperplasia, although induction of tumours is rare [15,16]. Thus *Int-2* acts as a potent growth factor in these epithelial cells. In double transgenic mice *Int-2* and *Wnt-1* cooperate in the induction of mammary tumours (see **WNT1, WNT2, WNT3**) and, in *Wnt-1* transgenic mice infected with MMTV, *Int-2* and *Hst-1* can cooperate with *Wnt-1* [17].

In animals

Int-2 is frequently activated by MMTV proviral insertion. In spontaneously arising murine mammary tumours *Int-2* may be activated together with other *Int* genes, for example, *Wnt-1*[18].

In vitro

Int-2 transforms NIH 3T3 cells with very low efficiency [19] but can substitute for FGFB in some cell lines [20].

GENE STRUCTURE

See *HSTF1/Hst*.

TRANSCRIPTIONAL REGULATION

In the mouse, *Int-2* gene transcription can initiate at multiple sites within three separate promoter domains and terminate distal to one of two polyadenylation signals [21,22]. An alternative non-coding first exon (exon 1a) occurs in minor classes of *Int-2* mRNA. Homology between murine *Int-2* and human *INT2* extends throughout the promoter domains, although there is no evidence for the use of exon 1a in *INT2* [23].

PROTEIN STRUCTURE

See *HSTF1/Hst*.

SEQUENCE OF INT2

```
  1  MGLIWLLLLS LLEPGWPAAG PGARLRRDAG GRGGVYEHLG GAPRRRKLYC
 51  ATKYHLQLHP SGRVNGSLEN SAYSILEITA VEVGIVAIRG LFSGRYLAMN
101  KRGRLYASEH YSAECEFVER IHELGYNTYA SRLYRTVSST PGARRQPSAE
151  RLWYVSVNGK GRPRRGFKTR RTQKSSLFLP RVLDHRDHEM VRQLQSGLPR
201  PPGKGVQPRR RRQKQSPDNL EPSHVQASRL GSQLEASAH (239)
```

Domain structure

1–17 Signal sequence (italics)
  65 Potential glycosylation site

Human and mouse INT2 proteins are 89% identical up to the C-terminus in which 22 amino acids of human INT2 are replaced by 27 unrelated residues in the mouse protein [23].

DATABASE ACCESSION NUMBERS

	PIR	SWISSPROT	EMBL/GENBANK	REFERENCE
Human INT2 (FGF3)	S04742	P11487	X14445	[22]

References

1 Peters, G. (1991) Semin. Virol. 2, 319–328.
2 Acland, P. et al. (1990) Nature 343, 662–665.
3 Dixon, M. et al. (1989) Mol. Cell. Biol, 9, 4896–4902.
4 Kiefer, P. et al. (1991) Mol. Cell. Biol. 11, 5929–5936.
5 Jakobovits, A. et al. (1986) Proc. Natl Acad. Sci. USA 83, 7806–7810.
6 Wilkinson, D.G. et al. (1989) Development 105, 131–136.
7 Paterno, G.D. et al. (1989) Development 106, 79–83.
8 Tsuda, H. et al. (1989) Cancer Res. 49, 3104–3108.
9 Theillet, C. et al. (1990) Oncogene 5, 147–149.
10 Meyers, S.L. et al. (1990) Cancer Res. 50, 5911–5918.
11 Tsuda, T. et al. (1989) Cancer Res. 49, 5505–5508.
12 Kitagawa, Y. et al. (1991) Cancer Res. 51, 1504–1508.
13 Wagata, T. et al. (1991) Cancer Res. 51, 2113–2117.
14 Somers, K.D. et al. (1990) Oncogene 5, 915–920.
15 Muller, W.J. et al. (1990) EMBO J. 9, 907–913.
16 Ornitz, D.M. et al. (1991) Proc. Natl Acad. Sci. USA 88, 698–702.
17 Shackleford, G.M. et al. (1993) Proc. Natl Acad. Sci. USA 90, 740–744.
18 Peters, G. et al. (1986) Nature 320, 628–631.
19 Goldfarb, M. et al. (1991) Oncogene 6, 65–71.
20 Venesio, T. et al. (1992) Cell Growth Differ. 3, 63–71.
21 Smith, R. et al. (1988) EMBO J. 7, 1013–1022.
22 Mansour, S.L. and Martin, G.R. (1988) EMBO J. 7, 2035–2041.
23 Brookes, S. et al. (1989) Oncogene 4, 429–436.

IDENTIFICATION

v-*jun* is the oncogene of avian sarcoma virus 17 (ASV 17) isolated from a spontaneous chicken sarcoma. It is specifically responsible for the oncogenicity of ASV 17 (*ju-nana* is Japanese for the number 17). *JUN* was identified by screening a human genomic library with a v-*jun* probe.

RELATED GENES

JUN is a member of the *JUN* gene family (*JUN*, *JUNB*, *JUND* and murine *Jund-2*) and of the helix–loop–helix/leucine zipper superfamily [1,2] JUN shares 44% and 45% identity with JUNB and JUND, respectively. The human and mouse JUN and JUNB proteins are 98% identical and human and mouse JUND are 77% identical.

	JUN	v-*jun*
Nucleotides (kb)	3.622	0.93
		3.5 (ASV17)
Chromosome	1p32–p31	
Mass (kDa): predicted	35.7	32
expressed	39	65$^{gag\text{-}jun}$

Cellular location

JUN: Nucleus. v-JUN: Nucleus.

Tissue distribution

JUN transcription, like that of *FOS*, is rapidly activated in mitogenically stimulated fibroblasts in which essentially all JUN protein exists as JUN/FOS heterodimers. Two other closely related genes *JUNB* and *JUND*, are also members of the group of "early response genes" [3-5]. *JUN* is expressed in human peripheral blood granulocytes [6]. mRNA expression in the mouse is maximal in the lung, ovary and heart and is very low in the intestine and liver [7]. *Jun* is also transiently expressed in IL2- and IL6-dependent mouse myeloma cell lines following withdrawal of growth factor and the onset of apoptosis [8].

PROTEIN FUNCTION

JUN forms heterodimers with FOS and with FOS-related antigens (FRA1, FRA2) that bind with high affinity to the AP-1 consensus site (the *cis*-acting TPA response element TRE, 5'-TGA^C/$_G$TCA-3'). Human JUN was originally termed AP-1 (PEA 1 in mice) [9] and was first identified by its selective binding to enhancer elements in the *cis* control regions of SV40 and human metallothionein IIA. AP-1 is a complex of polypeptides comprised predominantly of heterodimers of members of the JUN and FOS families [10]. The AP-1 complex binds to the same consensus sequence as GCN4 and in artificial constructs both v-JUN and JUN activate transcription via consensus AP-1 binding sites although they differ in their capacity to recognize AP-1-like and CREB-like target sequences [11]. JUN (and FOS) also interact with the NF-κB subunit p65 (RELA) through its REL homology domain to enhance binding to κB and AP-1 sites [12] and JUN dimers and JUN/FOS heterodimers also form complexes with the T cell transcription factor NFAT$_p$ [13] (see *FOS*).

JUN homodimers also bind to AP-1 sites with high affinity [14] and JUN *trans*-activates the human *MYB* promoter via an AP-1-like sequence [15]. However, JUN affinity depends on the flanking sequences (ATGACTCAPy>>ATGACTCAPu: for the sequence CTGACTCAT, more distant nucleotides may confer high or low affinity). Proteins of the FOS family enhance JUN binding to AP-1 in the order FOSB>FRA1>FOS, increasing the half-lives of the JUN/FOS/DNA complexes. JUN/JUN and JUN/FOS complexes also bind to CRE-containing nucleotides but with affinities that depend on the flanking sequences. The FOS/JUN and ATF/CREB families of transcription factors form selective cross-family heterodimers having distinct DNA binding specificities [16].

JUN acts as a negative regulator of insulin, MyoD and myogenin gene expression [17] and of MHC class I genes in L cells [18]. In Lewis lung carcinoma (3LL), B16 melanoma and K1735 melanoma cells, however, expression of either *Fos* and/or *Jun* by transfection upregulates MHC H-2 whereas expression of *JunB* causes downregulation [19]. Reduced expression of MHC H-2 correlates with high metastatic capacity and *Fos/Jun* overexpression with reduced metastatic potential. In mouse papilloma cells, the expression of v-*jun* suppresses TPA-induced stromelysin gene expression and this also inhibits metastasis [20].

JUN and JUND but not JUNB also form complexes with OCT-1 that activate transcription from an element in the IL2 promoter [21]. This mechanism of transcriptional activation occurs during T cell stimulation and is Ca^{2+}-sensitive and inhibited by cyclosporin A.

The IP-1 protein specifically blocks FOS/JUN binding to DNA when unphosphorylated but not after PKA-mediated phosphorylation. AP-1 DNA binding is increased in cells treated with A23187 or dibutyryl cAMP, consistent with an inhibition of IP-1 activity by phosphorylation [22,23].

A protein distinct from IP-1 and designated JUN interacting factor 1 (JIF-1) binds to the leucine zipper of viral and cellular JUN, inhibiting DNA binding and *trans*-activation by JUN [24]. JIF-1 is homologous to the product of the putative tumour suppressor gene *QM* (see **Tumour Suppressor Genes, WT1**).

JUN shares homology with GCN4 and can function as a transcriptional regulator in GCN4-deficient yeast strains. JUN, JUNB, JUND and GCN4 can each form homodimers that bind to DNA but the heterodimeric forms have greatly increased affinity and efficacy as transcriptional activators [10,25].

Jun transcription is transiently increased in rat aortic smooth muscle

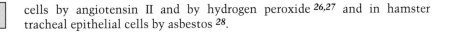

cells by angiotensin II and by hydrogen peroxide [26,27] and in hamster tracheal epithelial cells by asbestos [28].

Cancer

JUN overexpression has been detected in small cell and non-small cell lung cancers [29].

Transgenic animals

In mice carrying v-*jun* in the germline, wounding is a prerequisite for tumorigenesis, following which ~25% of animals homozygous for the transgene develop dermal fibrosarcomas. v-*jun* transgenic cells require TNFα or IL1 to become anchorage-independent for *in vitro* growth, indicating that these agents may act as cofactors in wound-induced carcinogenesis [30].

Murine *Jun* null embryos die at mid-gestation, exhibiting impaired hepatogenesis and fibroblasts from live mutant embryos have greatly reduced growth rates *in vitro* [31,32].

Bovine papilloma virus transgenic mice develop dermal fibrosarcoma and the enhanced expression of *Jun* and *Junb* but not of *Jund* or *Fos* correlates with the onset of an intermediate stage of tumour development [33].

In animals

Viruses carrying v-*jun* or a recombinant between v-*jun* and *Jun* induce tumours when injected into the wing web of chicks [34]. Embryonic stem (ES) cells induce teratocarcinomas when subcutaneously injected into syngeneic mice: however, the tumorigenicity of ES cells is drastically reduced when both copies of the *Jun* gene have been inactivated by homologous recombination, indicating that JUN may be necessary for efficient tumour growth [35].

In vitro

The cellular *Jun* gene, placed in an appropriate retroviral vector, is able by itself to transform immortalized rat fibroblasts and, in cooperation with *Hras*, primary rat fibroblasts [36]. *Jun* and *Hras* transforms more effectively than *Junb* and *Hras* and *Junb* inhibits *Jun/Ras* transformation, consistent with the differential DNA affinities of JUN and JUNB.

The transformation potential of v-*jun* in chick embryo fibroblasts is increased 10^3-fold relative to *Jun* by deletion of the δ region and further increased by loss of the 3' untranslated region [37,38]. v-*jun* cooperates with v-*erbB* to transform bone marrow cells and to enhance transformation of chick embryo fibroblasts caused by either oncogene alone [39].

Transformation by *Jun* of chick embryo fibroblasts is prevented (or reversed) by the expression of a synthetic *Fos* gene lacking a DNA binding domain [40], the mutant FOS protein forming heterodimers with JUN that are inactive as transcription factors.

GENE STRUCTURE

The single 3.4 kb exon (993 bp coding) has heterogeneous initiation and poly(A) sites that give rise to multiple transcripts all encoding the same protein.

TRANSCRIPTIONAL REGULATION

JUN expression is positively autoregulated by JUN binding to AP-1 sites. *JUN* promoters also contain NF-JUN [41], SP1, CTF, RSRF and E1A 13S RNA translation product binding sites. The cAMP responsive element binding protein can act as an inhibitor or an activator of *Jun* transcription, depending on its phosphorylation state [9, 42].

PROTEIN STRUCTURE

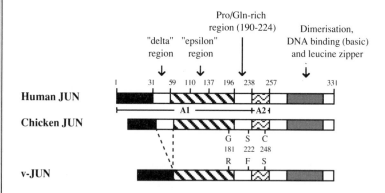

Region A1 is the activator domain, which confers transcriptional activity when fused to an heterologous DNA binding domain (e.g., Sp1 or GAL4). Residues 67–77 and 108–117 constitute the two homology box regions (HOB1 and HOB2) that are conserved in FOS and C/EBP (see **FOS**). Region A2 is the activation domain essential for *in vivo* activity. The δ domain (amino acids 28–54 in chicken JUN), missing in v-JUN, stabilizes the interaction of a cell-specific transcriptional inhibitor with A1 [43]. Expression of v-SRC or oncogenic RAS disrupts the JUN/inhibitor complex by interacting with the A1 domain, increasing transcriptional activity [44].

In v-JUN 220 residues encoding viral *gag* are joined in-frame to 296 *Jun*-encoded amino acids. There is a 27 amino acid deletion (the "δ region") in the N-terminal region of JUN and three non-conservative substitutions in the C-terminal half, two of which are in the DNA binding domain. A Ser222 to Phe mutation prevents the phosphorylation *in vitro* of the negative regulatory site by glycogen synthase kinase-3 and the mutation Cys248 to Ser may disrupt a regulatory mechanism involving the reversible oxidation of Cys248 which can inactivate DNA binding to AP-1 sites *in vitro* [45].

PHOSPHORYLATION OF JUN

Mutation of Ser243 to Phe blocks phosphorylation of all three sites *in vitro* and increases the *trans*-activation capability of JUN tenfold. In v-JUN the corresponding serine residue is not present and v-JUN binds to the AP-1 site to activate constitutive transcription of the gene [46].

Transforming oncogenes, including *Hras*, stimulate AP-1 activity: in rat embryo fibroblasts *Hras* increases JUN synthesis by 4.5-fold but causes a 35-fold increase in overall JUN phosphorylation [47] and similar increases in phosphorylation are caused by v-SIS, v-SRC and RAF-1 [48] and by ultraviolet light and the signals generated by each of these agents activate JUN N-terminal kinase (JNK) [49]. The N-terminal sites are phosphorylated *in vitro* and in U937 cells by MAP kinases [50]. *Hras* expression causes hypo-phosphorylation of the C-terminus of JUN, promoting binding to DNA (similar to the effect of TPA). These effects may underlie the cooperativity between *Ras* and *Jun* in transforming these cells.

Phosphorylation of sites in the N-terminal region of JUN is reversed by protein phosphatase 2A (PP2A), to which v-JUN is insensitive [51]. A possible PP2A-sensitive site lies in the δ domain, deleted from v-JUN, but other sites have not yet been mapped.

Chicken JUN is efficiently phosphorylated *in vitro* by p34^{cdc2}, ERK-1 (p44^{mapk}), protein kinase C or casein kinase II[52]. The major sites of phosphorylation are serines 63, 73 and 246 but, in contrast to the observations summarized above, the phosphorylation state of these residues does not affect FOS/JUN dimerization, DNA binding or *in vitro* transcription activity.

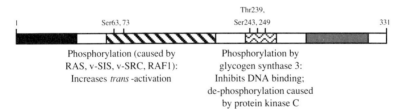

In unstimulated cells JUN mainly exists as a phosphorylated, inactive form in equilibrium with a hypo-phosphorylated form that is competent to bind to DNA. The equilibrium is maintained by a specific protein kinase and a phosphatase and shifted to the right by agents stimulating JUN-mediated transcription from AP-1 sites. The equilbrium is also shifted to the right in cells transfected so as to increase the number of AP-1 binding sites, which raises the concentration of bound dimer and causes a net dephosphorylation of JUN [53].

Different protein kinases can distinguish between the monomeric, homodimeric and heterodimeric forms of JUN and FOS proteins, as well as between DNA bound and unbound forms [54]. Thus JUN/JUN dimers are efficiently phosphorylated by casein kinase II and JUN/FOS dimers are not, whereas phosphorylation of FOS by cAMP-dependent protein kinase and by p34^{CDC2} is relatively insensitive to dimerization and DNA binding.

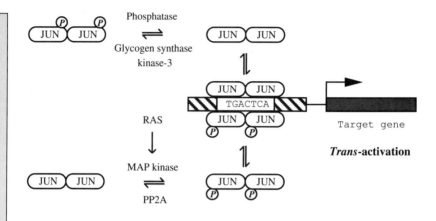

SEQUENCE OF JUN

```
  1  MTAKMETTFY DDALNASFLP SESGPYGYSN PKILKQSMTL NLADPVGSLK
 51  PHLRAKNSDL LTSPDVGLLK LASPELERLI IQSSNGHITT TPTPTQFLCP
101  KNVTDEQEGF AEGFVRALAE LHSQNTLPSV TSAAQPVNGA GMVAPAVASV
151  AGGSGSGGFS ASLHSEPPVY ANLSNFNPGA LSSGGGAPSY GAAGLAFPAQ
201  PQQQQQPPHH LPQQMPVQHP RLQALKEEPQ TVPEMPGETP PLSPIDMESQ
251  ERIKAERKRM RNRIAASKCR KRKLERIARL EEKVKTLKAQ NSELASTANM
301  LREQVAQLKQ KVMNHVNSGC QLMLTQQLQT F (331)
```

Domain structure

258–276	Basic DNA binding region
280–308	Leucine zipper domain (underlined)
63 and 73	Serine phosphorylation by MAP kinase and by JUN N-terminal kinase (JNK)
67–77	HOB1 domain
108–117	HOB2 domain
321 and 249	Threonine and serine phosphorylation by casein kinase II
239, 243 and 249	Threonine and serine phosphorylation by glycogen synthase kinase-3

The substitution of Glu293 and Asn299 by glycines, Ileu264 by Leu and Ser267 by Thr is responsible for the tenfold lower DNA binding activity of JUNB [55].

DATABASE ACCESSION NUMBERS

	PIR	SWISSPROT	EMBL/GENBANK	REFERENCES
Human *JUN*	A30009	P05412	J04111	[9,56]

References
1 Busch, S.J. and Sassone-Corsi, P. (1990) Trends Genet. 6, 36–40.
2 Kouzarides, T. and Ziff, E. (1989) Cancer Cells 1, 71–76.
3 Quantin, B. and Breathnach, R. (1988) Nature 334, 538–539.
4 Ryder, K. and Nathans, D. (1988) Proc. Natl Acad. Sci. USA 85, 8464–8467.
5 Ryseck, R.P. et al. (1988) Nature 334, 535–537.
6 Mollinedo, F. et al. (1991) Biochem. J. 273, 477–479.
7 Kovary, K. and Bravo, R. (1991) Mol. Cell. Biol. 11, 2451–2459.
8 Colotta, F. et al. (1992) J. Biol. Chem. 267, 18278–18283.
9 Bohmann, D. et al. (1987) Science 238, 1386–1392.
10 Chiu, R. et al. (1988) Cell 54, 541–552.
11 Hadman, M. et al. (1993) Oncogene 8, 1895–1903.
12 Stein, B. et al. (1993) EMBO J. 12, 3879–3891.
13 Jain, J. et al. (1993) Nature 365, 352–355.
14 Ryseck, R.-P. and Bravo, R. (1991) Oncogene 6, 533–542.
15 Nicolaides, N.C. et al. (1992) J. Biol. Chem. 267, 19665–19672.
16 Chatton, B. et al. (1994) Oncogene 9, 375–385.
17 Howcroft, T.K. et al. (1993) EMBO J. 12, 3163–3169.
18 Henderson, E. and Stein, R. (1994) Mol. Cell. Biol. 14, 655–662.
19 Yamit-Hezi, A. et al. (1994) Oncogene 9, 1065–1079.
20 Tsang, T.C. et al. (1994) Cancer Res. 54, 882–886.
21 Ullman, K.S. et al. (1993) Genes Devel. 7, 188–196.
22 Auwerx, J. and Sassone-Corsi, P. (1992) Oncogene 7, 2271–2280.
23 de Groot, R.P. and Sassone-Corsi, P. (1992) Oncogene 7, 2281–2286.
24 Monteclaro, F.S. and Vogt, P.K. (1993) Proc. Natl Acad. Sci. USA 90, 6726–6730.
25 Nakabeppu, Y. et al. (1988) Cell 55, 907–915.
26 Naftilan, A.J. et al. (1990) Mol. Cell. Biol. 10, 5536–5540.
27 Rao, G.N. et al. (1993) Oncogene 8, 2759–2764.
28 Heintz, N.H. et al. (1993) Proc. Natl Acad. Sci. USA 90, 3299–3303.
29 Schutte, J. et al. (1988) Proc. Am. Assoc. Cancer Res. Art. 1808, 455.
30 Vanhamme, L. et al. (1993) Cancer Res. 53, 615–621.
31 Hilberg, F. et al. (1993) Nature 365, 179–181.
32 Johnson, R.S. et al. (1993) Genes Devel. 7, 1309–1317.
33 Bossy-Wetzel, E. et al. (1992) Genes Devel. 6, 2340–2351.
34 Wong, W.-Y. et al. (1992) Oncogene 7, 2077–2080.
35 Hilberg, F. and Wagner, E.F. (1992) Oncogene 7, 2371–2380.
36 Schutte, J. et al. (1989) Proc. Natl Acad. Sci. USA 86, 2257–2261.
37 Bos, T.J. et al. (1990) Genes Devel. 4, 1677–1687.
38 Vogt, P.K. and Bos, T.J. (1990) Adv. Cancer Res. 55, 1–35.
39 Garcia, M. and Samarut, J. (1993) Proc. Natl Acad. Sci. USA 90, 8837–8841.
40 Okuno, H. et al. (1991) Oncogene 6, 1491–1497.
41 Brach, M.A. et al. (1993) Mol. Cell. Biol. 13, 4284–4290.
42 Angel, P. et al. (1988) Cell 55, 875–885.
43 Baichwal, V.R. and Tjian, R. (1990) Cell 63, 815–825.
44 Baichwal, V.R. et al. (1991) Nature 352, 165–168.
45 Frame, M.C. et al. (1991) Oncogene 6, 205–209.

⁴⁶ Hunter, T. and Karin, M. (1992) Cell 70, 375–387.

⁴⁷ Binetruy, B. et al. (1991) Nature 351, 122–127.

⁴⁸ Smeal, T. et al. (1992) Mol. Cell. Biol. 12, 3507–3513.

⁴⁹ Hibi, M. et al. (1993) Genes Devel. 7, 2135–2148.

⁵⁰ Pulverer, B.J. et al. (1993) Oncogene 8, 407–415.

⁵¹ Black, E.J. et al. (1991) Oncogene 6, 1949–1958.

⁵² Baker, S.J. et al. (1992) Mol. Cell. Biol. 12, 4694–4705.

⁵³ Papavassiliou, A.G. et al. (1992) Proc. Natl Acad. Sci. USA 89, 11562–11565.

⁵⁴ Abate, C. et al. (1993) Proc. Natl Acad. Sci. USA 90, 6766–6770.

⁵⁵ Deng, T. and Karin, M. (1993) Genes Devel. 7, 479–490.

⁵⁶ Hattori, K. et al. (1988) Proc. Natl Acad. Sci. USA 85, 9148–9152.

JUNB

IDENTIFICATION

JUNB was identified by screening a human genomic library with a v-*jun* probe.

RELATED GENES

JUNB is a member of the *JUN* gene family (see **JUN**). JUNB is 44% identical to JUN.

Nucleotides (bp)	2136
Chromosome	19p13.2
Mass (kDa): predicted	36
expressed	42

Cellular location

Nucleus.

Tissue distribution

JUNB is expressed in human peripheral blood granulocytes [1]. Murine *Junb* expression is ubiquitous but is particularly high in the testis, where *Jun* and *Jund* are barely detectable.

PROTEIN FUNCTION

JUNB is an "early response gene" induced by serum [2] but induction is attenuated in cells transformed by tyrosine kinase oncoproteins [3].

JUNB homodimers bind very weakly to AP-1 sites to which JUN binds with high affinity [4]. Proteins of the FOS family confer significant affinity for DNA on JUNB, increasing the half-lives of the protein/DNA complexes.

In vitro

Junb and *Hras* are less effective transforming agents than *Jun* and *Hras* and *Junb* inhibits *Jun/Ras* transformation [5], consistent with the differential DNA affinities of JUN and JUNB.

TRANSCRIPTIONAL REGULATION

Junb contains a serum response element (SRE) and a cAMP response element (CRE) located 3' of the gene that regulates its response to serum, PDGF, bFGF, TPA and forskolin [6]. The E1A 13S RNA product directly activates *Fos*, *Jun* and *Junb* promoters, inducing JUN/AP-1 binding to a TRE (TTACCTCA). E1A *trans*-activation is mediated by the JUN2 TRE sequence to which JUN/ATF-2 heterodimers bind [7]. E1A 12S RNA expression alone does not activate via TRE but, together with JUN does so: this activation is, in turn, blocked by expression of FOS [8]. Thus FOS modulates the dominance of E1A 12S or 13S products.

Junb transcription is specifically stimulated by the expression of v-SRC, the tyrosine kinase activity of which modulates binding of factors to a 121 bp region encompassing the CCAAT and TATAA elements [9].

SEQUENCE OF JUNB

```
  1  MCTKMEQPFY HDDSYTATGY GRAPGGLSLH DYKLLKPSLA VNLADPYRSL
 51  KAPGARGPGP EGGGGGSYFS GQGSDTGASL KLASSELERL IVPNSNGVIT
101  TTPTPPGQYF YPRGGGSGGG AGGAGGGVTE EQEGFADGFV KALDDLHKMN
151  HVTPPNVSLG ATGGPPAGPG GVYAGPEPPP VYTNLSSYSP ASASSGGAGA
201  AVGTGSSYPT TTISYLPHAP PFAGGHPAQL GLGRGASTFK EEPQTVPEAR
251  SRDATPPVSP INMEDQERIK VERKRLRNRL AATKCRKRKL ERIARLEDKV
301  KTLKAENAGL SSTAGLLREQ VAQLKQKVMT HVSNGCQLLL GVKGHAF  (347)
```

Domain structure

273–292 Basic DNA binding region
296–324 Leucine zipper domain (underlined)

DATABASE ACCESSION NUMBERS

	PIR	SWISSPROT	EMBL/GENBANK	REFERENCES
Human *JUNB*	S10183	P17275	M29039, X51345	*10, 11*

References
[1] Mollinedo, F. et al. (1991) Biochem. J. 273, 477–479.
[2] Ryder, K. et al. (1988) Proc. Natl Acad. Sci. USA 85, 1487–1491.
[3] Yu, C.-L. et al. (1993) Mol. Cell. Biol. 13, 2011–2019.
[4] Ryseck, R.-P. and Bravo, R. (1991) Oncogene 6, 533–542.
[5] Schutte, J. et al. (1989) Proc. Natl Acad. Sci. USA 86, 2257–2261.
[6] Perez-Albuerne et al. (1994) Proc. Natl Acad. Sci. USA 90, 11960–11964.
[7] van Dam, H. et al. (1993) EMBO J. 12, 479–487.
[8] de Groot, R. et al. (1991) Mol. Cell Biol. 11, 192–201.
[9] Apel, I. et al. (1992) Mol. Cell. Biol. 12, 3356–3364.
[10] Nomura, N. et al. (1990) Nucl. Acids Res. 18, 3047–3048.
[11] Schutte, J. et al. (1989) Cell 59, 987–997.

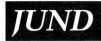

JUND

IDENTIFICATION

JUND was identified by screening a human genomic library with a v-*jun* probe.

RELATED GENES

JUND is a member of the *JUN* gene family (see **JUN**). JUND is 45% identical to JUN.

Nucleotides	Not fully mapped
Chromosome	19p13.2
Mass (kDa): predicted	35
expressed	40–50

Cellular location

Nucleus.

Tissue distribution

JUND mRNA is five- to tenfold more abundant than *JUN* mRNA and occurs in most tissues, being maximal in the intestine and thymus and readily detectable in human peripheral blood granulocytes [1,2]. It is present in serum-starved cells and is not significantly induced by the addition of serum [3]. *JunD*, together with *JunB* and *Fos*, is transcriptionally activated in mouse mammary epithelial cells after lactation. AP-1 DNA binding activity (primarily FOS/JUND) is transiently induced and may mediate the apoptosis of mammary cells during involution [4].

PROTEIN FUNCTION

JUND is an "early response gene", as are *JUN* and *JUNB*, although *JUND* is significantly expressed in quiescent cells.

JUND (and JUNB) homodimers bind very weakly to AP-1 sites to which JUN binds with high affinity [5]. JUND (and JUN) *trans*-activate the human *MYB* promoter *via* an AP-1-like sequence [6].

Cancer

JUND loci may be involved in chromosome translocations that occur in some cases of acute lymphocytic leukemia (ALL) and acute non-lymphocytic leukemia (19;11 and 19;1) [7].

In vitro

Mouse JUND negatively regulates fibroblast growth and antagonizes transformation by *Ras* [8]. The expression of *Jund* from a retroviral vector does not transform chick embryo fibroblasts but JUND is converted into a transforming protein in these cells by substitution of the 79 N-terminal amino acids of JUN [9] or by mutations in two of the N-terminal regions conserved within JUN proteins [10].

SEQUENCE OF JUND

```
  1   METPFYGDEA LSGLGGGASG SGGTFASPGR LFPGAPPTAA AGSMMKKDAL
 51   TLSLSEQVAA ALKPAPAPAS YPPAADGAPS AAPPDGLLAS PDLGLLKLAS
101   PELERLIIQS NGLVTTTPTS SQFLYPKVAA SEEQEFAEGF VKALEDLHKQ
151   NQLGAGRAAA AAAAAAGGPS GTATGSAPPG ELAPAAAAPE APVYANLSSY
201   AGGAGGAGGA ATVAFAAEPV PFPPPPPPGA LGPPRLAALK DEPQTVPDVP
251   SFGESPPLSP IDMDTQERIK AERKRLRNRI AASKCRKRKL ERISRLEEKV
301   KTLKSQNTEL ASTASLLREQ VAQLKQKVLS HVNSGCQLLP QHQVPAY (347)
```

Domain structure

158–166	Alanine-rich region
273–292	Basic DNA binding region
296–324	Leucine zipper domain (underlined)

DATABASE ACCESSION NUMBERS

	PIR	SWISSPROT	EMBL/GENBANK	REFERENCES
Human *JUND*	S10184	P17535	X51346, X56681	11,12

References

1 Mollinedo, F. et al. (1991) Biochem. J. 273, 477–479.
2 Ryder, K. et al. (1989) Proc. Natl Acad. Sci. USA 86, 1500–1503.
3 Hirai, S.-I. et al. (1989) EMBO J. 8, 1433–1439.
4 Marti, A. et al. (1994) Oncogene 9, 1213–1223.
5 Ryseck, R.-P. and Bravo, R. (1991) Oncogene 6, 533–542.
6 Nicolaides, N.C. et al. (1992) J. Biol. Chem. 267, 19665–19672.
7 Mattei, M.G. et al. (1990) Oncogene 5, 151–156.
8 Pfarr, C.M. et al. (1994) Cell 76, 747–760.
9 Metivier, C. et al. (1993) Oncogene 8, 2311–2315.
10 Kameda, T. et al. (1993) Proc. Natl Acad. Sci. USA 90, 9369–9373.
11 Berger, I. and Shaul, Y. (1991) Oncogene 6, 561–566.
12 Nomura, N. et al. (1990) Nucl. Acids Res. 18, 3047–3048.

KIT

IDENTIFICATION

v-*kit* is the oncogene of the Hardy–Zuckerman 4 strain of acutely transforming feline sarcoma virus (HZ4-FeSV). *KIT* was detected by screening cDNA with v-*kit* probes.

RELATED GENES

KIT is a member of receptor tyrosine kinase sub-class III which also includes *FLK2/FLT3*, PDGFRA, PDGFRB, and CSF1R, each having five Ig-like loops in an extracellular domain and a cytoplasmic region containing a 60–100 residue tyrosine kinase insert region. *KIT* also shares homology with the tyrosine-specific protein kinase family (ABL, FES, FGR, FMS and SRC), with the EGF and insulin receptors and with mouse *Flk-1* (*f*etal *l*iver *k*inase 1) and *Flk-2/Flt-3*.

	KIT	*v-kit*
Nucleotides (kb)	80	2.37 (HZ4-FeSV genome)
Chromosome	4q11–q21	
Mass (kDa): predicted	110	
expressed	gp124/gp160	p81*gag-kit*

Cellular location

Plasma membrane.

Tissue distribution

Expression of the KIT receptor and its ligand occurs in complementary tissues throughout the body from the early presomite stage to the mature adult. For example, the ligand (*steel*) is expressed in the follicular cells of the ovary and in Sertoli cells of the testes, the layers immediately surrounding the germ cells that express *Kit* [1-3].

KIT mRNA and protein are present in normal human neonatal and adult melanocytes and in the early stages of erythroid and myeloid cell differentiation [4,5] but are not detectable in most human melanoma-derived cell lines [6,7].

PROTEIN FUNCTION

KIT encodes a membrane tyrosine kinase receptor. In humans KIT is the receptor for stem cell factor (SCF, also called mast cell growth factor, MGF) [8-13].

The KIT receptor in mice is encoded by the dominant white spotting (*W*) locus. The ligand, KL (or SCF or MGF), is a growth factor encoded by the mouse *steel* (*Sl*) locus [14,16]. The phenotypes of *W* and *Sl* mutant mouse strains that bear germ line loss of function mutations in *Kit* and its ligand, respectively, demonstrate roles for *Kit* in haematopoiesis, melanogenesis and germ cell development [17–20]. Furthermore, SCF acts synergistically with other cytokines to stimulate *in vitro* growth of a number of committed hematopoietic precursors [21–26]. These activities can be blocked by antibodies directed against KIT [27] or by anti-sense oligodeoxynucleotides that block *Kit* expression [28]. Anti-KIT antibodies also block melanoblast migration and prevent melanocyte activation in post-natal mice [29]. SCF promotes germ cell survival *in vitro* [30,31] and anti-KIT antibodies inhibit survival and/or proliferation of mature type-A spermatogonia [32].

The interaction of the ligand KL with its receptor causes receptor dimerization [33] that leads to enhanced KIT tyrosine autophosphorylation and association with PtdIns 3-kinase and PLCγ although not detectably with GAP [34]. KL causes protein kinase C-mediated phosphorylation of KIT, which inhibits tyrosine autophosphorylation of the receptor [35], and an increase in the cellular concentration of RAS–GTP [36] and the serine phosphorylation of RAF1 [37]. Activated KIT also transiently associates with the tyrosine phosphatase haematopoietic cell phosphatase (HCP or PTP1C) that can dephosphorylate KIT *in vitro* [38].

Cancer

KIT and its ligand are highly expressed in small cell lung cancer [39,40], on acute myeloblastic leukaemia blast cells [41] and in a significant proportion of testicular germ cell tumours [42]. The level of expression of *KIT* declines during the progression of cutaneous melanoma [43].

Transgenic animals

Mice expressing the dominant negative *W*[42] mutation show effects on pigmentation and the number of tissue mast cells that are characteristic of some *W* phenotypes. Germ cell development and erythropoiesis are not affected [44].

In animals

HZ4-FeSV induces fibrosarcomas in the domestic cat but does not cause tumours in kittens.

In vitro

v-*kit* transforms NIH 3T3 cells. Tumour cells bearing HZ4-FeSV transform feline embryo fibroblasts and CCL64 mink cells [45,46].

GENE STRUCTURE OF *KIT*

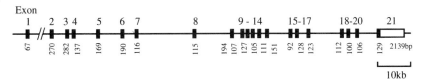

The overall structure closely resembles that of *FMS* including the large first intron and identical exon/intron boundaries in their two kinase domains. There are two *KIT* isoforms in both mice and humans distinguished by alternative splicing of the final 12 bp of exon 9, immediately upstream of the region encoding the transmembrane domain. The inclusion of this exon gives rise to *KitA+* [47–49].

PROTEIN STRUCTURE OF MOUSE KIT

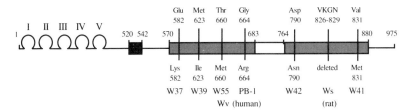

Point mutations and deletions occurring in mutated *Kit* alleles are shown below the diagram. The third immunoglobulin domain is essential for rodent SCF binding whereas the major binding determinant for human SCF is the second domain [50]. In the mouse, W^{55} and W^v arise from the same substitution in independent alleles giving identical phenotypes. The W^{42} mutation, which is particularly severe in its effects in both the homozygous and heterozygous states, arises from a missense mutation [20]. The original W mutant bears a deletion of the transmembrane domain and part of the kinase domain [48]. The product of this gene is not expressed at the cell surface, kinase activity is lost and the homozygous mutation is lethal. For the other mutations indicated in the diagram immunoprecipitable KIT protein is synthesized: its kinase activity is reduced in W^{39}, W^{55}, W^v and W^{41} mutants and abolished in W^{37} and W^{42} mutants [18–20]. The W^v,W^{41} and W^{42} mutations also differentially affect the binding of p145^{kit} to PLCγ, GAP and the p85 subunit of PtdIns 3-kinase[51]. W^f, W^{lic} and W^n mutants arise from point mutations in the kinase-encoding region [52].

PB-1 refers to a substitution at Gly664 in the human sequence detected in a case of piebaldism, a condition similar to the dominant white spotting (*W*) disorder in mice [53]. Truncation of KIT has also been detected in piebaldism [54]. Ws refers to a mutant rat strain having a four amino acid deletion in the conserved phosphotransferase region [55].

Human, mouse and feline KIT share >80% sequence identity. v-KIT differs in six scattered point mutations from the corresponding region of human KIT and its oncogenicity appears to derive from the removal of the extracellular and transmembrane domains, together with 50 amino acids from the C-terminus of KIT [56].

SEQUENCE OF KIT

```
  1  MRGARGAWDF LCVLLLLLRV QTGSSQPSVS PGEPSPPSIH PGKSDLIVRV
 51  GDEIRLLCTD PGFVKWTFEI LDETNENKQN EWITEKAEAT NTGKYTCTNK
101  HGLSNSIYVF VRDPAKLFLV DRSLYGKEDN DTLVRCPLTD PEVTNYSLKG
151  CQGKPLPKDL RFIPDPKAGI MIKSVKRAYH RLCLHCSVDQ EGKSVLSEKF
201  ILKVRPAFKA VPVVSVSKAS YLLREGEEFT VTCTIKDVSS SVYSTWKREN
251  SQTKLQEKYN SWHHGDFNYE RQATLTISSA RVNDSGVFMC YANNTFGSAN
301  VTTTLEVVDK GFINIFPMIN TTVFVNDGEN VDLIVEYEAF PKPEHQQWIY
351  MNRTFTDKWE DYPKSENESN IRYVSELHLT RLKGTEGGTY TFLVSNSDVN
401  AAIAFNVYVN TKPEILTYDR LVNGMLQCVA AGFPEPTIDW YFCPGTEQRC
451  SASVLPVDVQ TLNSSGPPFG KLVVQSSIDS SAFKHNGTVE CKAYNDVGKT
501  SAYFNFAFKG NNKEQIHPHT LFTPLLIGFV IVAGMMCIIV MILTYKYLQK
551  PMYEVQWKVV EEINGNNYVY IDPTQLPYDH KWEFPRNRLS FGKTLGAGAF
601  GKVVEATAYG LIKSDAAMTV AVKMLKPSAH LTEREALMSE LKVLSYLGNH
651  MNIVNLLGAC TIGGPTLVIT EYCCYGDLLN FLRRKRDSFI CSKQEDHAEA
701  ALYKNLLHSK ESSCSDSTNE YMDMKPGVSY VVPTKADKRR SVRIGSYIER
751  DVTPAIMEDD ELALDLEDLL SFSYQVAKGM AFLASKNCIH RDLAARNILL
801  THGRITKICD FGLARDIKND SNYVVKGNAR LPVKWMAPES IFNCVYTFES
851  DVWSYGIFLW ELFSLGSSPY PGMPVDSKFY KMIKEGFRML SPEHAPAEMY
901  DIMKTCWDAD PLKRPTFKQI VQLIEKQISE STNHIYSNLA NCSPNRQKPV
951  VDHSVRINSV GSTASSSQPL LVHDDV (976)
```

Domain structure

1–22	Signal sequence (italics)
23–520	Extracellular domain
521–543	Transmembrane domain (underlined)
544–976	Intracellular domain
596–601 and 623	ATP binding region
792	Active site
823	Autophosphorylation site
130, 145, 283, 293, 300, 320, 352, 367, 463, 486	Potential carbohydrate attachment sites

The insertion in murine *KitA+* encodes Gly–Asn–Asn–Lys between amino acids 512 and 513 [49]. This insert is also present in human KIT.

DATABASE ACCESSION NUMBERS

	PIR	SWISSPROT	EMBL/GENBANK	REFERENCES
Human *KIT*	S01426	P10721	X06182	47,57,58

References

1 Keshet, E. et al. (1991) EMBO J. 10, 2425–2435.
2 Matsui, Y. et al. (1990) Nature 347, 667–669.
3 Motro, B. et al. (1991) Development 113, 1207–1222.
4 Andre, C. et al. (1989) Oncogene 4, 1047–1049.
5 Nocka, K. et al. (1989) Genes Devel. 3, 816–826.
6 Lassam, N. and Bickford, S. (1992) Oncogene 7, 51–56.
7 Zakut, R. et al. (1993) Oncogene 8, 2221–2229.
8 Anderson, D.M. et al. (1990) Cell 63, 235–243.
9 Huang, E. et al. (1990) Cell 63, 225–233.
10 Martin, F.H. et al. (1990) Cell 63, 203–211.
11 Nocka, K. et al. (1990) EMBO J. 9, 3287–3294.
12 Williams, D.E. et al. (1990) Cell 63, 167–174.
13 Zsebo, K.M. et al. (1990) Cell 63, 195–201.
14 Copeland, N.G. et al. (1990) Cell 63, 175–183.
15 Brannan, C.I. et al. (1991) Proc. Natl Acad. Sci. USA 88, 4671–4674.
16 Zsebo, K.M. et al. (1990) Cell 63, 213–224.
17 Silvers, W.K. (1979) In The Coat Colors of Mice: a Model for Mammalian Gene Action and Interaction, Springer-Verlag, New York, pp.206–241.
18 Nocka, K. et al. (1990) EMBO J. 9, 1805–1813.
19 Reith, A.D. et al. (1990) Genes Devel. 4, 39 0–400.
20 Tan, J.C. et al. (1990) Science 247, 209–212.
21 Bernstein, I.D. et al. (1991) Blood 77, 2316–2321.
22 Briddell, R.A. et al. (1991) Blood 78, 2854–2859.
23 Broxmeyer, H.E. et al. (1991) Blood 77, 2142–2149.
24 McNeice, I.K. et al. (1991) Exp. Hematol. 19, 226–231.
25 Metcalf D. and Nicola, N.A. (1991) Proc. Natl Acad. Sci. USA 88, 6239–6243.
26 Migliaccio, G. et al. (1991) Proc. Natl Acad. Sci. USA 88, 7420–7424.
27 Ogawa, M. et al. (1991) J. Exp. Med. 174, 63–71.
28 Ratajczak, M.Z. et al. (1992) Proc. Natl Acad. Sci. USA 89, 1710–1714.
29 Nishikawa, S. et al. (1991) EMBO J. 10, 2111–2118.
30 Dolci, S. et al. (1991) Nature 352, 809–811.
31 Godin, I. et al. (1991) Nature 352, 807–809.
32 Yoshinaga, K. et al. (1991) Development 113, 689–699.
33 Lev, S. et al. (1992) J. Biol. Chem. 267, 15970–15977.
34 Shearman, M.S. et al. (1993) EMBO J. 12, 3817–3826.
35 Blume-Jensen, P. et al. (1993) EMBO J. 12, 4199–4209.
36 Duronio, V. et al. (1992) Proc. Natl Acad. Sci. USA 89, 1587–1591.
37 Lev, S. et al. (1991) EMBO J. 10, 647–654.
38 Yi, T. and Ihle, J.N. (1993) Mol. Cell. Biol. 13, 3350–3358.
39 Hibi, K. et al. (1991) Oncogene 6, 2291–2296.
40 Sekido, Y. et al. (1991) Cancer Res. 51, 2416–2419.
41 Buhring, H.-J. et al. (1993) Cancer Res. 53, 4424–4431.
42 Strohmeyer, T. et al. (1991) Cancer Res. 51, 1811–1816.
43 Natali, P.G. et al. (1992) Int. J. Cancer 52, 197–201.
44 Ray, P. et al. (1991) Genes Devel. 5, 2265–2273.
45 Besmer, P. et al. (1986) Nature 320, 415–421.
46 Hampe, A. et al. (1984) Proc. Natl Acad. Sci. USA 81, 85–89.

[47] Vandenbark, G.R. et al. (1992) Oncogene 7, 1259–1266.
[48] Hayashi, S.-I. et al. (1991) Nucl. Acids Res. 19, 1267–1271.
[49] Reith, A.D. et al. (1991) EMBO J. 10, 2451–2459.
[50] Lev , S. et al. (1993) Mol. Cell. Biol. 13, 2224–2234.
[51] Herbst, R. et al. (1992) J. Biol. Chem. 267, 13210–13216.
[52] Koshimizu, U. et al. (1994) Oncogene 9, 157–162.
[53] Giebel, L.B. and Spritz, R.A. (1991) Proc. Natl Acad. Sci. USA 88, 8696–8699.
[54] Spritz, R. A. et al. (1993) Hum. Mol. Genet. 2, 1499–1500.
[55] Tsujimura, T. et al. (1991) Blood 78, 1942–1946.
[56] Qiu, F. et al. (1988) EMBO J. 7, 1003–1011.
[57] Yarden, Y. et al. (1987) EMBO J. 6, 3341–3351.
[58] Giebel, L.B. et al. (1992) Oncogene 7, 2207–2217.

IDENTIFICATION

Lck encodes a cellular tyrosine kinase (formerly *lsk*[T] or *tck*), detected originally in the LSTRA murine lymphoma cell line derived from MuLV-induced thymomas [1].

RELATED GENES

LCK is a member of the *SRC* tyrosine kinase family (*Blk, FGR, FYN, HCK, LCK/Tkl, LYN, SRC, YES*). Murine BMK has 70% homology with murine LCK. A *Lck*-related gene is expressed in murine eggs. *Tkl* is the avian cellular tyrosine kinase homologue of *L*ck.

Nucleotides (kb)	2.2
Chromosome	1p35-p32
Mass (kDa): predicted	58
expressed	56

Cellular location

Plasma membrane.

Tissue distribution

LCK, FGR, LYN and *HCK* are expressed only in haematopoietic cells and *LCK* is found specifically only in lymphoid cells, T cells, NK cells and some B cells. Chicken *Tkl* is abundantly expressed in the thymus with less expression in the spleen [2].

PROTEIN FUNCTION

LCK is a lymphocyte-specific tyrosine kinase associated with the cytoplasmic domains of CD4 and CD8α (CD8 can exist as αα or αβ dimers) that bind to class II and class I MHC molecules, respectively [3]. The intracellular domain of CD4 negatively regulates the replicative rate of HIV-1 in T cells and its association with LCK is necessary for this effect [4].

LCK also co-precipitates with PtdIns 3-kinase, PtdIns 4-kinase, the IL-2R β chain [5], CD5 [6] and CD2 [7], and also with GAP and immunoglobulin receptors in LSTRA cells and B cells, respectively [8-12].

Stimulation of the T cell receptor (TCR) activates LCK but it is FYN, rather than LCK, that co-precipitates with the TCR [13]. Furthermore, T cells from LCK-deficient mice proliferate in response to activation of the TCR or to IL-2 [14]. Cross-linking CD4 enhances the autophosphorylation of LCK, which may cause the phosphorylation of the ζ chain of the CD3/TCR complex, although ζ has only been shown to be a direct substrate *in vitro*. RAF1 and MAP kinase are substrates for LCK [15,16]. Thus MAP kinases may be directly regulated by LCK (and other members of the SRC family) and participate in cell signalling cascades that may activate substrates such as ribosomal S6 kinases (RSKs).

An alternative role for LCK may be in regulating T cell maturation and differentiation: it is expressed before CD4/8 in developing T cells and is present in complexes with CD4 and CD8 in immature CD4+/CD8+ cells. The expression in transgenic mice of a catalytically inactive form of LCK that functions in a dominant negative manner indicates that normal LCK plays a critical role in CD4+8+ thymocyte development for which FYN cannot substitute [17,18]. However, this role may be independent of association between LCK and CD4 or CD8.

Cancer

Greatly reduced expression of LCK has been detected in T cells infiltrating renal cell carcinoma, correlating with reduced anti-tumour activity [19]. LCK is expressed in B cells from patients with chronic lymphocytic leukaemia (CLL) though not in normal B cells [20]. A translocation breakpoint within the first LCK intron has been detected in a T cell acute lymphoblastic leukaemia (T cell ALL) cell line with a t(1;7)(p34;q34). This separates the two LCK promoters (see below) and juxtaposes the constant region of the TCR β chain gene to the proximal promoter and protein-coding region of LCK [21].

Transgenic animals

Transgenic mice that do not express LCK show considerable thymic atrophy with a marked decrease in the number of CD4+/CD8+ thymocytes [14]. Transgenic mice expressing high levels of a catalytically inactive form of LCK are defective in the production of virtually all T lymphocytes [17].

In animals

A significant proportion (14%) of primary tumours induced in rats by Mo-MuLV have a proviral insertion upstream of Lck that increases Lck transcription, generating three different hybrid transcripts [22].

In vitro

The phenotype of LSTRA murine lymphoma cells appears to be caused by the enhanced expression of Lck caused by promoter insertion [23]. Substitution of Phe for Tyr505 increases the apparent kinase activity and this mutant form of LCK transforms NIH 3T3 cells [24]. The overexpression of Lck promotes tumorigenesis in otherwise normal thymocytes [25].

GENE STRUCTURE

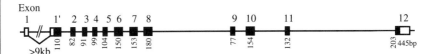

Exon

The structures of the human and murine *LCK* genes are closely similar. They have identical exon sizes except for the untranslated region of exon 12 [26]. There are at least two *LCK* mRNAs expressed in human and mouse cells, types I and II [27]. These have different 5′ untranslated regions arising from the use of alternative promoters [28].

TRANSCRIPTIONAL REGULATION

The type I promoter in Jurkat cells and in the colon carcinoma cell line SW620 contains an ETS binding element that is essential for its activity [29]. Type II *LCK* transcripts initiate from a promoter ~9 kb from the downstream promoter and have an alternative 5′ UTR. The sequence between −584 and +37 with respect to the proximal promoter transcription start site directs tissue-specific and temporally appropriate transcription of *LCK* [30]. The type II promoter is used in both normal, mature T cells and in transformed T cells and an alternatively spliced transcript utilizing this promoter is also expressed in both types of cell [31]. In this Type IIB mRNA the deletion of exon 1′ results in the use of a different AUG codon in exon 1. In the Type IIB translation product 10 residues encoded by exon 1 replace the first 35 residues encoded by exon 1′.

PROTEIN STRUCTURE

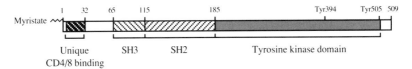

LCK has 65% sequence homology to SRC in the C-terminal 450 amino acids; the N-termini are unrelated. Deletion of the SH2 or SH3 domains increases LCK tyrosine kinase activity and phosphorylation of the autophosphorylation site Tyr394 [32]. The structure of the SH2 domain of LCK complexed with an 11 amino acid peptide derived from hamster polyoma middle T antigen has been analysed by high-resolution crystallography [33].

The regulatory site, phosphorylated in resting T cells, is Tyr505 (equivalent to Tyr527 in SRC). Site-directed mutagenesis of Tyr505 activates the oncogenic potential of LCK, as does deletion of the C-terminal region containing Tyr505 [34]. The SH2 but not the SH3 domain is required for full oncogenic activity in LCK from which Tyr505 has been removed [35] and the SH2 domain binds *in vitro* to several TCR-regulated tyrosine phosphorylation substrates [36]. Tyr505 is specifically phosphorylated by the human p50^{CSK} tyrosine kinase which thus negatively regulates LCK kinase activity. However, p50^{CSK} also phosphorylates the CD45 tyrosine phosphatase which promotes its binding to LCK via the SH2 domain of the kinase and increases the activity of the phosphatase [37]. The non-transmembrane phosphatase SH-PTP1, expressed primarily in haematopoietic cells, including T cells, undergoes tyrosyl phosphorylation in response to LCK activation via CD4 or CD8 [38].

Tyr505 is dephosphorylated by CD45 when cells are activated *via* surface receptors, thus permitting the phosphorylation of Tyr394 (equivalent to Tyr416 in SRC) which represents the switch to the activated enzyme form. Physical association between LCK and CD45 occurs independently of the TCR [39]. Oxidative reagents induce phosphorylation of Tyr394 and Tyr505 in LCK, indicating that a redox-sensitive signalling mechanism in T cells is in part mediated by LCK [40].

SEQUENCE OF LCK

```
  1  MGCGCSSHPE  DDWMENIDVC  ENCHYPIVPL  DGKGTLLIRN  GSEVRDPLVT
 51  YEGSNPPASP  LQDNLVIALH  SYEPSHDGDL  GFEKGEQLRI  LEQSGEWWKA
101  QSLTTGQEGF  IPFNFVAKAN  SLEPEPWFFK  NLSRKDAERQ  LLAPGNTHGS
151  FLIRESESTA  GSFSLSVRDF  DQNQGEVVKH  YKIRNLDNGG  FYISPRITFP
201  GLHELVRHYT  NASDGLCTRL  SRPCQTQKPQ  KPWWEDEWEV  PRETLKLVER
251  LGAGQFGEVW  MGYYNGHTKV  AVKSLKQGSM  SPDAFLAEAN  LMKQLQHQRL
301  VRLYAVVTQE  PIYIITEYME  NGSLVDFLKT  PSGIKLTINK  LLDMAAQIAE
351  GMAFIEERNY  IHRDLRAANI  LVSDTLSCKI  ADFGLARLIE  DNEYTAREGA
401  KFPIKWTAPE  AINYGTFTIK  SDVWSFGILL  TEIVTHGRIP  YPGMTNPEVI
451  QNLERGYRMV  RPDNCPEELY  QLMRLCWKER  PEDRPTFDYL  RSVLEDFFTA
501  TEGQYQPQP  (509)
```

Domain structure

2	Myristate attachment site
42, 59	Major sites for TPA-induced phosphorylation. Ser59 phosphorylation by MAP kinase *in vitro* reduces LCK activity [41]
232–493	Tyrosine kinase domain
251–259 and 273	ATP binding region
364	Active site
394	Autophosphorylation site
505	Phosphorylation site
66–117	SH3 domain (underlined)

DATABASE ACCESSION NUMBERS

	PIR	SWISSPROT	EMBL/GENBANK	REFERENCES
Human LCK	JQ0152	P06239, P07100	X13529, X04476	42, 43
			X14055, X06369	26, 44
			X05027, M21510	45

References

1 Sefton, B.M. (1991) Oncogene 6, 683–686.
2 Chow, L.M.L. et al. (1992) Mol. Cell. Biol. 12, 1226–1233.
3 Thompson, P.A. et al. (1992) Oncogene 7, 719–725.
4 Tremblay, M. et al. (1994) EMBO J. 13, 774–783.
5 Hatakeyama, M. et al. (1991) Science 252, 1523–1528.
6 Burgess, K.E. et al. (1992) Proc. Natl Acad. Sci. USA 89, 9311–9315.
7 Bell, G.M. et al. (1992) Mol. Cell. Biol. 12, 5548–5554.
8 Ellis, C. et al. (1991) Oncogene 6, 895–901.
9 Amrein, K.E. et al. (1992) Proc. Natl Acad. Sci. USA 89, 3343–3346.
10 Campbell, M.A. and Sefton, B.M. (1992) Mol. Cell. Biol. 12, 2315–2321.
11 Taieb, J. et al. (1993) J. Biol. Chem. 268, 9169–9171.
12 Prasad, K.V.S. et al. (1993) Mol. Cell. Biol. 13, 7708–7717.
13 Samelson, L.E. et al. (1990) Proc. Natl Acad. Sci. USA 87, 4358–4362.
14 Molina, T.J. et al. (1992) Nature 357, 161–164.
15 Thompson, P.A. et al. (1991) Cell Growth Differ. 2, 609–617.
16 Prasad, K.V.S. and Rudd, C.E. (1992) Mol. Cell. Biol. 12, 5260–5267.
17 Levin, S.D. et al. (1993) EMBO J. 12, 1671–1680.
18 Anderson, S.J. et al. (1993) Nature 365, 552–554.
19 Finke, J.H. et al. (1993) Cancer Res. 53, 5613–5616.
20 Abts, H. et al. (1991) Leukemia Res. 15, 987–997.
21 Burnett, R.C. et al. (1991) Genes Chromosom. Cancer 3, 461–467.
22 Shin, S. and Steffen, D.L. (1993) Oncogene 8, 141–149.
23 Marth, J.D. et al. (1985) Cell 43, 393–404.
24 Marth, J.D. et al. (1988) Mol. Cell. Biol. 8, 540–550.
25 Abraham, K.M. et al. (1991) Proc. Natl Acad. Sci. USA 88, 3977–3981.
26 Rouer, E. et al. (1989) Gene 84, 105–113.
27 Garvin, A.M. et al. (1988) Mol. Cell. Biol. 8, 3058–3064.
28 Adler, H.T. et al. (1988) J. Virol. 62, 4113–4122.
29 Leung, S. et al. (1993) Oncogene 8, 989–997.
30 Allen, J.M. et al. (1992) Mol. Cell. Biol. 12, 2758–2768.
31 Rouer, E. and Benarous, R. (1992) Oncogene 7, 2535–2538.
32 Reynolds, P.J. et al. (1992) Oncogene 7, 1949–1955.
33 Eck, M.J. et al. (1993) Nature 362, 87–91.
34 Adler, H.T. and Sefton, B.M. (1992) Oncogene 7, 1191–1199.
35 Veillette, A. et al. (1992) Oncogene 7, 971–980.
36 Peri, K.G. et al. (1993) Oncogene 8, 2765–2772.
37 Autero, M. et al. (1994) Mol. Cell. Biol. 14, 1308–1321.
38 Lorenz, U. et al. (1994) Mol. Cell. Biol. 14, 1824–1834.
39 Koretzky, G.A. et al. (1993) J. Biol. Chem. 268, 8958–8964.
40 Nakamura , K. et al. (1993) Oncogene 8, 3133–3139.
41 Winkler, D.G. et al. (1993) Proc. Natl Acad. Sci. USA 90, 5176–5180.

42 Perlmutter, R.M. et al. (1988) J. Cell. Biochem. 38, 117–126.
43 Koga, Y. et al. (1986) Eur. J. Immunol. 16, 1643–1646.
44 Trevillyan, J.M. et al. (1986) Biochim. Biophys. Acta 888, 286–295.
45 Veillette, A. et al. (1987) Oncogene Res. 1, 357–374.

LYN

IDENTIFICATION

LYN (<u>L</u>CK/<u>Y</u>ES-related <u>n</u>ovel tyrosine kinase, formerly *SYN*) was initially cloned from a placental cDNA library using a v-*yes* probe.

RELATED GENES

LYN is a member of the *SRC* tyrosine kinase family (*Blk, FGR, FYN, HCK, LCK/Tkl, LYN, SRC, YES*). Highly homologous in the kinase domain to LCK and YES.

Nucleotides	Not fully mapped
Chromosome	8q13–qter
Mass (kDa): predicted	58.5
expressed	53/56

Cellular location

Cytoplasm.

Tissue distribution

Expressed in brain and in B lymphocytes. Related forms of *LYN* have been detected in the spleen [1].

PROTEIN FUNCTION

p53^{LYN} and p56^{LYN} are physically associated with IgM on B cells and cross-linking IgM increases the kinase activity of LYN. LYN kinase activity is also stimulated by IL2 or IL3. LYN activates PtdIns 3-kinase (binding via its SH3 domain) and PLCγ2, MAP kinase and GAP via its N-terminal 27 amino acids [2,3]. LYN may modulate receptor-mediated changes in $[Ca^{2+}]_i$ [4].

In the rat basophilic leukaemia cell line RBL-2H3 the kinase activity of both LYN and SRC is increased after cellular stimulation via the high-affinity IgE receptor [5]. LYN immunoprecipitates with both the activated IgE and Thy-1 receptors [6] and may therefore be responsible for the tyrosine phosphorylation of the β and γ subunits of the activated receptor. Association of LYN, together with YES and FYN, with a major signalling receptor also occurs in human platelets and in some cell lines (see **YES**).

GENE STRUCTURE

Common splicing patterns indicate that *LYN, SRC, FGR, FYN* and *YES* are derived from a common gene but each differs in C-terminus and tissue-specific expression and thus, presumably, in function.

TRANSCRIPTIONAL REGULATION

The *LYN* promoter lacks TATA or CAAT boxes but contains four GC-rich regions, a cAMP-responsive element, an octamer-binding motif, PEA 3-like motifs and an NF-κB-binding sequence. In T cells transcription is induced by the HTLV 1-encoded p40[tax] protein [7].

PROTEIN STRUCTURE

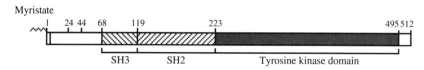

SEQUENCE OF LYN

```
  1  MGCIKSKGKD  SLSDDGVDLK  TQPVRNTERT  IYVRDPTSNK  QQRPVPESQL
 51  LPGQRFQTKD  PEEQGDIVVA  LYPYDGIHPD  DLSFKKGEKM  KVLEEHGEWW
101  KAKSLLTKKE  GFIPSNYVAK  LNTLETEEWF  FKDITRKDAE  RQLLAPGNSA
151  GAFLIRESET  LKGSFSLSVR  DFDPVHGDVI  KHYKIRSLDN  GGYYISPRIT
201  FPCISDMIKH  YQKQADGLCR  RLEKACISPK  PQKPWDKDAW  EIPRESIKLV
251  KRLGAGQFGE  VWMGYYNNST  KVAVKTLKPG  TMSVQAFLEE  ANLMKTLQHD
301  KLVRLYAVVT  REEPIYIITE  YMAKGSLLDF  LKSDEGGKVL  LPKLIDFSAQ
351  IAEGMAYIER  KNYIHRDLRA  ANVLVSESLM  CKIADFGLAR  VIEDNEYTAR
401  EGAKFPIKWT  APEAINFGCF  TIKSDVWSFG  ILLYEIVTYG  KIPYPGRTNA
451  DVMTALSQGY  RMPRVENCPD  ELYDIMKMCW  KEKAEERPTF  DYLQSVLDDF
501  YTATEGQYQQ  QP  (512)
```

Domain structure

2	Myristate attachment site
24–44	Region deleted in the alternative form of LYN[8,9] (underlined)
253–261 and 275	ATP binding site
367	Active site
397, 508	Autophosphorylation site
68–119	SH3 domain (or A box: italics)

DATABASE ACCESSION NUMBERS

	PIR	*SWISSPROT*	*EMBL/GENBANK*	*REFERENCES*
Human *LYN*	A26719	P07948	M16038	*10*

References
1 Brunati, A.M. et al. (1991) Biochim. Biophys. Acta 1091, 123–126.
2 Yamanashi, Y. et al. (1992) Proc. Natl Acad. Sci USA 89, 1118–1122.

3 Pleiman, C.M. et al. (1993) Mol. Cell. Biol. 13, 5877–5887.
4 Takata, M. et al. (1994) EMBO J. 13, 1341–1349.
5 Eiseman, E. and Bolen, J.B. (1992) Nature 355, 78–80.
6 Draberova, L. and Draber, P. (1993) Proc. Natl Acad. Sci. USA 90, 3611–3615.
7 Uchiumi, F. et al. (1992) Mol. Cell. Biol. 12, 3784–3795.
8 Stanley, E. et al. (1991) Mol. Cell. Biol. 11, 3399–3406.
9 Yi, T. et al. (1991) Mol. Cell. Biol. 11, 2391–2398.
10 Yamanashi, Y. et al. (1987) Mol. Cell. Biol. 7, 237–243.

MAS

IDENTIFICATION

MAS is a human transforming gene having no homology with known viral oncogenes that was originally detected by NIH 3T3 fibroblast transfection of DNA from an epidermoid carcinoma.

RELATED GENES

<u>R</u>at <u>t</u>horacic <u>a</u>orta (*Rta*); human <u>m</u>as-<u>r</u>elated <u>g</u>ene (*MRG*). MAS is a member of the seven transmembrane-spanning receptor family that includes the visual opsins, α_2-, β_1- and β_2-adrenergic receptors, M1 and M2 muscarinic acetylcholine receptors and substance K receptor.

Nucleotides	Not fully mapped
Chromosome	6q24–q27
Mass (kDa): predicted	37
expressed	45

Cellular location

Transmembrane cell surface protein.

Tissue distribution

Rat *Mas* is strongly expressed in the hippocampus and cerebral cortex [1,2]. The related RTA protein is significantly expressed in the gut, vas deferens, uterus and aorta [3]. *MRG* expression has not been detected [4].

PROTEIN FUNCTION

Receptor for neuronal type angiotensin III. Its action is mediated by G proteins that activate PtdInsP_2 hydrolysis causing increase in $[Ca^{2+}]_i$ [5]. *MAS* is activated oncogenically by rearrangement of 5′ non-coding regions in which human centromeric alpha satellite repeat DNA (alphoid sequences) are juxtaposed upstream of *MAS* [6].

In animals

MAS renders NIH 3T3 fibroblasts tumorigenic in nude mice and has a weak focus-inducing activity in NIH 3T3 cells [7].

SEQUENCE OF MAS

```
  1  MDGSNVTSFV VEEPTNISTG RNASVGNAHR QIPIVHWVIM SISPVGFVEN
 51  GILLWFLCFR MRRNPFTVYI THLSIADISL LFCIFILSID YALDYELSSG
101  HYYTIVTLSV TFLFGYNTGL YLLTAISVER CLSVLYPIWY RCHRPKYQSA
151  LVCALLWALS CLVTTMEYVM CIDREEESHS RNDCRAVIIF IAILSFLVFT
201  PLMLVSSTIL VVKIRKNTWA SHSSKLYIVI MVTIIIFLIF AMPMRLLYLL
251  YYEYWSTFGN LHHISLLFST INSSANPFIY FFVGSSKKKR FKESLKVVLT
301  RAFKDEMQPR RQKDNCNTVT VETVV (325)
```

Domain structure

1–30, 98–104, 173–185, 251–257	Extracellular domains
31–61, 66–97, 105–135, 150–172, 186–214, 225–250, 258–286	Seven transmembrane domains (underlined)
62–65, 136–149, 215–224, 287–325	Cytoplasmic domains
5, 16, 22	Potential carbohydrate attachment sites

DATABASE ACCESSION NUMBERS

	PIR	SWISSPROT	EMBL/GENBANK	REFERENCE
Human *MAS*	A01375	P04201	M13150	7

References

1 Young, D. et al. (1988) Proc. Natl Acad. Sci. USA 85, 5339–5342.
2 Bunnemann, B. et al. (1990) Neurosci. Lett. 114, 147–153.
3 Ross, P.C. et al. (1990) Proc. Natl Acad. Sci. USA 87, 3052–3056.
4 Monnot, C. et al. (1991) Mol. Endocrinol. 5, 1477–1487.
5 Jackson, T.R. et al. (1988) Nature 335, 437–440.
6 van't Veer, L.J. et al. (1993) Oncogene 8, 2673–2681.
7 Young, D. et al. (1986) Cell 45, 711–719.

MAX

IDENTIFICATION

MAX was detected by screening a cDNA expression library with the C-terminus of human MYC.

RELATED GENES

MAX is a member of the helix–loop–helix/leucine zipper superfamily. ΔMAX is a truncated form. The murine homologue is *Myn*. Variant forms of *Xmax* occur in *Xenopus laevis*.

Nucleotides	Not fully mapped
Chromosome	14q22–q24
Mass (kDa): predicted	18
expressed	21/22
	16.5 (ΔMAX)

Cellular location

Nucleus. Translocation from the cytosol is dependent on association with MYC. The steady-state concentration of MAX is constant throughout the cell cycle [1] and intracellular MYC is always complexed with MAX.

Tissue distribution

MAX and MYN, its murine homologue to which human MYCN also binds, occur in many cell types of diverse origin: MAX has been detected in NIH 3T3 fibroblasts, HeLa cells and neuroblastoma-derived cell lines. The ratio of MAX to ΔMAX is cell-line specific [2].

PROTEIN FUNCTION

MAX is a helix–loop–helix protein that forms sequence-specific DNA binding homodimers and also heterodimerizes with MYC [3,4]. The core consensus sequence is CACGTG but the complete 12 bp consensus binding sites are RACCACGTGGTY (MYC/MAX) and RANCACGTGNTY (MAX/MAX) where R represents purine and Y pyrimidine [5,6]. MYC/MAX does not bind when the core is flanked by a 5′T or 3′A whereas MAX/MAX readily binds such sequences. Thus the flanking motif can strongly inhibit MYC/MAX *trans*-activation. The leucine zipper domain is critical to the formation of heterodimers with MAX [7]. Unlike MYC, MAX can homodimerize efficiently to bind to the same DNA sequence as the MYC/MAX heterodimer, the homodimers acting as transcriptional repressors.

MYC/MAX heterodimers are required for the induction of both cell cycle progression and apoptosis [8]. Phosphorylation of the N-terminus of MAX by casein kinase II inhibits DNA binding of the homodimer *in vitro* but does not affect that of MYC/MAX heterodimers [9]. ΔMAX retains the capacity to form heterodimers with MYC that bind to the CACGTG motif but lacks the putative regulatory domain of MAX [2,10].

The basic helix–loop–helix/leucine zipper proteins MAD and MXI1 [11,12] form heterodimers with MAX that bind efficiently to the MYC/MAX consensus sequence to repress transcription. MAD protein is rapidly induced upon differentiation of cells of the myeloid lineage and MAD/MAX complexes replace MYC/MAX complexes found in undifferentiated cells. Thus the relative abundance of these binding partners may determine the extent of formation of the transcriptionally active MYC/MAX complex.

TRANSCRIPTIONAL REGULATION BY MYC AND MAX

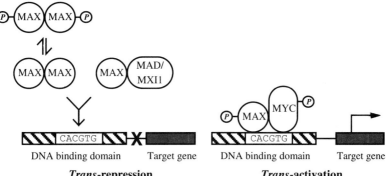

Trans-repression　　　　　**Trans-activation**

MAX homodimers phosphorylated by casein kinase II do not interact with binding domains. Unphosphorylated MAX homodimers repress transcription of genes that are targets for MYC, for example, in quiescent cells in which the concentration of MYC is low. Phosphorylated MAX/MYC heterodimers *trans*-activate target genes, for example, in proliferating cells [9].

STRUCTURES OF MYC, MAX AND DMAX PROTEINS

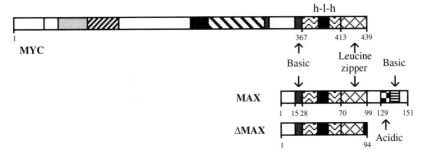

The helix–loop–helix/leucine zipper domain mediates the interaction between MYC and MAX and these regions are critical for transforming potential, autoregulation of *MYC* expression, and inhibition of differentiation [13,14]. Artificial deletion of the N-terminus generates a dominant-negative mutant of MAX [15]. X-Ray structural analysis of the MAX homodimer has revealed a symmetrical, parallel, left-handed, four-helix bundle in which each monomer contributes two α-helical segments separated by a loop [16].

SEQUENCE OF MAX

```
  1  MSDNDDIEVE SDADKRAHHN ALERKRRDHI KDSFHSLRDS VPSLQGEKAS
 51  RAQILDKATE YIQYMRRKNH THQQDIDDLK RQNALLEQQV RALGKARSSA
101  QLQTNYPSSD NSLYTNAKGS TISAFDGGSD SSSESEPEEP QSRKKLRMEA
151  S (151)
```

Domain structure

15–28	Basic motif
13–21	The alternative forms of MAX and ΔMAX contain a nine amino acid insertion (EEQPRFQSA) after Asp12
30–41 and 48–66	Helix I and helix II of the basic helix–loop–helix region (underlined)
79–93	Three leucines spaced seven residues apart (underlined)
90–151	C-Terminal 62 amino acids of MAX replaced in ΔMAX by GESES
90–151	An alternative 36 residue C-terminus is predicted to be encoded by the 5′ region of the first intron of *MAX* (GEHPSSWGSW PCCAPARSGF GTWACRVRAS HGVCAQ) [17]
2, 11, 20, 140, 142, 144	Potential casein kinase II phosphorylation sites
129–139	Acidic region
140–147	Nuclear localization signal (italics) [10]

DATABASE ACCESSION NUMBERS

	PIR	SWISSPROT	EMBL/GENBANK	REFERENCES
Human *MAX*		P25912	M64240	3
Human Δ*MAX*			X60287	2
Human Δ*MAX* (3.5 kb mRNA)			X66867	17

References
1 Blackwood, E.M. et al. (1992) Genes Devel. 6, 71–80.
2 Makela, T.P. et al. (1992) Science 256, 373–377.
3 Blackwood, E.M. and Eisenman, R.N. (1991) Science 251, 1211–1217.
4 **Cole, M.D. et al. (1991) Cell 65, 715–716.**
5 Solomon, D.L.C. et al. (1993) Nucl. Acids Res. 21, 5372–5376.
6 Fisher, F. et al. (1993) EMBO J. 12, 5075–5082.

7   Reddy, C.D. et al. (1992) Oncogene 7, 2085–2092.
8   Amati, B. et al. (1993) EMBO J. 12, 5083–5087.
9   Berberich, S.J. and Cole, M.D. (1992) Genes Devel. 6, 166–176.
10 Prendergast, G.C. et al. (1992) Genes Devel. 6, 2429–2439.
11 Ayer, D.E. and Eisenman, R.N. (1993) Genes Devel. 7, 2110–2119.
12 Larsson, L.-G. et al. (1994) Oncogene 9, 1247–1252.
13 Penn, L.J.Z. et al. (1990) Mol. Cell. Biol. 10, 4961–4966.
14 Crouch, D.H. et al. (1990) Oncogene 5, 683–689.
15 Billaud, M. et al. (1993) Proc. Natl Acad. Sci. USA 90, 2739–2743.
16 Ferre-D'Amare, A.R. et al. (1993) Nature 363, 38–45.
17 Vastrik, I. et al. (1993) Oncogene 8, 503–507.

MET

IDENTIFICATION

Identified as an activated oncogene in an N-methyl-N′-nitro-N-nitrosoguanidine-treated human osteosarcoma cell line (MNNG-HOS) and in MNNG-treated human xeroderma pigmentosum cells. *MET* was activated as an oncogene by the formation of a chimeric gene generated by chromosomal rearrangement fusing the *TPR* gene (translocated promoter region) to the N-terminally truncated *MET* kinase domain.

RELATED GENES

MET has homology with *SEA* and with *RON*. *TPR* has weak homology in α-helical regions to tropomyosin, spectrin, laminin B1, myosin heavy chain and *Drosophila glued* protein and to vimentin. The C-terminus of the larger TPR protein (TPR-L) is homologous to *Drosophila engrailed* protein, *E. coli* RNA polymerase σ subunit and nucleolin.

	MET	*TPR*	*TPR–MET*
Nucleotides	Not fully mapped	Not fully mapped	
Chromosome	7q31	1	
Mass (kDa): predicted	155.5	84	
expressed	gp190		p65$^{TPR\text{-}MET}$
	(p50α/p145β disulphide-linked, heterodimer)		
	gp140 (p50α/p85β)/gp130 (p50α/p75β)		
	(alternative splicing)		

Cellular location

MET β subunit (p145): Transmembrane. MET α subunit (p50): Extracellular. Multimeric forms of the α/β heterodimer occur, suggesting that the receptors exist as patches on the cell surface [1]. TPR/MET: Probably cytoplasmic [2].

Tissue distribution

High levels of *MET* mRNA occur in liver, gastrointestinal tract, thyroid and kidney and gp140 is present in the microglial cells of the human CNS [3]. Low levels are expressed in normal colorectal mucosa [4,5]. *TPR* is expressed in tumour cell lines of epithelial and mesenchymal origin and in T and B cell neoplasia [6]. The alternatively spliced *Tpr-l* is expressed in rat testis, lung, thymus and spleen [7].

PROTEIN FUNCTION

MET is a tyrosine kinase receptor that binds hepatocyte growth factor (HGF, also called scatter factor) [8-10]. The activity of MET may be greatly enhanced by autophosphorylation of the cytoplasmic domain [11]. HGF causes rapid tyrosine phosphorylation of the β subunit of MET [8,12]. HGF is a potent mitogen for hepatocytes *in vitro* and is an hepatotrophic factor possibly involved in liver regeneration [13]. In epithelial cells HGF stimulates the RAS guanine nucleotide exchanger and increases the proportion of RAS–GTP [14].

HGF was originally discovered as an activity that causes MDCK epithelial cells to change shape and become motile and invasive in *in vitro* assays [15]. HGF exerts similar effects on NIH 3T3 cells transfected to express p190^{MET} [16]. Responses to HGF are cell-dependent and it can exert mitogenic, motogenic or morphogenic effects [13]. HGF is a co-mitogen for normal human melanocytes, acting synergistically with basic fibroblast growth factor (FGFB) or mast cell growth factor (MGF). Melanocytes express the MAP2 kinases ERK1 and ERK2, the latter being phosphorylated in response to HGF [17].

TPR is a protein of unknown function but it activates the oncogenic potential of both *MET, RAF* and *TRK* [18]. The *TPR–MET* oncogene appears to be activated by an insertion of chromosome 1 (*TPR*) DNA into the *MET* locus on chromosome 7, both upstream and downstream portions of *MET* being conserved. This is similar to the mechanism of activation of *RAF* by *TPR* [19]. Both *TPR–MET* and *TPR–RAF* rearrangements occur within introns but there is no sequence homology between the sites.

A second *MET* allele is rearranged in the chemically treated human cell line MNNG-HOS. der(7)t(1;7)(q23;q32) represents a deletion of the N-terminus of the MET extracellular ligand binding domain but the rearranged allele also includes sequences derived from chromosome 2 [18].

Cancer

MET mRNA and protein concentrations are increased in some human carcinomas and in epithelial tumour cell lines [5,20]. In thyroid papillary carcinomas MET protein concentration is increased by 100-fold [21] but it is not detectably overexpressed in breast carcinomas. *MET* is amplified and overexpressed in cell lines from human tumours of non-haematopoietic origin, particularly gastric tumours [22].

In animals

NIH 3T3 fibroblasts that overexpress the human *MET* proto-oncogene are only weakly tumorigenic in nude mice but cells co-transfected with *MET* and *HGF* are highly tumorigenic, indicating that an autocrine transformation mechanism occurs [23].

In vitro

Overexpression of *MET* transforms NIH 3T3 fibroblasts [24] and HGF transforms immortalized mouse liver epithelial cells [25].

PROTEIN STRUCTURE

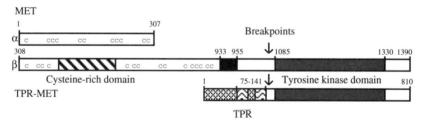

MET

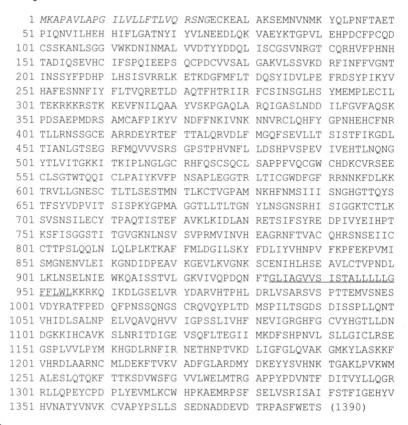

307 N-terminal amino acids of the MET precursor are cleaved to release the α subunit which then associates with the membrane-bound β subunit. The alternatively spliced isoform of MET is also expressed as a membrane tyrosine kinase but does not undergo cleavage to yield α and β subunits [26]. In TPR–MET the tyrosine kinase domain of MET is fused to 142 N-terminal amino acids of TPR. This region of TPR includes two leucine zipper motifs that mediate dimerization of TPR–MET and are essential for transforming activity [27]. The arrow indicates the breakpoint involved in the formation of TPR–MET. C: cysteine.

SEQUENCE OF MET

```
   1 MKAPAVLAPG ILVLLFTLVQ RSNGECKEAL AKSEMNVNMK YQLPNFTAET
  51 PIQNVILHEH HIFLGATNYI YVLNEEDLQK VAEYKTGPVL EHPDCFPCQD
 101 CSSKANLSGG VWKDNINMAL VVDTYYDDQL ISCGSVNRGT CQRHVFPHNH
 151 TADIQSEVHC IFSPQIEEPS QCPDCVVSAL GAKVLSSVKD RFINFFVGNT
 201 INSSYFPDHP LHSISVRRLK ETKDGFMFLT DQSYIDVLPE FRDSYPIKYV
 251 HAFESNNFIY FLTVQRETLD AQTFHTRIIR FCSINSGLHS YMEMPLECIL
 301 TEKRKKRSTK KEVFNILQAA YVSKPGAQLA RQIGASLNDD ILFGVFAQSK
 351 PDSAEPMDRS AMCAFPIKYV NDFFNKIVNK NNVRCLQHFY GPNHEHCFNR
 401 TLLRNSSGCE ARRDEYRTEF TTALQRVDLF MGQFSEVLLT SISTFIKGDL
 451 TIANLGTSEG RFMQVVVSRS GPSTPHVNFL LDSHPVSPEV IVEHTLNQNG
 501 YTLVITGKKI TKIPLNGLGC RHFQSCSQCL SAPPFVQCGW CHDKCVRSEE
 551 CLSGTWTQQI CLPAIYKVFP NSAPLEGGTR LTICGWDFGF RRNNKFDLKK
 601 TRVLLGNESC TLTLSESTMN TLKCTVGPAM NKHFNMSIII SNGHGTTQYS
 651 TFSYVDPVIT SISPKYGPMA GGTLLTLTGN YLNSGNSRHI SIGGKTCTLK
 701 SVSNSILECY TPAQTISTEF AVKLKIDLAN RETSIFSYRE DPIVYEIHPT
 751 KSFISGGSTI TGVGKNLNSV SVPRMVINVH EAGRNFTVAC QHRSNSEIIC
 801 CTTPSLQQLN LQLPLKTKAF FMLDGILSKY FDLIYVHNPV FKPFEKPVMI
 851 SMGNENVLEI KGNDIDPEAV KGEVLKVGNK SCENIHLHSE AVLCTVPNDL
 901 LKLNSELNIE WKQAISSTVL GKVIVQPDQN FTGLIAGVVS ISTALLLLLG
 951 FFLWLKKRKQ IKDLGSELVR YDARVHTPHL DRLVSARSVS PTTEMVSNES
1001 VDYRATFPED QFPNSSQNGS CRQVQYPLTD MSPILTSGDS DISSPLLQNT
1051 VHIDLSALNP ELVQAVQHVV IGPSSLIVHF NEVIGRGHFG CVYHGTLLDN
1101 DGKKIHCAVK SLNRITDIGE VSQFLTEGII MKDFSHPNVL SLLGICLRSE
1151 GSPLVVLPYM KHGDLRNFIR NETHNPTVKD LIGFGLQVAK GMKYLASKKF
1201 VHRDLAARNC MLDEKFTVKV ADFGLARDMY DKEYYSVHNK TGAKLPVKWM
1251 ALESLQTQKF TTKSDVWSFG VVLWELMTRG APPYPDVNTF DITVYLLQGR
1301 RLLQPEYCPD PLYEVMLKCW HPKAEMRPSF SELVSRISAI FSTFIGEHYV
1351 HVNATYVNVK CVAPYPSLLS SEDNADDEVD TRPASFWETS (1390)
```

Domain structure

1–24	Signal sequence (italics)
25–932	Extracellular domain
933–955	Transmembrane domain (underlined)
956–1390	Intracellular domain
1009–1010	Breakpoint for the translocation to form TPR–MET
1085–1330	Tyrosine kinase domain
1084–1092 and 1110	ATP binding site
1204	Active site
307–308	Potential cleavage site
1234–1235	Autophosphorylation sites critical for activation of *MET* [28]
45, 106, 149, 202, 399, 405, 607, 635, 785, 879, 930	Potential carbohydrate attachment sites
755	S→STWWKEPLNIVSFLFCFAS [29]

SEQUENCE OF TPR

```
  1  MAAVLQQVLE RTELNKLPKS VQNKLEKFLA DQQSEIDGLK GRHEKFKVES
 51  EQQYFEIEKR LSHSQERLVN ETRECQSLRL ELEKLNNQLK ALTEKNKELE
101  IAQDRNIAIQ SQFTRTKEEL EAEKRDLIRT NERLSQELEY LTEDVKRLNE
151  KLKESNTTKG ELQLKLDELQ ASDVSVKYRE KRLEQEKELL HSQNTWLNTE
201  LKTKTDELLA LGREKGNEIL ELKCNLENKK EEVSRLEEQM NGLKTSNEHL
251  QKHVEDLLTK LKEAKEQQAS MEEKFHNELN AHIKLSNLYK SAADDSEAKS
301  NELTRAVEEL HKLLKEAGEA NKAIQDHLLE VEQSKDQMEK EMLEKIGRLE
351  KELENANDLL SATKRKGAIL SEEELAAMSP TAAAVAKIVK PGMKLTELYN
401  AYVETQDQLL LEKLENKRIN KYLDEIVKEV EAKAPILKRQ REEYERAQKA
451  VASLSVKLEQ AMKEIQRLQE DTDKANKQSS VLERDNRRME IQVKDLSQQI
501  RVLLMELEEA RGNHVIRDEE VSSADISSSS EVISQHLVSY RNIEELQQQN
551  QRLLVALREL GETREREEQE TTSSKITELQ LKLESALTEL EQLRKSRQHQ
601  MQLVDSIVRQ RDMYRILLSQ TTGVAIPLHA SSLDDVSLAS TPKRPSTSQT
651  VSTPAPVPVI ESTEAIEAKA ALKQLQEIFE NYKKEKAENE KIQNEQLEKL
701  QEQVTDLRSQ NTKISTQLDF ASKRYL (726)
                         EMLQD NVEGYRREIT SLHERNQKLT
751  ATTQKQEQII NTMTQDLRGA NEKLAVAEVR AENLKKEKEM LKLSEVRLSQ
801  QRESLLAEQR (810)
```

Domain structure

75–99 and 117–141	Leucine zipper domains (underlined)
726–810	The 30 bp deletion that extends the ORF to 810 amino acids causes the deletion of the C-terminal leucine from p84^{TPR} and the substitution of 85 amino acids

DATABASE ACCESSION NUMBERS

	PIR	SWISSPROT	EMBL/GENBANK	REFERENCES
Human *MET*	A40175	P08581	J02958	29
			X54559	8, 30, 31
Human *TPR-S*			X63105	32
Human *TPR-L*			M15326, X66397	7

References

1   Faletto, D.L. et al. (1992) Oncogene 7, 1149–1157.
2   **Cooper, C.S. (1992) Oncogene 7, 3–7.**
3   Di Renzo, M.F. et al. (1993) Oncogene 8, 219–222.
4   Iyer, A. et al. (1990) Cell Growth Differ. 1, 87–95.
5   Liu, C. et al. (1992) Oncogene 7, 181–185.
6   Park, M. et al. (1986) Cell 45, 895–904.
7   Mitchell, P.J. and Cooper, C.S. (1992) Oncogene 7, 2329–2333.
8   Bottaro, D.P. et al. (1991) Science 251, 802–804.
9   Naldini, L. et al. (1991) EMBO J. 10, 2867–2878.
10 Hartmann, G. et al. (1992) Proc. Natl Acad. Sci. USA 89, 11574–11578.
11 Naldini, L. et al. (1991) Mol. Cell. Biol. 11, 1793–1803.
12 Naldini, L. et al. (1991) Oncogene 6, 501–504.
13 **Vande Woude, G. (1992) Jpn. J. Cancer Res. 83, cover article.**
14 Graziani, A. et al. (1993) J. Biol. Chem. 268, 9165–9168.
15 Rosen, E.M. et al. (1991) Cell Growth Differ. 2, 603–607.
16 Giordano, S. et al. (1993) Proc. Natl Acad. Sci. USA 90, 649–653.
17 Halaban, R. et al. (1992) Oncogene 7, 2195–2206.
18 Testa, J.R. et al. (1990) Oncogene 5, 1565–1571.
19 Ishikawa, F. et al. (1987) Mol. Cell. Biol. 7, 1226–1232.
20 Di Renzo, M.F. et al. (1991) Oncogene 6, 1997–2003.
21 Di Renzo, M.F. et al. (1992) Oncogene 7, 2549–2553.
22 Soman, N.R. et al. (1991) Proc. Natl Acad. Sci. USA 88, 4892–4896.
23 Rong, S. et al. (1992) Mol. Cell. Biol. 12, 5152–5158.
24 Cooper, C.S. et al. (1984) Nature 311, 29–33.
25 Kanda, H. et al. (1993) Oncogene 8, 3047–3053.
26 Rodrigues, G.A. et al. (1991) Mol. Cell. Biol. 11, 2962–2970.
27 Rodrigues, G.A. and Park, M. (1993) Mol. Cell. Biol. 13, 6711–6722.
28 Longati, P. et al. (1994). Oncogene 9, 49–57.
29 Park, M. et al. (1987) Proc. Natl Acad. Sci. USA 84, 6379–6383.
30 Chan, A.M.L. et al. (1987) Oncogene 1, 229–233.
31 Dean, M. et al. (1985) Nature 318, 385–388.
32 Mitchell, P.J. and Cooper, C.S. (1992) Oncogene 7, 383–388.

IDENTIFICATION

v-*mil* (also v-*mht*) is the oncogene of avian retrovirus Mill-Hill-2 (MH2), which also carries v-*myc*. v-*Rmil* is the oncogene of the IC10 and IC11 retroviruses generated during *in vitro* passaging of RAV-1 in chicken NR cells. *Mil* was detected by screening chicken DNA with a v-*mil* probe.

RELATED GENES

Mil is the avian homologue of mammalian *RAF1*. v-*Rmil* is the avian homologue of human *RAFB1*. *Mil* has homology with *Src, Fes, Fms, Mos, Yes, Fps, ErbB*, the catalytic subunit of cAMP-dependent protein kinase and protein kinase C.

	Mil (chicken)	*Rmil*	v-*mil*
Nucleotides (bp)	Not fully mapped	Not fully mapped	1154 (MH2 genome)
Mass (kDa): predicted	73	42.8	
expressed	71/73	93.5/95	P100*gag-mil*

Cellular location

MIL: Unknown. RMIL: Unknown. v-MIL: Cytoplasm

Tissue distribution

In most chicken tissues *Mil* mRNA lacking exon 7a is expressed: mRNA containing E7a occurs only in heart, skeletal muscle and brain [1]. *Rmil* is expressed at much higher levels in neural cells, neuroretinas and brain than in other embryonic tissues.

PROTEIN FUNCTION

MIL is a serine/threonine kinase of unknown function belonging to the RAF/MOS subfamily [2]. P100*gag-mil* binds RNA and DNA *in vitro* [3].

In animals

MH2 induces monocytic leukaemias and liver tumours in chickens [4].

In vitro

MH2 rapidly transforms chick haematopoietic cells (macrophages) and fibroblasts [4]. In contrast to its mammalian homologue v-*raf*, v-*mil* alone does not fully transform avian primary fibroblasts, probably because v-*mht/mil* contains an extra 5′ segment relative to v-*raf* that affects substrate recognition [5].

GENE STRUCTURE

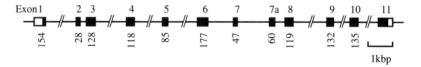

PROTEIN STRUCTURE

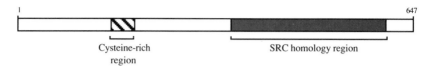

SEQUENCE OF CHICKEN MIL

```
  1  MEHIQGAWKT  ISNGFGLKDS  VFDGPNCISP  TIVQQFGYQR  RASDDGKISD
 51  TSKTSNTIRV  FLPNKQRTVV  NVRNGMTLHD  CLMKALKVRG  LQPECCAVFR
101  LVTEPKGKKV  RLDWNTDAAS  LIGEELQVDF  LDHVPLTTHN  FARKTFLKLA
151  FCDICQKFLL  NGFRCQTCGY  KFHEHCSTKV  PTMCVDWSNI  RQLLLFPNSN
201  ISDSGVPALP  PLTMRRMRES  VSRIPVSSQH  RYSTPHVFTF  NTSNPSSEGT
251  LSQRQRSTST  PNVHMVSTTM  PVDSRIIEDA  IRNHSESASP  SALSGSPNNM
301  SPTGWSQPKT  PVPAQRERAP  GTNTQEKNKI  RPRGQRDSSY  YWEIEASEVM
351  LSTRIGSGSF  GTVYKGKWHG  DVAVKILKVV  DPTPEQFQAF  RNEVAVLRKT
401  RHVNILLFMG  YMTKDNLAIV  TQWCEGSSLY  KHLHVQETKF  QMFQLIDIAR
451  QTAQGMDYLH  AKNIIHRDMK  SNNIFLHEGL  TVKIGDFGLA  TVKSRWSGSQ
501  QVEQPTGSIL  WMAPEVIRMQ  DSNPFSFQSD  VYSYGIVLYE  LMTGELPYSH
551  INNRDQIIFM  VGRGYASPDL  SKLYKNCPKA  MKRLVADCLK  KVREERPLFP
601  QILSSIELLQ  HSLPKINRSA  SEPSLHRASH  TEDINSCTLT  STRLPVF  (647)
```

Domain structure

139–184	Phorbol ester and diacylglycerol binding region (underlined)
355–363 and 375	ATP binding site
468	Active site
269–647	v-MIL (379 amino acids) differs from this region in two point mutations (Ser293 and Leu350 (italics))

DATABASE ACCESSION NUMBERS

	PIR	SWISSPROT	EMBL/GENBANK	REFERENCES
Chicken *Mil*	S00644	P05625	X07017	*6*
Chicken *Mil* exon E7a			X55430	*1*

References

1 Dozier, C. et al. (1991) Oncogene 6, 1307–1311.
2 Moelling, K. et al. (1984) Nature 312, 558–561.
3 Bunte, T. et al. (1983) EMBO J. 2, 1087–1092.
4 Graf, T. et al. (1986) Cell 45, 357–364.
5 Kan, N.C. et al. (1991) Avian Dis. 35, 941–949.
6 Koenen, M. et al. (1988) Oncogene 2, 179–185.

MOS

IDENTIFICATION

v-*mos* is the oncogene of the acutely transforming murine <u>Mo</u>loney <u>s</u>arcoma virus (Mo-MuSV). Isolated from a rhabdosarcoma in BALB/c mice infected with Moloney murine leukaemia virus. *MOS* was detected by screening placental DNA with a v-*mos* probe.

RELATED GENES

MOS is a member of the *RAF–MOS* subfamily and has homology with *SRC* but is not a tyrosine kinase.

	MOS	**v-mos**
Nucleotides (kb)	1.2	>1.2
Chromosome	8q11	
Mass (kDa): predicted	37.8	
expressed	39	P37/39*env-mos*
	24, 29, 42 and 44 in transformed cells	P85*gag-mos*

Cellular location

MOS: Cytoplasm. v-MOS: Nucleus (mainly).

Tissue distribution

Mos mRNA is only expressed at relatively high levels in germ cells in testes [1] and ovaries [2,3]. Human *MOS* is expressed at low levels in normal T and B lymphocytes and in neuroblastoma and cervical carcinoma cell lines [4].

PROTEIN FUNCTION

MOS is a serine/threonine kinase and the protein from *Xenopus* eggs exhibits autophosphorylation activity *in vitro* [5]. *Mos* expression is sufficient to cause meiosis I [6] and is required for meiosis II [7,8]. MOS is an active component of cytostatic factor [9, 10], an activity responsible for arrest in metaphase at the end of meiosis II [11]. The inactivation of maturation promoting factor (MPF (p34^{CDC2} and cyclin)) is required to allow oocytes to complete nuclear division, thus, MOS directly or indirectly activates and/or stabilizes MPF. Proteins other than MOS contribute to CSF and are not required for meiosis I [6]. MOS is an upstream activator of MAP kinase and may directly phosphorylate MAP kinase kinase during *Xenopus* oocyte entry into meiosis [12,13].

In unfertilized eggs and transformed cells MOS associates with tubulin and the p35^{CDK} isoform of p34^{CDC2}. MOS phosphorylates tubulin *in vitro* [14–16] and may promote the reorganization of microtubules that leads to meiotic spindle formation. The transforming capacity of MOS probably derives from expression of its M phase activity during interphase [9,10,12,17].

Cancer

MOS and the flanking regions of its gene are mutated in some benign pleomorphic adenomas of the salivary glands [18].

Transgenic animals

Transgenic mice expressing *Mos* develop pheochromocytomas and medullary C-cell carcinomas of the thyroid resembling the human syndrome multiple endocrine neoplasia type II [19].

In animals

MOS causes fibrosarcomas in mice following Mo-MuSV infection and can also cause osteosarcomas in other species [20,21]. Activation of *Mos* by insertion of an endogenous intracisternal A-particle has been detected in some mouse plasmacytomas [22].

In vitro

Mos/LTR or v-*mos*/LTR hybrid genes transform NIH 3T3 fibroblasts [23]. The expression of v-MOS in 3T3 fibroblasts blocks PDGF-mediated signalling by inhibiting PDGFβR autophosphorylation [24].

GENE STRUCTURE

Human, mouse, rat and chicken *MOS* genes contain a single contiguous ORF of ~1050 bp.

TRANSCRIPTIONAL REGULATION

Transcription of *Mos* in mouse oocytes is directed by a simple promoter (consensus PyPyCAPyPyPyPyPy) comprising sequences within 20 bp of the transcription start site [25]. A negative regulatory region between 400 and 500 bp upstream from the *Mos* ATG inhibits transcription in somatic cells [26]. In rat and mouse a 200 bp region upstream of the *Mos* exon has *cis*-inhibitory activity (e.g., can block the transforming activity of v-*mos*). The region contains two poly(A) signals and when located downstream of a gene causes termination of transcription [27].

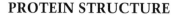

PROTEIN STRUCTURE

v-MOS from the earliest Mo-MuSV isolated (HT1 Mo-MuSV) is identical in amino acid sequence to murine MOS [28]. A number of other MuSV isolates show some sequence changes in transduced v-*mos* [29]. Human and mouse MOS are 77% identical in sequence.

SEQUENCE OF MOS

```
  1  MPSPLALRPY  LRSEFSPSVD  ARPCSSPSEL  PAKLLLGATL  PRAPRLPRRL
 51  AWCSIDWEQV  CLLQRLGAGG  FGSVYKATYR  GVPVAIKQVN  KCTKNRLASR
101  RSFWAELNVA  RLRHDNIVRV  VAASTRTPAG  SNSLGTIIME  FGGNVTLHQV
151  IYGAAGHPEG  DAGEPHCRTG  GQLSLGKCLK  YSLDVVNGLL  FLHSQSIVHL
201  DLKPANILIS  EQDVCKISDF  GCSEKLEDLL  CFQTPSYPLG  GTYTHRAPEL
251  LKGEGVTPKA  DIYSFAITLW  QMTTKQAPYS  GERQHILYAV  VAYDLRPSLS
301  AAVFEDSLPG  QRLGDVIQRC  WRPSAAQRPS  ARLLLVDLTS  LKAELG (346)
```

Domain structure

66–74 and 87   ATP binding site (underlined)
       201   Active site

DATABASE ACCESSION NUMBERS

	PIR	SWISSPROT	EMBL/GENBANK	REFERENCE
Human *MOS*	A00649	P00540	J00119	30

References

1 Propst, F. and Vande Woude, G.F. (1985) Nature 315, 516–518.
2 Goldman, D.S. et al. (1988) Proc. Natl Acad. Sci. USA 84, 4509–4513.
3 Keshet, E. et al. (1987) Oncogene 2, 234–240.
4 Li, C.-C.H. et al. (1993) Oncogene 8, 1685–1691.
5 Watanabe, N. et al. (1989) Nature 342, 505–511.
6 Yew, N. et al. (1992) Nature 355, 649–652.
7 Kanki, J.P. and Donoghue, D.J. (1991) Proc. Natl Acad. Sci. USA 88, 5794–5798.
8 Daar, I. et al. (1991) J. Cell Biol. 114, 329–335.
9 Sagata, N. et al. (1989) Science 245, 643–646.
10 Sagata, N. et al. (1989) Nature 342, 512–518.
11 Lorca, T. et al. (1991) EMBO J. 10, 2087–2093.
12 Posada, J. et al. (1993) Mol. Cell. Biol. 13, 2546–2553.
13 Nebreda, A.R. and Hunt, T. (1993) EMBO J. 12, 1979–1986.
14 Zhou, R. et al. (1992) Mol. Cell. Biol. 12, 3583–3589.
15 Bai, W. et al. (1992) Oncogene 7, 493–500.
16 Bai, W. et al. (1992) Oncogene 7, 1757–1763.
17 Daar, I. et al. (1991) Science 253, 74–76.
18 Stenman, G. et al. (1991) Oncogene 6, 1105–1108.

19 Schulz, N. et al. (1992) Cancer Res. 52, 450–455.
20 Fefer, A. et al. (1967) Cancer Res. 27, 1626–1631.
21 Fujinaga, S. et al. (1970) Cancer Res. 30, 1698–1708.
22 Horowitz, M. et al. (1984) EMBO J. 3, 2937–2941.
23 Freeman, R.S. et al. (1989) Proc. Natl Acad. Sci. USA 86, 5805–5809.
24 Faller, D.V. et al. (1994) J. Biol. Chem. 269, 5022–5029.
25 Pal, S.K. et al. (1991) Mol. Cell. Biol. 11, 5190–5196.
26 Zinkel, S.S. et al. (1992) Mol. Cell. Biol. 12, 2029–2036.
27 McGeady, M.L. et al. (1986) DNA 5, 289–298.
28 Seth, A. and Vande-Woude, G.F. (1985) J. Virol. 56, 144–152.
29 Brow, M.A. et al. (1984) J. Virol. 49, 579–582.
30 Watson, R. et al. (1982) Proc. Natl Acad. Sci. USA 79, 4078–4082.

MYB

IDENTIFICATION

v-*myb* is the oncogene of the acutely transforming avian myeloblastosis virus (AMV) and E26 leukaemia virus [1]. *MYB* was identified by screening a cDNA library with a v-*myb* probe.

RELATED GENES

Human *MYBA* and *MYBB* and *MYB*-like genes *MYBL1* and *MYBL2*; chicken *B-myb*. MYB related proteins also occur in *Schizosaccharomyces pombe* (*cdc5*+), *Xenopus laevis*, *Drosophila melanogaster*, yeast (BAS1, REB1), *D. discoideum*, *Zea mays*, barley and *Arabidopsis thaliana*.

	MYB	v-*myb*
Nucleotides (kb)	>25	7.14 (AMV genome)
		5.7 (E26 genome)
Chromosome	6q22–q23	
Mass (kDa): predicted	72.5	43*v-myb*
		75*gag-myb-ets*
expressed	75	48*v-myb* (AMV)
	90	P135*gag-myb-ets* (E26)

Cellular location

MYB: Nucleus. v-MYB: Nucleus.

Tissue distribution

MYB is expressed in immature cells of the lymphoid, erythroid and myeloid lineages [2–4]. It is also strongly expressed in CD4+ thymocytes, induced in T lymphocytes and fibroblasts by mitogenic stimulation [5] and is detectable in vascular smooth muscle cells [6,7]. *Myb* is co-expressed with *Mim-1* during granulopoiesis in the chicken pancreas and spleen [8]. *B-myb* is strongly expressed only during the late G_1 and S phases of the cell cycle.

PROTEIN FUNCTION

MYB contains DNA binding, transcriptional activation and negative regulatory domains and binds directly to double-stranded DNA, inducing DNA bending [9–12]. The consensus binding site is YAAC^G/$_T$G; most commonly: CCTAACTG [13] or YAAC^T/(C)/$_G$GYCA [14], from which intact MYB or v-MYB activates transcription.

MYB is essential for normal haematopoiesis. Cellular differentiation is accompanied by suppression of *MYB* expression and MYB is probably an important regulator of cell differentiation [5,15,16]. The generation in normal cells of multiple isoforms of *MYB* by alternative splicing and/or alternative initiation indicates that the protein products may have differing, tissue-specific roles [17].

There is a dramatic increase in *MYB* expression associated with generalized autoimmune diseases, which appears to occur in the greatly expanded population of CD4-8- cells. Studies in MRL-*lpr/lpr* mice, which carry the same defect, indicate the existence of specific nuclear DNA binding proteins that regulate *Myb* expression [18].

Regulation of gene expression by MYB

Genes *trans*-activated by MYB:

> *Mim-1* (*M*yb *i*nduced *m*yeloid protein-*1* – the only cellular gene known to be a direct target of MYB) [19]
> *MYB* [20]
> *MYC* [21]
> *CDC2* [22]
> *CD4* [23]
> T cell receptor δ enhancer [24]
> DNA polymerase α [25]
> Epstein–Barr virus (EBV) transcription factor Z (BZLF1) [26]
> Insulin-like growth factor I (IGF-I) [27,28]
> Human HSP70 [29]
> Ribonuclease A-related gene [30]
> *GATA-1* [31]
> HIV-1 and HTLV-1 LTRs [32–34]
> SV40 enhancer [35].

Cancer

Amplification of *MYB* has been detected in acute myeloblastic leukaemia (AML), chronic myelogenous leukaemia (CML), acute lymphoblastic leukaemia (ALL), T cell leukaemias, colon carcinomas and melanomas [36–43]. The stability of *MYB* and *MYC* mRNAs is increased in the cells of some AML patients [44]. Malignant haematopoietic colony forming units can be removed from the cells of CML patients by exposure to *MYB* antisense oligodeoxynucleotides (ODNs) [45] and proliferation of a variety of malignant cell lines is inhibited by *MYB* antisense ODNs [41,46]. Abnormal MYB expression has also been detected in some ovarian and breast carcinomas [47,48] and *MYB* mRNA is detectable in human neuroblastoma [16] and teratocarcinoma cell lines [49]. *MYBA* and *MYBB* are expressed in carcinoma and sarcoma-derived cell lines [50].

In animals

AMV induces acute myeloid leukaemia in chickens [51]. The recombinant avian leukosis virus (ALV) EU-8, injected into chicken embryos, induces a high incidence of B cell lymphomas [52], caused by proviral integration of EU-8 in the *Myb* locus. A similar metastatic lymphoma develops when chicken embryos are infected with the RAV-1 isolate of ALV [53]. The induction of lymphomas following infection of embryos, rather than the classic lymphoid leukosis caused by ALV in adult animals, implies that the target cells in which *Myb* is activated occur only in embryos. Chemically induced rat colon tumours have frequent rearrangements, insertions or deletions in the *Myb* and *Hras* loci [54].

Transgenic animals

Homozygous *Myb* mutant mice appear normal at day 13 of gestation but by day 15 are severely anaemic. Embryonic erythropoiesis is not impaired but adult-type erythropoiesis is greatly diminished [55]. This indicates that *Myb* is not essential for early development but may be required to maintain the proliferative state of haematopoietic progenitor cells

In vitro

AMV transforms macrophage precursors (monoblasts) *in vivo* and *in vitro*, chicken bone marrow cells and avian yolk-sac cells. It does not transform fibroblasts and may be a unique oncogene in this respect. E26 transforms fibroblasts (quail) and erythroid or myeloid cells. Erythroid cell transformation by E26 is caused by v-*ets* which has a cooperative effect with v-*myb* in this lineage, although neither the DNA binding domain nor the *trans*-activating domain of v-MYB is required [56,57]. E26 stimulates the proliferation of chicken neuroretina cells, as does AMV in the presence of basic fibroblast growth factor [58]. v-MYB appears to block differentiation [59] and, in normal or v-*myc* transformed macrophages, AMV or E26 cause "de-differentiation", inducing changes characteristic of immature cells [60].

GENE STRUCTURE

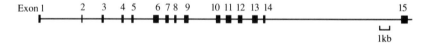

The organization of *MYB* sequences is not completely resolved. The complete chicken and human *MYB* genes are expressed as the result of an intermolecular recombination process involving coding sequences from transcription units on different chromosomes and a putative splicing factor (PR264) is encoded by the opposite strand of the *Myb trans*-spliced E_T exon [61]. As E_T bears 85% homology to the equivalent human and mouse exons and human E_T maps to a different chromosome to that carrying the remainder of *MYB*, it seems probable that the complex organization of the chicken gene reflects a general property of mammalian *MYB*.

TRANSCRIPTIONAL REGULATION

The promoters of chicken and mouse *Myb* contain GC-rich upstream regions with no TATA box (mouse) or with a TATA box that is not associated with a CAAT box (chicken). In murine *Myb* a positive intragenic regulatory mechanism operates via two tandem repeats of AP-1 sites in the first intron [62] (see also *FOS* and *MYC*). Thus the decrease in the level of *Myb* mRNA that accompanies differentiation of mouse erythroleukaemic cells correlates with a decrease in sequence-specific protein binding to this region. Transcriptional attenuation is also the major mechanism of regulation of human *MYB* during retinoic acid- or vitamin D$_3$-induced differentiation of HL-60 cells [63]. However, DMSO or phorbol ester regulate *MYB* expression by an additional, post-translational mechanism that, for DMSO, requires continuous transcription.

B-Myb transcription is maximal during the G$_1$ and S phases of the cell cycle. Transcription is regulated by p107/E2F and HPV16 E7 activates *B-Myb* transcription by directly interfering with this complex [64].

PROTEIN STRUCTURE

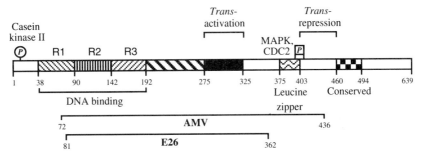

The overall identity between human and chicken MYB is 82%. AMV p45^{v-myb} is derived from chicken *Myb* via extensive 5' and 3' deletions, generating *myb*^{A} (lacking 71 N-terminal amino acids and 198 C-terminal amino acids of MYB, and with 11 point mutations). v-*myb* replaces 26 codons of the 3' end of *pol* and most of *env*. There are six *gag*-encoded amino acids and 33 bp of *env* give rise to 11 C-terminal amino acids [65]. E26 v-*myb* (*myb*^{E}) lacks 80 N-terminal and 278 C-terminal amino acids of p75^{myb}, has one point mutation and is expressed as p135$^{gag\text{-}myb\text{-}ets}$.

SEQUENCE OF MYB

```
  1   MARRPRHSIY SSDEDDEDFE MCDHDYDGLL PKSGKRHLGK TRWTREEDEK
 51   LKKLVEQNGT DDWKVIANYL PNRTDVQCQH RWQKVLNPEL IKGPWTKEED
101   QRVIELVQKY GPKRWSVIAK HLKGRIGKQC RERWHNHLNP EVKKTSWTEE
151   EDRIIYQAHK RLGNRWAEIA KLLPGRTDNA IKNHWNSTMR RKVEQEGYLQ
201   ESSKASQPAV ATSFQKNSHL MGFAQAPPTA QLPATGQPTV NNDYSYYHIS
251   EAQNVSSHVP YPVALHVNIV NVPQPAAAAI QRHYNDEDPE KEKRIKELEL
301   LLMSTENELK GQQVLPTQNH TCSYPGWHST TIADHTRPHG DSAPVSCLGE
351   HHSTPSLPAD PGSLPEESAS PARCMIVHQG TILDNVKNLL EFAETLQFID
401   SFLNTSSNHE NSDLEMPSLT STPLIGHKLT VTTPFHRDQT VKTQKENTVF
451   RTPAIKRSIL ESSPRTPTPF KHALAAQEIK YGPLKMLPQT PSHLVEDLQD
501   VIKQESDESG FVAEFQENGP PLLKKIKQEV ESPTDKSGNF FCSHHWEGDS
551   LNTQLFTQTS PVRDAPNILT SSVLMAPASE DEDNVLKAFT VPKNRSLASP
601   LQPCSSTWEP ASCGKMEEQM TSSSQARKYV NAFSARTLVM (640)
```

Domain structure

1–200	Dispersed nuclear localization signal
11–12	Casein kinase II phosphorylation sites which, when phosphorylated, reduce MYB binding to DNA [66]
34–86, 87–138, 139–189	Repeat regions R1 and R2 (essential for MYB binding to the MYB recognition element (pyAAC^G/$_T$G)) and R3 [67,68]. Deletion of R1 diminishes DNA binding and activates transformation of myeloid cells *in vitro* [69].
66–454	Homologous to the region of chicken MYB incorporated in AMV v-MYB (388 amino acids: underlined)
186–363	Homologous to chicken MYB expressed in P135*gag-myb-ets* with the substitution of Met152 for Arg337
43, 63, 82, 95, 115, 134, 166, 185	Conserved tryptophan residues in the R1, R2 and R3 domains (bold)
130	Cys130 is conserved in all MYB-related proteins. Its reduction is essential for MYB to bind to DNA and for transformation of myeloid cells [70,71]. The equivalent amino acid in v-MYB (Cys65) is essential for the transcription factor activity of v-MYB
275–325	Transcription activation domain that interacts with the MYB response element in the promoters of *Myc* and *Mim-1* [72,73]
383, 389, 396, 403	Leucine zipper [74] domain (bold) that interacts with cellular proteins, including the nuclear proteins p67 and p160 [75] (bold). Mutations in this region increase both the *trans*-activating and transforming capacities of MYB.

DATABASE ACCESSION NUMBERS

	PIR	*SWISSPROT*	*EMBL/GENBANK*	*REFERENCES*
Human *MYB*	A26661	P10242	M15024	[76]
			M13665, M13666	[77]
Human *MYBA*	S03423	P10243	X13294	[49]
Human *MYBB*	S01991	P10244	X13293	[49]
Human *MBM2*			X52125, X52126	[78]

References

1 **Shen-Ong, G.L.C. (1990) Biochim. Biophys. Acta 1032, 39–52.**
2 Gonda, T.J. and Metcalf, D. (1984) Nature 310, 249–251.
3 Sheiness, D. and Gardinier, M. (1984) Mol. Cell. Biol. 4, 1206–1212.
4 Duprey, S.P. and Boettiger, D. (1985) Proc. Natl Acad. Sci. USA 82, 6937–6941.
5 Thompson, C.B. et al. (1986) Nature 319, 374–380.
6 Brown, K.E. et al. (1992) J. Biol. Chem. 267, 4625–4630.
7 Simons, M. and Rosenberg, R.D. (1992) Circ. Res. 70, 835–843.
8 Queva, C. et al. (1992) Development 114, 125–133.
9 **Luscher, B. and Eisenman, R.N. (1990) Genes Devel. 4, 2235–2241.**
10 **Graf, T. (1992) Curr. Opin. Genetics Devel. 2, 249–255.**
11 Sakura, H. et al. (1989) Proc. Natl Acad. Sci. USA 86, 5758–5762.
12 Saikumar, P. et al. (1994) Oncogene 9, 1279–1287.
13 Biedenkapp, H. et al. (1988) Nature 335, 835–837.
14 Weston, K. (1992) Nucl. Acids Res. 20, 3043–3049.
15 Westin, E.H. et al. (1982) Proc. Natl Acad. Sci. USA 79, 2194–2198.
16 Thiele, C.J. et al. (1988) Mol. Cell. Biol. 8, 1677–1683.
17 Ramsay, R.G. et al. (1989) Oncogene Res. 4, 259–269.
18 Mountz, J.D. and Steinberg, A.D. (1989) J. Immunol. 142, 328–335.
19 Ness, S.A. et al. (1993) Genes Devel. 7, 749–759.
20 Nicolaides, N.C. et al. (1991) Mol. Cell. Biol. 11, 6166–6176.
21 Nakagoshi, H. et al. (1992) Oncogene 7, 1233–1239.
22 Ku, D.-H. et al. (1993) J. Biol. Chem. 268, 2255–2259.
23 Siu, G. et al. (1992) Mol. Cell. Biol. 12, 1592–1604.
24 Hernandez-Munain, C. and Krangel, M.S. (1994) Mol. Cell. Biol. 14, 473–483.
25 Sudo, T. et al. (1992) Oncogene 7, 1999–2006.
26 Kenney, S.C. et al. (1992) Mol. Cell. Biol. 12, 136–146.
27 Reiss, K. et al. (1991) Cancer Res. 51, 5997–6000.
28 Travali, S. et al. (1991) Mol. Cell. Biol. 11, 731–736.
29 Foos, G. et al. (1993) Oncogene 8, 1775–1782.
30 Nakano, T. and Graf, T. (1992) Oncogene 7, 527–534.
31 Aurigemma, R.E. et al. (1992) J. Virol. 66, 3056–3061.
32 Dasgupta, P. et al. (1990) Proc. Natl Acad. Sci. USA 87, 8090–8094.
33 Bosselut, R. et al. (1992) Virology 186, 764–769.
34 Dasgupta, P. et al. (1992) J. Virol. 66, 270–276.
35 Nishina, Y. et al. (1989) Nucl. Acids Res. 17, 107–117.
36 Alitalo, K. et al. (1984) Proc. Natl Acad. Sci. USA 81, 4534–4538.
37 Balaban, G.B. et al. (1984) Cancer Genet. Cytogenet. 11, 429–439.
38 Barletta, C. et al. (1987) Science 235, 1064–1067.
39 Griffin, C.A. and Baylin, S.B. (1985) Cancer Res. 45, 272–275.
40 Pellici, P.G. et al. (1984) Science 224, 1117–1121.
41 Slamon, D.J. et al. (1984) Science 224, 256–262.
42 Melani, C. et al. (1991) Cancer Res. 51, 2897–2901.
43 Tesch, H. et al. (1992) Leuk. Res. 16, 265–274.
44 Baer, M.R. et al. (1992) Blood 79, 1319–1326.
45 Ratajczak, M.Z. et al. (1992) Blood 79, 1956–1961.
46 Citro, G. et al. (1992) Proc. Natl Acad. Sci. USA 89, 7031–7035.

47 Guerin, M. et al. (1990) Oncogene 5, 131–135.

48 Barletta, C. et al. (1992) Eur. J. Gynaecol. Oncol. 13, 53–59.

49 Janssen, J.W.G. et al. (1986) Cytogenet. Cell. Genet. 41, 129–135.

50 Nomura, N. et al. (1988) Nucl. Acids Res. 16, 11075–11090.

51 Baluda, M.A. and Goetz, I.E. (1961) Virology 15, 185–199.

52 Kanter, M.R. et al. (1988) J. Virol. 62, 1423–1432.

53 Pizer, E. and Humphries, E.H. (1989) J. Virol. 63, 1630–1640.

54 Alexander, R.J. et al. (1992) Am. J. Med. Sci. 303, 16–24.

55 Mucenski, M.L. et al. (1991) Cell 65, 677–689.

56 Domenget, C. et al. (1992) Oncogene 7, 2231–2241.

57 Metz, T. and Graf, T. (1991) Genes Devel. 5, 369–380.

58 Garrido, C. et al. (1992) J. Virol. 66, 160–166.

59 Patel, G. et al. (1993) Mol. Cell. Biol. 13, 2269–2276.

60 Ness, S.A. et al. (1987) Cell 51, 41–50.

61 Vellard, M. et al. (1992) Proc. Natl Acad. Sci. USA 89, 2511–2515.

62 Reddy, C.D. and Reddy, E.P. (1989) Proc. Natl Acad. Sci. USA 86, 7326–7330.

63 Boise, L.H. et al. (1992) Oncogene 7, 1817–1825.

64 Lam, E.W.-F. et al. (1994) EMBO J. 13, 871–878.

65 Klempnauer, K.-H. et al. (1983) Cell 33, 345–355.

66 Luscher, B. et al. (1990) Nature 344, 517–522.

67 Howe, K.M. et al. (1990) EMBO J. 9, 161–169.

68 Oehler, T. et al. (1990) Nucl. Acids Res. 18, 1703–1710.

69 Dini, P.W. and Lipsick, J.S. (1993) Mol. Cell. Biol. 13, 7334–7348.

70 Grasser, F.A. et al. (1992) Oncogene 7, 1005–1009.

71 Guehmann, S. et al. (1992) Nucl. Acids Res. 20, 2279–2286.

72 Evans, J.L. et al. (1990) Mol. Cell. Biol. 10, 5747–5752.

73 Zobel, A. et al. (1991) Oncogene 6, 1397–1407.

74 Kanei-Ishii, C. et al. (1992) Proc. Natl Acad. Sci. USA 89, 3088–3092.

75 Favier, D. and Gonda, T. (1994) Oncogene 9, 305–311.

76 Majello B. et al. (1986) Proc. Natl Acad. Sci. USA 83, 9636–9640.

77 Slamon, D.J. et al. (1986) Science 233, 347–351.

78 Westin, E.H. et al. (1990) Oncogene 5, 1117–1124.

MYC

IDENTIFICATION

The v-*myc* oncogene was first detected in avian <u>my</u>elo<u>c</u>ytomatosis virus MC29 [1]. *Myc* has also been transduced by the acutely transforming avian retroviruses CMII, OK10, MH2 and FH3. *MYC* was detected by screening human DNA with an MC29 *myc* probe [2].

RELATED GENES

MYC is a member of the helix–loop–helix/leucine zipper superfamily. The *MYC* gene family contains at least seven closely related genes, *MYC, MYCN, MYCL, PMYC, RMYC, SMYC* and *BMYC*, together with *LMYC*Ψ, an inactive pseudogene.

	MYC	*MYCN*	*MYCL*	*v-myc* (MC29)
Nucleotides (kb)	6–7	6–7	6–7	5.7
Chromosome	8q24	2p24.1	1p32 (*MYCL1*) 7p15 (*MYCLK1*)	
Mass (kDa): predicted	49	49.5	40	96
expressed	64/67	66	60/66/68	P110$^{\Delta gag\text{-}myc}$

Cellular location

Nucleus.

Tissue distribution

MYC is expressed during proliferation in a wide variety of adult tissues and at all stages of embryonal development. *MYCN* and *MYCL* expression is generally restricted to embryonic brain, kidney and lung, suggesting their possible involvement in differentiation [3]. *Myc* is not expressed in invertebrates.

MYC protein concentration: undetectable in quiescent Swiss 3T3 fibroblasts; ~10^5 molecules/cell in Burkitt's lymphoma and other tumour cells [4,5].

PROTEIN FUNCTION

MYC, MYCN and MYCL are helix–loop–helix/leucine zipper (HLH/LZ) proteins that form sequence-specific (core consensus sequence CACGTG), DNA binding heterodimers with MAX [6] (see **MAX**). MYCN also binds to asymmetric (CATGTG) sequences [7]. MYC proteins do not dimerize with other HLH/LZ proteins (e.g. FOS, JUN, MyoD or E12).

Regulation of gene expression by MYC

Genes *trans*-activated directly or indirectly by highly expressed MYC or MYCN:

> Cyclins A and E [8]
> Human heat shock protein 70
> Ornithine decarboxylase [9]
> Adenovirus E4 (via the E1A activation region)
> α-Prothymosin and serum-inducible genes
> *Mr1* (plasminogen activator inhibitor-1) and *Mr2* fibroblast genes
> *ECA39*.

Genes *trans*-repressed directly or indirectly by highly expressed MYC or MYCN:

> MHC class I antigens [10]
> Lymphocyte function-related antigen-1 (LFA-1)
> Neural cell adhesion molecule (N-CAM)
> Collagen genes
> Mouse metallothionein I promoter.

Cell regulation

MYC is implicated in the control of normal proliferation, transformation and differentiation. Expression of *MYC* in untransformed cells is growth factor dependent and essential for progression through the cell cycle [11]. High levels of expression accelerate growth. Downregulation of *MYC* expression usually correlates with the onset of differentiation and constitutive expression interferes with normal differentiation. *MYCN* expression correlates with metastatic potential [12], consistent with the repressive effects of MYC on genes coding for MHC class I antigens and N-CAM.

In haematopoietic cells sustained expression of *MYC* accelerates apoptosis [13–16]. Genes that are known to cooperate with *MYC* in transformation, e.g. *Pim-1*, *BCL2*, *HRAS* and v-*raf*, may maintain cell viability without being directly mitogenic: in the absence of any of these gene products MYC may accelerate programmed cell death.

Cancer

MYC may be activated to become a transforming gene by proviral insertion, chromosomal translocation, or gene amplification. In general the result is to elevate expression of *MYC*, rather than to change the structure of the protein itself, although mutations may enhance pathogenicity [17]. Deletions 3′ of the *MYC* gene have been detected in *MYC* amplicons in some human tumour cell lines [18].

Deregulated *MYC* expression correlates with the occurrence of many types of human tumours, particularly small cell lung carcinoma (SCLC) [19], breast [20–22] and cervical carcinomas [23]. Enhanced transcription arising from translocation of *MYC* occurs in some but not all Burkitt's lymphomas, following translocation of the gene to the vicinity of the immunoglobulin enhancer [24-26]. In many such rearrangements the first (non-coding) exon is lost from the gene: mutations may occur in the *trans*-activation domain but are not typical [27].

MYC is induced during vitamin K_3-stimulated apoptosis of naso-pharyngeal carcinoma cells [28] and the high rate of apoptosis in Burkitt's lymphoma cells is suppressed when MYC protein levels are lowered [29].

MYCN is frequently amplified in neuroblastomas [30], retinoblastomas and SCLC. Expression correlates with appearance of the more severe forms of cervical intraepithelial carcinoma (CIN types II and III) and with increased metastasis in the advanced stages of neuroblastoma.

MYCL1 displays two allele polymorphism that can give rise to three genotypes (LL, LS and SS). Loss of heterozygosity at the *MYCL1* locus has been detected in breast and colon cancers and the SS genotype may contribute to the progression of colorectal cancer [31].

Transgenic animals

Myc can cause mammary carcinomas in transgenic mice [32,33]. Nevertheless excessive expression of *Myc* in transgenic mice does not prevent normal development and mammary tumours and lymphomas develop in a stochastic manner, indicating that overexpression of *Myc* is necessary but not sufficient for tumorigenesis.

In Eµ transgenics B cell tumour formation is accelerated by retroviral infection with Mo-MuLV. Identification of loci occupied by the integrated provirus (*Pim-1, Pim-2, Bmi-1, Pal-1, Bla-1* and *Emi-1*, see Table 2, page 33) shows that *Bmi-1* and *Pim-1* cooperate with *Myc* in tumour formation [34-37].

These observations are generally consistent with *in vitro* data indicating that alteration in the *Myc* content of cells, rather than mutation, activates its oncogenic potential and that transformation probably requires cooperation between MYC and other oncogene products including RAS.

Homozygous deletion of *Nmyc* results in embryonic lethality [38,39]. In these animals the lung airway epithelium is underdeveloped and death results from inability to oxygenate their blood.

In animals

Viruses expressing *Myc* cause myeloid leukaemias, sarcomas and carcinomas [40,41].

In vitro

Primary fibroblasts are immortalized by *Myc, Nmyc* or v-*myc* but are rendered tumorigenic only when activated *Ras* is also expressed [42]. Fibroblast cell lines, however, show reduced growth factor requirements and are tumorigenic when transfected with *Myc* alone. *Lmyc* also co-transforms primary cells with an activated *Ras* gene but is <10% as effective as *Myc*, a difference that reflects the relative potencies of the activation domains of the MYC proteins [43].

GENE STRUCTURE

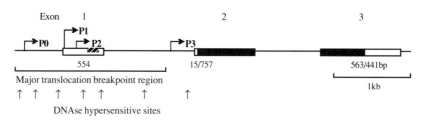

Exons 2 and 3 are 70%–90% identical between species and exon 1 is 70% conserved between the human and mouse genes. The three exon gene organization is similar in *MYCN* and *MYCL*.

The 5′ end of exon 1 (non-coding) includes two major transcriptional initiation sites (TATAA boxes), P1 and P2. Two minor promoters, P0 (upstream of P1) and P3 (near the 3′ end of intron 1) lack TATAA boxes. Cross-hatched bar: sequence upstream of the P2 initiation site that is the site of the conditional block to transcriptional elongation [44,45]. Two MYC proteins with different N-termini (p64/p67) arise from alternative translation initiation between AUG in exon 2 and a CUG codon near the 3′ end of exon 1.

The chicken *Myc* promoter has a high (~80%) GC content and binding sites for an SP1-like factor and a zinc finger CCCTC-binding factor (CTCF) [46].

TRANSCRIPTIONAL REGULATION

Regulatory elements mapped in the 5′ untranslated regions of *Myc* comprise AP-1 and AP-2 sites and the murine P2 promoter elements ME1a2, E2F and ME1a1 [47]. Murine *Myc* also has two NF-κB sites [48] and binding sites for MYC-associated zinc finger protein (MAZ) [49], MYC/PRF and MYC/CF1 (common factor 1, also identical to the zinc finger protein yin-yang 1 (YY1)) [50]. In addition to these sites regulatory elements upstream from −3500 (with respect to the mouse P1 promoter) and 1500 bp 3′ of the poly(A) sites are required for correct transcription *in vivo* [51].

Factors shown to bind within the human *MYC* promoter are nuclear factor 1 (NF1) [52], PuF and a ribonucleoprotein [53], FUSE-binding protein (FBP) that activates the far upstream element (FUSE) at −1500 relative to the P1 promoter [54], MSSP [55], TGFβ$_1$ and p105^{RB1} [56], E2F and p55 [57], *MYC* binding protein 1 (MBP1) [58], v-MYB and MYB [59] (see **MYB**), SP1, NF1 and CCAAT binding protein (CBP) [60] and the terminator binding factor TBF I [61].

The rapid increase in fibroblast mRNA from very low levels in G$_0$ cells that occurs on stimulation with EGF is due to relief of a block to transcriptional elongation, as evidenced by the high concentration of RNA polymerase II in the exon 1 region in G$_0$ cells. *In vitro* studies have defined a 95 bp 5′ region of exon 1 of the human *MYC* gene that specifies premature termination and the deletion of the first exon/intron region of *Myc* genes elevates the levels of mRNA and oncogenic activity [62,63]. The efficiency of premature termination sites declines markedly when they are placed >~400 bp from the start site [45]. A transcriptional inhibitor binds within intron 1 [64]. Point mutations that abolish binding occur in some Burkitt's lymphomas. Intragenic regulatory regions also occur in the *Fos* and *Myb* genes but the sequence in *MYC* is unrelated to the FIRE sequence of *Fos* [65].

Transcription of *MYC* and *MYCN* occurs in both the sense and antisense directions although the role of antisense transcription is unknown [66–68].

RNA STABILITY

Two regions within *MYC* mRNA regulate the half-life of the molecule: one is within the 3' untranslated region (three copies of AUUUA at the 3' end of exon 3) and the other is the C-terminal portion of the coding region (see also **FOS**). The 3' UTR is the stronger destabilizing element. Two proteins (37 kDa and 40 kDa) bind to AU-rich regions in the 3'-UTR of *MYC* and other unstable mRNAs and increase the *in vitro* rate of RNA degradation [69]. The C-terminal coding region determinant of stability requires translation for its efficient action [70]. A 75 kDa protein binds to this region of *Myc* mRNA and appears to confer stability on the transcript. In transgenic mice deletion of both the 5' and 3' non-coding sequences of the *MYC* gene do not affect MYC expression, indicating that in this system sequences of exon 2 and/or exon 3 are critical in post-transcriptional regulation [69].

In contrast to the effect of EGF, serum stimulation (which causes up to 40-fold elevation of *Myc* mRNA) increases initiation by stabilizing mRNA [71]. A human T cell leukaemia-derived cell line carries a translocation 24 nucleotides 5' of the first poly(A) addition signal of *MYC*. This replaces a 61 bp AU-rich region with sequences derived from chromosome 2 and causes a fivefold increase in *MYC* expression due to enhanced mRNA stability. The hybrid gene transforms rat fibroblasts to a tumorigenic phenotype [72]. This *MYC* rearrangement contrasts with those occurring in Burkitt's lymphoma and other cancers in that it does not involve TCR or Ig loci.

HUMAN MYC PROTEIN STRUCTURE

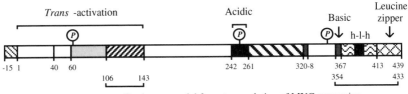

Regions essential for auto-regulation of MYC expression
and co-transformation with RAS

Cross-hatched box (–15 to 1): additional N-terminal region of p64 translated from a CUG codon in exon 1. Circles: phosphorylation sites. The major site for casein kinase II (CKII) phosphorylation, hyperphosphorylated during mitosis, is in the central acidic domain. MYCN is also phosphorylated by CKII. The acidic domain resembles those of other transcriptional activators. Deletions in this region have little effect on MYC/RAS co-transformation but in v-MYC they influence the transforming host range [73].

The v-MYC protein encoded by the CMII virus is identical to chicken MYC. Other viral forms contain scattered mutations including that of Thr61 (corresponding to human Thr58) [74].

SEQUENCE OF MYC

```
  1   MPLNVSFTNR NYDLDYDSVQ PYFYCDEEEN FYQQQQQSEL QPPAPSEDIW
 51   KKFELLPTPP LSPSRRSGLC SPSYVAVTPF SLRGDNDGGG GSFSTADQLE
101   MVTELLGGDM VNQSFICDPD DETFIKNIII QDCMWSGFSA AAKLVSEKLA
151   SYQAARKDSG SPNPARGHSV CSTSSLYLQD LSAAASECID PSVVFPYPLN
201   DSSSPKSCAS QDSSAFSPSS DSLLSSTESS PQGSPEPLVL HEETPPTTSS
251   DSEEEQEDEE EIDVVSVEKR QAPGKRSESG SPSAGGHSKP PHSPLVLKRC
301   HVSTHQHNYA APPSTRKDYP AAKRVKLDSV RVLRQISNNR KCTSPRSSDT
351   EENVKRRTHN VLERQRRNEL KRSFFALRDQ IPELENNEKA PKVVILKKAT
401   AYILSVQAEE QKLISEEDLL RKRREQLKHK LEQLRNSCA (439)
```

Domain structure

–15–1	15 amino acid N-terminal extension in p67 (MDFFRVVENQQPPAT)
58	MAP kinase and glycogen synthase 3-kinase phosphorylation site [75]. Thr58 is mutated to a non-phosphorylatable residue in the MC29, MH2 and OK10 v-MYC proteins and is also frequently mutated in Burkitt's lymphoma [27, 76]
33–245	Region over which point mutations occur in Burkitt's lymphoma [27, 77]
62	Ser62 is phosphorylated by MAP kinases (ERK, ERT (EGF receptor Thr699) and MAP2 protein kinase). Ser62 is within a p34^{CDC2} kinase recognition motif but MYC is not phosphorylated by p34^{CDC2} *in vitro* [78]. Phosphorylation of Thr58 and Ser62 is necessary for high levels of *trans*-activation by MYC [79]
355–367	Basic region (underlined)
413–437	Leucine zipper (underlined)
290–318	Non-specific DNA binding region
359	His359 corresponds to avian His336 that contacts or is close to the thymine 5-methyl group at position 2 of the DNA half site [80]: the homologous residue in MAX recognizes the same site

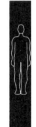

364–374 Incomplete nuclear localization signal: highly conserved between MYC, MYCN and MYCL and essential for oncogenicity

106–143 and 354–433 Essential for *Ras* complementation in transforming normal rat embryo cells: these domains are conserved in MYCN and MYCL (MYC box proteins). Deletion of 106–143 dominantly inhibits the cooperation of normal MYC with oncogenic RAS to transform rat embryo fibroblasts

SEQUENCE OF MYCL

```
  1  MDYDSYQHYF YDYDCGEDFY RSTAPSEDIW KKFELVPSPP TSPPWGLGPG
 51  AGDPAPGIGP PEPWPGGCTG DEAESRGHSK GWGRNYASII RRDCMWSGFS
101  ARERLERAVS DRLAPGAPRG NPPKASAAPD CTPSLEAGNP APAAPCPLGE
151  PKTQACSGSE SPSDSENEEI DVVTVEKRQS LGIRKPVTIT VRADPLDPCM
201  KHFHISIHQQ QHNYAARFPP ESCSQEEASE RGPQEEVLER DAAGEKEDEE
251  DEEIVSPPPV ESEAAQSCHP KPVSSDTEDV TKRKNHNFLE RKRRNDLRSR
301  FLALRDQVPT LASCSKAPKV VILSKALEYL QALVGAEKRM ATEKRQLRCR
351  QQQLQKRIAY LSGY (364)
```

Domain structure

343–361   Leucine zipper (underlined)

SEQUENCE OF MYCN

```
  1  MPSCSTSTMP GMICKNPDLE FDSLQPCFYP DEDDFYFGGP DSTPPGEDIW
 51  KKFELLPTPP LSPSRGFAEH SSEPPSWVTE MLLENELWGS PAEEDAFGLG
101  GLGGLTPNPV ILQDCMWSGF SAREKLERAV SEKLQHGRGP PTAGSTAQSP
151  GAGAASPAGR GHGGAAGAGR AGAALPAELA HPAAECVDPA VVFPFPVNKR
201  EPAPVPAAPA SAPAAGPAVA SGAGIAAPAG APGVAPPRPG GRQTSGGDHK
251  ALSTSGEDTL SDSDDEDDEE EDEEEIDVV TVEKRRSSSN TKAVTTFTIT
301  VRPKNAALGP GRAQSSELIL KRCLPIHQQH NYAAPSPYVE SEDAPPQKKI
351  KSEASPRPLK SVIPPKAKSL SPRNSDSEDS ERRRNHNILE RQRRNDLRSS
401  FLTLRDHVPE LVKNEKAAKV VILKKATEYV HSLQAEEHQL LLEKEKLQAR
451  QQQLLKKIEH ARTC (464)
```

Domain structure

262–278   AU-rich (acidic)
433–454   Leucine zipper (underlined)
261, 263 Phosphorylation by casein kinase II

DATABASE ACCESSION NUMBERS

	PIR	SWISSPROT	EMBL/GENBANK	REFERENCES
Human *MYC*	A10349	P01106; P01107	X00196, X00364	81
	A10350		V00568	82–86
Human *MYCL1*	A27675	P12524	M19720	87
			X07262, X07263	
Human *MYCL2*	A30146	P12525	J03069	88
Human *MYCN*	A01355	P04198	M13228, M13241	89
	A22937		X03294, X03295	90
	A25744		X02363	91
	S02249		Y00664	92, 93
AMV-MC 29	A01353	P01110	V01173, V01174	94, 95
v-*myc*				

References

1 Sheiness, D. and Bishop, M.J. (1979) J. Virol. 31, 514–521.
2 Eva, A. et al. (1982) Nature 295, 116–119.
3 Zimmerman, K.A. et al. (1986) Nature 319, 780–783.
4 Moore, J.P. et al. (1987) Oncogene Res. 2, 65–80.
5 Waters, C.M. et al. (1991) Oncogene 6, 797–805.
6 Blackwood, E.M. and Eisenman, R.N. (1991) Science 251, 1211–1217.
7 Ma, A. et al. (1993) Oncogene 8, 1093–1098.
8 Jansen-Durr, P. et al. (1993) Proc. Natl Acad. Sci. USA 90, 3685–3689.
9 Bello-Fernandez, C. et al. (1993) Proc. Natl Acad. Sci. USA 90, 7804–7808
10 Schrier, P.I. and Peltenburg, L.T.C. (1993) Adv. Cancer Res. 60, 181–246.
11 Seth, A. et al. (1993) Mol. Cell. Biol. 13, 4125–4136.
12 Bernards, R. et al. (1986) Cell 47, 667–674.
13 Askew, D.S. et al. (1991) Oncogene 6, 1915–1922.
14 Williams, G.T. (1991) Cell 65, 1097–1098.
15 Shi, Y. et al. (1992) Science 257, 212–214.
16 Evan, G.I. et al. (1992) Cell 69, 119–128.
17 Symonds, G. et al. (1989) Oncogene 4, 285–294.
18 Feo, S. et al. (1994) Oncogene 9, 955–961.
19 Gazdar, A.F. et al. (1985) Cancer Res. 45, 2924–2930.
20 Guerin, M. et al. (1988) Oncogene Res. 3, 21–31.
21 Tsuda, H. et al. (1989) Cancer Res. 49, 3104–3108.
22 Mariani-Costantini, R. et al. (1988) Cancer Res. 48, 199–205.
23 Ocadiz, R. et al. (1987) Cancer Res. 47, 4173–4177.
24 DePinho, R.A. et al. (1991) Adv. Cancer Res. 57, 1–46.
25 MaGrath, I. (1990) Adv. Cancer Res. 55, 133–270.
26 Polack, A. et al. (1993) EMBO J. 12, 3913–3920.
27 Albert, T. et al. (1994) Oncogene 9, 759–763.
28 Wu, F.Y.-H. et al. (1993) Oncogene 8, 2237–2244.
29 Milner, A.E. et al. (1993) Oncogene 8, 3385–3391.
30 Schwab, M. et al. (1983) Nature 305, 245–248.
31 Young, J. et al. (1994) Oncogene 9, 1053, 1056.
32 Sinn, E. et al. (1987) Cell 49, 465–475.

33 Schoenenberger, C.A. et al. (1988) EMBO J. 7, 169–175.
34 van Lohuizen, M. et al. (1991) Cell 65, 737–752.
35 Haupt, Y. et al. (1991) Cell 65, 753–763.
36 Verbeek, S. et al. (1991) Mol. Cell. Biol. 11, 1176–1179.
37 Moroy, T. et al. (1991) Oncogene 6, 1941–1948.
38 Sawai, S. et al. (1991) New Biol. 3, 861–869.
39 Moens, C.B. et al. (1992) Genes Devel. 6, 691–704.
40 Bister, K. and Jansen, H.W. (1986) Adv. Cancer Res. 47, 99–188.
41 Chen, C. et al. (1989) J. Virol., 63, 5092–5100.
42 Schreiber-Agus, N. et al. (1993) Mol. Cell. Biol. 13, 2765–2775.
43 Barrett, J. et al. (1992) Mol. Cell. Biol. 12, 3130–3137.
44 Krumm, A. et al. (1992) Genes Devel. 6, 2201–2213.
45 Roberts, S. and Bentley, D.L. (1992) EMBO J. 11, 1085–1093.
46 Klenova, E.M. et al. (1993) Mol. Cell. Biol. 13, 7612–7624.
47 Dufort, D. et al. (1993) Oncogene 8, 165–171.
48 Kessler, D.J. et al. (1992) Oncogene 7, 2447–2453.
49 Bossone, S.A. et al. (1992) Proc. Natl Acad. Sci. USA 89, 7452–7456.
50 Lee, T.C. et al. (1994) Oncogene 9, 1047–1052.
51 Lavenu, A. et al. (1994) Oncogene 9, 527–536.
52 Siebenlist, U. et al. (1984) Cell 37, 381–391.
53 Spencer, C.A. and Groudine, M. (1990) Adv. Cancer Res. 56, 1–48.
54 Duncan, R. et al. (1994) Genes Devel. 8, 465–480.
55 Negishi, Y. et al. (1994) Oncogene 9, 1133–1143.
56 Pietenpol, J.A. et al. (1991) Proc. Natl Acad. Sci. USA 88, 10227–10231.
57 Parkin, N.T. and Sonenberg, N. (1989) Oncogene 4, 815–822.
58 Ray, R. and Miller, D.M. (1991) Mol. Cell. Biol. 11, 2154–2161.
59 Cogswell, J.P. et al. (1993) Mol. Cell. Biol. 13, 2858–2869.
60 Lang, J.C. et al. (1991) Oncogene 6, 2067–2075.
61 Roberts, S. et al. (1992) Genes Devel. 6, 1562–1574.
62 Xu, L. et al. (1993) Oncogene 8, 2547–2553.
63 Strobl, L.J. et al. (1993) Oncogene 8, 1437–1447.
64 Zajac-Kaye, M. et al. (1988) Science 240, 1776–1780.
65 Tourkine, N. et al. (1989) Oncogene 4, 973–978.
66 Nepveu, A. and Marcu, K.B. (1986) EMBO J. 5, 2859–2865.
67 Krystal, G.W. et al. (1990) Mol. Cell. Biol. 10, 4180–4191.
68 Celano, P. et al. (1992) J. Biol. Chem. 267, 15092–15096.
69 Morello, D. et al. (1993) Oncogene 8, 1921–1929.
70 Herrick, D.J. and Ross, J. (1994) Mol. Cell. Biol. 14, 2119–2128.
71 Nepveu, A. et al. (1987) Oncogene 1, 243–250.
72 Aghib, D.F. and Bishop, M.J. (1991) Oncogene 6, 2371–2375.
73 Heaney, M.L. et al. (1986) J. Virol. 60, 167–176.
74 Frykberg, L. et al. (1987) Oncogene 1, 415–421.
75 Henriksson, M et al. (1993) Oncogene 8, 3199–3209.
76 Pulverer, B.J. et al. (1994) Oncogene 9, 59–70.
77 Bhatia, K. et al. (1993) Nature, Genetics 5, 56–61.
78 Luscher, B. and Eisenman, R.N. (1992) J. Cell Biol. 118, 775–784.
79 Gupta, S. et al. (1993) Proc. Natl Acad. Sci. USA 90, 3216–3220.
80 Dong, Q., et al. (1994) EMBO J. 13, 200–204.
81 Colby, W.W. et al. (1983) Nature 301, 722–725.

82 Saito, H. et al. (1983) Proc. Natl Acad. Sci. USA 80, 7476–7480.

83 Watt, R. et al. (1983) Nature 303, 725–728.

84 Bernard, O. et al. (1983) EMBO J. 2, 2375–2383.

85 Rabbitts, T.H. et al. (1983) Nature 306, 760–765.

86 Gazin, C. et al. (1984) EMBO J. 3, 383–387.

87 Kaye, F. J. et al. (1988) Mol. Cell. Biol. 8, 186–195.

88 Morton, C.C. et al. (1989) Genomics 4, 367–375.

89 Slamon, D.J. et al. (1986) Science 232, 768–772.

90 Stanton, L.W. et al. (1986) Proc. Natl Acad. Sci. USA 83, 1772–1776.

91 Kohl, N.E. et al. (1986) Nature 319, 73–77.

92 Ibson, J.M. and Rabbitts, P.H. (1988) Oncogene 2, 399–402.

93 Michitsch, R.W. et al. (1985) Nucl. Acids Res. 13, 2545–2558.

94 Alitalo, K. et al. (1983) Proc. Natl Acad. Sci. USA. 80, 100–104.

95 Reddy, E.P. et al. (1983) Proc. Natl Acad. Sci. USA 80, 2500–2504.

IDENTIFICATION

v-*sis* is the acutely transforming oncogene of <u>si</u>mian <u>s</u>arcoma virus (SSV) isolated from woolly monkey sarcoma and derived from the platelet-derived growth factor B chain gene (*Pdgfb*).

RELATED GENES

The 3' untranslated regions of *PDGFB* share sequence homology with the corresponding regions of human *IL2*, human IFNβ₁, human and mouse NGFβ and proenkephalin. PDGFB is 60% similar to PDGFA.

	PDGFB	**v-*sis***
Nucleotides (kb)	24	5.1 (SSV)
Chromosome	22q12.3–212	212q13.1
Mass (kDa): predicted	27	33
expressed	26	28

Cellular location

PDGFB: Secreted. v-SIS: PDGFR-associated.

Tissue distribution

PDGF is a disulphide-bonded dimer of two chains (A and B) that occurs in three forms (AA, BB and AB). PDGFB is generated by proteolytic cleavage of a precursor. PDGF is released from the α granules of platelets during blood clotting but is also synthesized by many other types of cell and all three forms occur in both normal and transformed cells [1].

v-SIS is detectable in SSV-transformed NRK cells [2]. It is retained at the cell surface by virtue of a hydrophilic membrane retention domain located at the C-terminus and functions by interaction with the PDGF receptor [3].

PROTEIN FUNCTION

PDGF is the major growth factor in human serum and is a potent mitogen *in vitro*.

Cancer

PDGF and *PDGF* receptor genes are co-expressed in primary human astrocytomas [4] and *PDGFB* transcription occurs in fibrosarcomas and glioblastomas. Malignant mesothelioma cell lines express primarily PDGFB receptors (and PDGFB) whereas the equivalent normal cells express only PDGFA receptors [5] and synthesize only PDGFA. This suggests that both types of cell may undergo autocrine stimulation, PDGF-AA acting via the α receptor and PDGF-BB via the β receptor [6].

PDGFB is translocated to chromosome 9 in CML (i.e. the reciprocal translocation to that undergone by *ABL*). There is no evidence that the translocated gene is transcribed, however, and *PDGFB* probably does not play a role in CML.

In animals

SSV induces fibrosarcomas and glioblastomas in monkeys [7]. In human WM9 melanoma cells expression of PDGF-BB promotes vascularization of the tumours that arise when the cells are injected into mice.

In vitro

SSV transforms rat kidney cells into a fibroblastic morphology unusual for cells infected by acute transforming viruses and also transforms fibroblasts. Suramin, a polyanionic drug used clinically for parasitic infections, disrupts PDGF ligand–receptor binding and induces reversion of fibroblasts transformed by v-*sis* [8].

Murine cell lines overexpressing v-*sis*/*Pdgfb* are highly tumorigenic: *in vitro* their growth is independent of the presence of PDGF and they show constitutively high expression of *Myc*, *Fos*, *Jun* and *Jund* but not of other early response genes (*Fra-1*, *Fosb*, *Junb* and *Krox20*) [9], emphasizing the probable importance of *Myc*, *Fos*, *Jun* and *Jund* in the regulation of growth.

STRUCTURE OF THE HUMAN *PDGFB* GENE

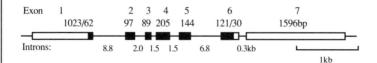

STRUCTURE OF v-SIS AND HUMAN PDGFB

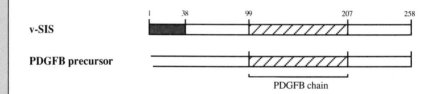

The PDGFB precursor undergoes proteolytic cleavage to generate a final form in which the N- and C-termini correspond to amino acids 99 and 207 of v-SIS, respectively [10]. Residues 99–207 of v-SIS (220 amino acids) differ in only four positions from the 108 residues of PDGFB.

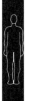

SEQUENCE OF PDGFB PRECURSOR

```
  1  MNRCWALFLS LCCYLRLVSA EGDPIPEELY EMLSDHSIRS FDDLQRLLHG
 51  DPGEEDGAEL DLNMTRSHSG GELESLARGR RSLGSLTIAE PAMIAECKTR
101  TEVFEISRRL IDRTNANFLV WPPCVEVQRC SGCCNNRNVQ CRPTQVQLRP
151  VQVRKIEIVR KKPIFKKATV TLEDHLACKC ETVAAARPVT RSPGGSQEQR
201  AKTPQTRVTI RTVRVRRPPK GKHRKFKHTH DKTALKETLG A (241)
```

Domain structure

1–20	Signal sequence (italics)
21–81 and 191–241	Propeptide
82–190	PDGFB (underlined)
108 and 111	Involved in receptor binding
97–141, 130–178, 134–180	Disulphide bonds
124–133	Interchain disulphide bond

DATABASE ACCESSION NUMBERS

	PIR	SWISSPROT	EMBL/GENBANK	REFERENCES
Human *PDGFB*	A94276	P01127	M12783	11
(*PDGF2* or *SIS*)				12
			K01913 to K01916	13, 14
			M16288	15
			X03702	16–18
Human *SIS*			V00504	19
(v-*sis* homologous region)				
Human *SIS* (3′ flank)			M32009	20
Human *SIS* (clone pSM-1)			X02744	16

References

1 **Heldin, C.-H. and Westermark, B. (1990) J. Cell Sci. 96, 193–196.**
2 Devare, S.G. et al. (1983) Proc. Natl Acad. Sci. USA 80, 731–735.
3 LaRochelle, W.J. et al. (1991) Genes Devel. 5, 1191–1199.
4 Maxwell, M. et al. (1990) J. Clin. Invest. 86, 131–140.
5 Versnel, M.A. et al. (1991) Oncogene 6, 2005–2011.
6 **Heldin, C.-H. (1992) EMBO J., 11, 4251–4259.**
7 Wolfe, L.G. et al. (1972) J. Natl Cancer Inst. 48, 1905–1907.
8 Fleming, T.P. et al. (1989) Proc. Natl Acad. Sci. USA 86, 8063–8067.
9 Sonobe, M.H. et al. (1991) Oncogene 6, 1531–1537.
10 Robbins, K.C. et al. (1983) Nature 305, 605–608.
11 Rao, C.D. et al. (1986) Proc. Natl Acad. Sci. USA 83, 2392–2396.
12 Antoniades, H.N. and Hunkapiller, M.W. (1983) Science 220, 963–965.
13 Chiu, I.-M. et al. (1984) Cell 37, 123–129.
14 Collins, T. et al. (1985) Nature 316, 748–750.
15 Josephs, S.F. et al. (1984) Science 225, 636–639.
16 Ratner, L. et al. (1985) Nucl. Acids Res. 13, 5007–5018.
17 Waterfield, M.D. et al. (1983) Nature 304, 35–39.

18 Weich, H.A. et al. (1986) FEBS Letts 198, 344–348; erratum in FEBS Letts (1986) 201, 180.

19 Josephs, S.F. et al. (1983) Science 219, 503–505.

20 Tong, B.D. et al. (1986) Mol. Cell. Biol. 6, 3018–3022.

PIM1

IDENTIFICATION

Pim-1 was first identified as a common proviral integration site in MuLV-induced murine T cell lymphomas.

RELATED GENES

PIM1 has extensive homology with the protein kinase gene family, high homology with the γ subunit of phosphorylase kinase, C-terminal homology with ABL and N-terminal homology with MOS.

Nucleotides (kb)	5
Chromosome	6p21
Mass (kDa): predicted	35.7
expressed	35

Cellular location

Cytoplasm.

Tissue distribution

PIM1 is expressed at high concentrations in haematopoietic tissues, testes and ovaries and in embryonic stem cells [1,2]. Alternative gene products arise in rodents from variable polyadenylation and the use of different translational initiation codons [3,4].

PROTEIN FUNCTION

PIM1 is a serine/threonine protein kinase that may be involved in early B and T cell lymphomagenesis [5]. However, physiological substrates have not been identified and Pim-1-deficient mice are apparently normal in all respects other than in having a decreased erythrocyte mean cell volume [6].

Cancer

Enhanced PIM1 transcription occurs in some acute myeloid and lymphoid leukaemias [1,7] although the 6;9 translocation is not the direct cause [8]. Thus, although the PIM1 human chromosome site (6p21) is fragile, elevated PIM1 protein synthesis occurs in many human leukaemias by mechanisms other than translocation or amplification.

Transgenic animals

Pim-1 is the integration locus of Mo-MuLV in 35% of B cell lymphomas generated in Eμ-myc transgenic mice [9]. Transgenic animals overexpressing Pim-1 in lymphoid cells show a low frequency of predisposition to lymphomagenesis but have a greatly increased susceptibility to tumour induction by MuLV or by *N*-ethyl-nitrosourea [10]. Tumours overexpressing *Pim-1* also show activation of *Myc*, *Nmyc* and *Pal-1* (see **MYC**: Transgenic animals).

In animals

Pim-1 and *Myc* are the most frequently occupied insertion sites in MuLV-induced tumours and both may be activated within the same cell lineage [11,12]. Activation of *Pim-1* also occurs in B cell lymphomas [13] and in murine thymomas induced by NMU [14].

In vitro

Pim-1 alone does not transform 3T3 fibroblasts but causes transformation in cooperation with *Myc* or *Ras*. *Pim-1* does not appear to be necessary for proliferation or differentiation of embryonic stem cells *in vitro* [15].

GENE STRUCTURE OF *PIM1*

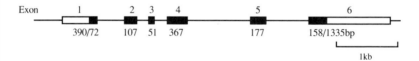

The human and murine genes share >80% identity and the proteins are 94% identical.

TRANSCRIPTIONAL REGULATION

The *PIM1* promoter does not contain TATA or CAAT box sequences but has consensus binding sites for AP1, AP2, SP1, NF-κB, NF-A2 (Oct2) and PIM1 promoter factor-348.

Proviral activation of murine *Pim-1* involves elevated transcription by enhancer insertion and, usually, removal of 3′ untranslated (ATTT)$_5$ sequences that destabilize mRNAs. The protein coding domain is unaffected by insertions and the transforming effects of *Pim-1* are thus due to abnormally high expression of the gene.

In most lymphomas the provirus is integrated within the *Pim-1* gene and has duplicated or triplicated enhancer regions within their LTRs. Integrations within the gene (in the 3′ untranslated region) or 3′ of the gene are all in the same transcriptional orientation as *Pim-1*. The concentration of *Pim-1* mRNA is higher in such tumours than when integration is outside the transcription unit: transcription is terminated at the poly(A) signal in the 5′ LTR, generating truncated *Pim-1* transcripts lacking up to 1300 bases.

Proviruses integrated upstream of *Pim-1* and in the same transcriptional orientation have intact 5′ and 3′ LTRs but major internal deletions. Such integrations do not provide a promoter for *Pim-1*, nor do they alter the transcript size: thus transcriptional enhancement appears to be the mechanism of activation for integrations outside coding regions of *Pim-1*.

SEQUENCE OF PIM

```
  1  MLLSKINSLA HLRAAPCNDL HATKLAPGKE KEPLESQYQV GPLLGSGGFG
 51  SVYSGIRVSD NLPVAIKHVE KDRISDWGEL PNGTRVPMEV VLLKKVSSGF
101  SGVIRLLDWF ERPDSFVLIL ERPEPVQDLF DFITERGALQ EELARSFFWQ
151  VLEAVRHCHN CGVLHRDIKD ENILIDLNRG ELKLIDFGSG ALLKDTVYTD
201  FDGTRVYSPP EWIRYHRYHG RSAAVWSLGI LLYDMVCGDI PFEHDEEIIR
251  GQVFFRQRVS SECQHLIRWC LALRPSDRPT FEEIQNHPWM QDVLLPQETA
301  EIHLHSLSPG PSK (313)
```

Domain structure

44–52 and 67   ATP binding site (underlined)
        167   Active site

DATABASE ACCESSION NUMBERS

	PIR	SWISSPROT	EMBL/GENBANK	REFERENCES
Human *PIM1*	A27476, JU0327	P11309	M27903	16
			M16750, M54915	17, 18

References
1 Amson, R. et al. (1989) Proc. Natl Acad. Sci. USA 86, 8857–8861.
2 Meeker, T.C. et al. (1990) Mol. Cell. Biol. 10, 1680–1688.
3 Saris, C.J.M. et al. (1991) EMBO J. 10, 655–664.
4 Wingett, D. et al. (1992) Nucl. Acids Res. 20, 3183–3189.
5 Dautry, F. et al. (1988) J. Biol. Chem. 263, 17615–17620.
6 Laird, P.W. et al. (1993) Nucl. Acids Res. 21, 4750–4755.
7 Nagarajan, L. et al. (1986) Proc. Natl Acad. Sci. USA 83, 2556–2560.
8 von Lindern, M. et al. (1989) Oncogene 4, 75–79.
9 van Lohuizen, M. et al. (1991) Cell 65, 737–752.
10 Breuer, M. et al. (1991) Cancer Res. 51, 958–963.
11 Selten, G. et al. (1984) EMBO J. 3, 3215–3222.
12 O'Donnell, P.V. et al. (1985) J. Virol. 55, 500–503.
13 Mucenski, M.L. et al. (1987) Oncogene Res. 2, 33–48.
14 Warren, W. et al. (1987) Carcinogenesis 8, 163–172.
15 te Riel, H. et al. (1990) Nature 348, 649–651.
16 Reeves, R. et al. (1990) Gene 90, 303–307.
17 Zakut-Houri, R. et al. (1987) Gene 54, 105–111.
18 Domen, J. et al. (1987) Oncogene Res. 1, 103–112.

IDENTIFICATION

v-*raf* is the oncogene of murine transforming retrovirus (MSV) 3611. 3611-MSV arose after transforming gene rescue in culture with MuLV followed by infection of a mouse treated with butylnitrosourea (BNU). This mouse developed histiocytic lymphoma and lung adenocarcinoma.

The mammalian *RAF* family (*RAF1*, *RAFA1* and *RAFB1* (murine *Raf-1*, *Araf-1* and *Braf-1*)) were detected by screening genomic libraries with v-*raf* probes.

RELATED GENES

RAF1, *RAFA1* and *RAFB1* are members of the *RAF–MOS* subfamily and the *SRC* super-family of protein kinases [1]. *RAF1P1/RAF2*, *ARAF2* and *BRAF2* are pseudogenes. The avian homologue of *Raf* is v-*mil* (see **Mil**). Other *RAF1*-related genes are: *PKS*, Xe-*raf* (*Xenopus laevis*) D-*raf-1*, D-*raf-2* (*Drosophila melanogaster*) and *Elegans raf-1* (*Caenorhabditis elegans*).

		RAFA1	RAFB1	RAF1	v-raf
Nucleotides (kb)		11	Not fully mapped	>100	1.1 7.6 (3611-MSV)
Chromosome		Xp11.2	7q33–36	3p25	
Mass (kDa):	**predicted**	67.5	84/72.5	73	37 (v-*raf*)
	expressed	68	73/95	70–74 (pp74–pp78) 150 (activated)	gp90*gag-raf* P75*gag-raf*

Cellular location

Cytosolic.

Tissue distribution

RAFA1: Predominantly urogenital tissues. RAFB1: Cerebrum, testes. RAF1: Ubiquitous.

PROTEIN FUNCTION

RAF genes encode serine/threonine protein kinases. RAF1 is positively regulated by serine/tyrosine phosphorylation [2] and has no auto-phosphorylating protein kinase activity (unlike Δ*gag-v-raf* and Δ*gag-v-mil*) [3]. The ubiquitous distribution of RAF1 suggests that it may have a basic regulatory function. *Xenopus* RAF1 appears to mediate the developmental effects of basic fibroblast growth factor during mesoderm induction [4].

In NIH 3T3 cells RAF1 undergoes rapid phosphorylation, mainly on serine and threonine, in response to PDGF, EGF, insulin, thrombin, endothelin, acidic FGF, CSF1 or TPA, and also in response to the oncoproteins of v-*fms*, v-*src*, v-*sis*, *Hras* or polyoma middle T antigen [5–10]. RAF1 protein complexes with the activated PDGF β receptor and with RAS–GTP in intact, stimulated cells [11–13]. The activated enzyme is translocated to the perinuclear region and the nucleus. RAF1 is also activated in mitogenically stimulated epithelial and lymphoid cells [14–18].

RAF1 activates MAP kinase kinase (MAPK-K) in NIH 3T3 cells which in turn stimulates the MAP kinases ERK1 and ERK2, resulting in phosphorylation of p62^{TCF} (see **FOS**) and JUN (see ***JUN***). MAPK-K, ERK1 and ERK2 are constitutively active in v-*raf*-transformed cells [19–23] and RAF1 is itself an *in vitro* substrate for MAPK-K [19].

RAF oncoproteins *trans*-activate expression of genes driven by AP-1, ETS and NF-κB binding motifs [24–26]. Transfection of a v-*raf* expression vector into NIH 3T3 cells induces transcription of the growth factor-regulated early response genes *Egr-1*, *Fos* and β-actin [27–30]. The expression of v-*raf* or *RAF1* activates transcription of the *MDR1* multidrug resistance genes in human and rodent cells [31].

Revertant cell lines that suppress transformation by v-*ras* carrying viruses and by v-*fes* or v-*src* are transformed by v-*fms*, v-*mos* or v-*sis* and by 3611-MSV or *Araf*-MSV [32,33]. Furthermore, neither microinjection of anti-RAS antibody nor block of RAS activity by mutation affects growth in cells transformed by *Raf* or *Mos*. Thus *Raf*, *Fms*, *Mos* and *Sis* are the only oncogenes that appear to function independently of *Ras*. In NIH 3T3 cells expression of *Raf-1* antisense RNA inhibits proliferation, causes reversion of *Raf*-transformed cells and blocks transformation by *Kras* or *Hras* [34]. Thus RAF1 functions downstream of *Ras*.

Ras and *Raf-1* cooperate to transform NIH 3T3 cells and dominant negative mutants of *Ras* inhibit the activation of RAF1 kinase in NIH 3T3 cells stimulated by serum or TPA and of both RAF1 and BRAF1 in NGF-stimulated PC-12 cells [35], indicating that RAS may control the coupling of growth factor receptors and protein kinase C to cytosolic RAF kinases. This

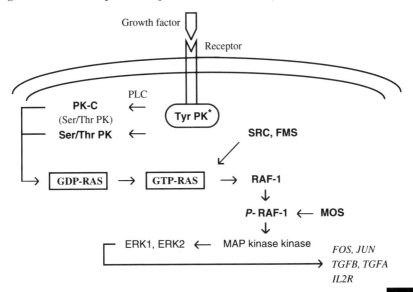

is consistent with the finding that N-terminally truncated, oncogenic RAF activates the MAP kinase ERK2 independently of RAS function [20] and that the kinase activity of RAF-1 is enhanced as a result of direct phosphorylation by protein kinase Cα, β or γ [36,37].

The generalized scheme summarizes the above data, indicating that RAF1 kinase may be activated by a wide variety of receptors with intrinsic tyrosine kinase activity or by receptors that interact with tyrosine kinases (e.g. CD4). RAS may mediate coupling to RAF1 of pathways that either require or are independent of protein kinase C.

Cancer

Oncogenic *RAF1* has been detected by transfection of DNA from a primary stomach cancer [38], laryngeal [39], lung and other carcinomas and sarcomas [40] and a glioblastoma cell line [41]. High levels of *RAF1* expression occur in many small cell lung cancers (SCLC) and derived cell lines [42]. *RAF1* is also amplified in some non-small cell lung cancers [43].

In animals

The oncogenically active v-*raf*, derived from mouse *Raf-1*, induces a defined spectrum of tumours *in vivo* [33]. The differences in tumour spectra induced by *Raf*- and *Myc*-expressing retroviruses suggest that the preferred *Myc* targets (lymphoid) differ from the preferred *Raf* targets (erythroid, fibroblast) in the rate-limiting pathways through which their growth is normally controlled.

In vitro

Raf-1 preferentially transforms erythroid cells and also transforms fibroblasts and epithelial cells [44]. *Raf* and *Myc* act synergistically to transform cells of all haematopoietic lineages: their co-expression in lymphoid and erythroid cells induces differentiation to a myeloid form [45]. *Araf-1* transforms NIH 3T3 fibroblasts after incorporation into the genome of murine leukaemia virus and expression of the *gag–raf* gene product [46].

GENE STRUCTURE OF *RAF1*

Open boxes: Exons homologous to those in the mouse genome that are transduced in v-*raf*.

Exon:

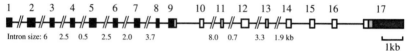

TRANSCRIPTIONAL REGULATION

The human *RAF1* promoter is located in an HTF-island (CpG-rich, non-methylated) and lacks TATA and CAAT boxes [47]. The 5' untranslated exon 1 is located at least 55 kb upstream of the body of the gene which spans

45 kb [48]. The last *RAF1* exon (17) contains 905 bp of 3' untranslated sequence. The large size of the gene may account for the relatively high frequency with which truncation-activated oncogenic versions of *RAF1* have been obtained.

PROTEIN STRUCTURE OF RAF1

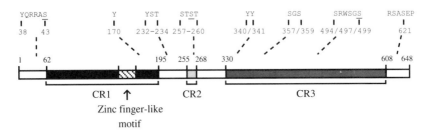

Conserved region 1 (CR1) contains a zinc finger-like motif; CR2 is conserved in virtually all forms of RAF and interacts directly with RAS proteins, binding GTP–RAS in preference to GDP–RAS and inhibiting RAS/GAP activity [11,12]. CR3 comprises the minimal transforming element [49]. CR1, CR2 and CR3 are between 61% and 100% homologous in RAF1, RAFA1 and RAFB1. Potential phosphorylation sites are shown above the figure. RAF1 is phosphorylated at multiple sites in the N-terminus that are deleted in the transforming protein. Underlines: major phosphorylation sites.

Deletion of residues 245–261 in CR2 causes oncogenic activation [49,50] but mutation of Ser259 alone is not sufficient to activate transforming potential: the additional deletion of the region 283–309 activates weak transforming power but the complete removal of the N-terminal 303 residues (which includes nine serines) is required for maximal activity [51].

SEQUENCE OF RAF1

```
  1  MEHIQGAWKT ISNGFGFKDA VFDGSSCISP TIVQQFGYQR RASDDGKLTD
 51  PSKTSNTIRV FLPNKQRTVV NVRNGMSLHD CLMKALKVRG LQPECCAVFR
101  LLHEHKGKKA RLDWNTDAAS LIGEELQVDF LDHVPLTTHN FARKTFLKLA
151  FCDICQKFLL NGFRCQTCGY KFHEHCSTKV PTMCVDWSNI RQLLLFPNST
201  IGDSGVPALP SLTMRRMRES VSRMPVSSQH RYSTPHAFTF NTSSPSSEGS
251  LSQRQRSTST PNVHMVSTTL PVDSRMIEDA IRSHSESASP SALSSSPNNL
301  SPTGWSQPKT PVPAQRERAP VSGTQEKNKI RPRGQRDSSY YWEIEASEVM
351  LSTRIGSGSF GTVYKGKWHG DVAVKILKVV DPTPEQFQAF RNEVAVLRKT
401  RHVNILLFMG YMTKDNLAIV TQWCEGSSLY KHLHVQETKF QMFQLIDIAR
451  QTAQGMDYLH AKNIIHRDMK SNNIFLHEGL TVKIGDFGLA TVKSRWSGSQ
501  QVEQPTGSVL WMAPEVIRMQ DNNPFSFQSD VYSYGIVLYE LMTGELPYSH
551  INNRDQIIFM VGRGYASPDL SKLYKNCPKA MKRLVADCVK KVKEERPLFP
601  QILSSIELLQ HSLPKINRSA SEPSLHRAAH TEDINACTLT TSPRLPVF (648)
```

Domain structure

139–184	Phorbol ester and DAG binding
355–363 and 375	ATP binding
340, 341	Major tyrosine phosphorylation sites. The introduction of negative charge at these sites appears essential for enzymatic activation of RAF1 by tyrosine kinases [52].
378	Mutation of corresponding v-RAF residue (Lys53) eliminates transforming capacity.
468	Active site

RAF proteins can be oncogenically activated by N-terminal fusion, truncation or point mutations [40,50,53]. The generation of an activated oncoprotein by removal of the N-terminus of RAF1 indicates that myristylation and *gag* sequences are not essential for transformation [54].

The v-*raf* gene encodes amino acids 326–648 of mouse RAF1 linked to *gag* sequences. The sequence of v-RAF is identical to residues 326–648 of human RAF1 with the substitutions GluIle343/344→LysMet; Phe387→Leu; Thr543→Ala; Ser549→Ala; Lys572→Arg; Met581→Ile; Ser621→Pro.

SEQUENCE OF RAFA1

```
  1  MEPPRGPPAN  GAEPSRAVGT  VKVYLPNKQR  TVVTVRDGMS  VYDSLDKALK
 51  VRGLNQDCCV  VYRLIKGRKT  VTAWDTAIAP  LDGEELIVEV  LEDVPLTMHN
101  FVRKTFFSLA  FCDFCLKFLF  HGFRCQTCGY  KFHQHCSSKV  PTVCVDMSTN
151  RQQFYHSVQD  LSGGSRQHEA  PSNRPLNELL  TPQGPSPRTQ  HCDPEHFPFP
201  APANAPLQRI  RSTSTPNVHM  VSTTAPMDSN  LIQLTGQSFS  TDAAGSRGGS
251  DGTPRGSPSP  ASVSSGRKSP  HSKSPAEQRE  RKSLADDKKK  VKNLGYRXSG
301  YYWEVPPSEV  QLLKRIGTGS  FGTVFRGRWH  GDVAVKVLKV  SQPTAEQAQA
351  FKNEMQVLRK  TRHVNILLFM  GFMTRPGFAI  ITQWCEGSSL  YHHLHVADTR
401  FDMVQLIDVA  RQTAQGMDYL  HAKNIIHRDL  KSNNIFLHEG  LTVKIGDFGL
451  ATVKTRWSGA  QPLEQPSGSV  LWMAAEVIRM  QDPNPYSFQS  DVYAYGVVLY
501  ELMTGSLPYS  HIGCRDQIIF  MVGRGYLSPD  LSKISSNCPK  AMRRLLSDCL
551  KFQREERPLF  PQILATIELL  QRSLPKIERS  ASEPSLHRTQ  ADELPACLLS
601  AARLVP  (606)
```

Domain structure

99–144	Phorbol ester and DAG binding
316–324 and 336	ATP binding
429	Active site

SEQUENCE OF RAFB1

```
  1  MDTVTSSSSS SLSVLPSSLS VFQNPTDVAR SNPKSPQKPI VRVFLPNKQR
 51  TVVPARCGVT VRDSLKKALM MRGLIPECCA VYRIQDGEKK PIGWDTDISW
101  LTGEELHVEV LENVPLTTHN FVRKTFFTLA FCDFCRKLLF QGFRCQTCGY
151  KFHQRCSTEV PLMCVNYDQL DLLFVSKFFE HHPIPQEEAS LAETALTSGS
201  SPSAPASDSI GPQILTSPSP SKSIPIPQPF RPADEDHRNQ FGQRDRSSSA
251  PNVHINTIEP VNIDDLIRDQ GFRGDGGSTT GLSATPPASL PGSLTNVKAL
301  QKSPGPQRER KSSSSSEDRN RMKTLGRRDS SDDWEIPDGQ ITVGQRIGSG
351  SFGTVYKGKW HGDVAVKMLN VTAPTPQQLQ AFKNEVGVLR KTRHVNILLF
401  MGYSTKPQLA IVTQWCEGSS LYHHLHIIET KFEMIKLIDI ARQTAQGMDY
451  LHAKSIIHRD LKSNNIFLHE DLTVKIGDFG LATVKSRWSG SHQFEQLSGS
501  ILWMAPEVIR MQDKNPYSFQ SDVYAFGIVL YELMTGQLPY SNINNRDQII
551  FMVGRGYLSP DLSKVRSNCP KAMKRLMAEC LKKKRDERPL FPQILASIEL
601  LARSLPKIHR SASEPSLNRA GFQTEDFSLY ACASPKTPIQ AGGYGAFPVH (650)
```

Domain structure

6–11	Poly serine
119–164	Phorbol ester and DAG binding
347–355 and 367	ATP binding
460	Active site

DATABASE ACCESSION NUMBERS

	PIR	SWISSPROT	EMBL/GENBANK	REFERENCES
Human *RAF1*	A00637	P04049	X03484	*48,55*
Human *RAFA1*	A26439	P10398	X04790	*56*
Human *RAFB1*	A31850	P15056	M95712,	*57*
	S13798		M95721, X54072,	
			M21001	*58, 59, 60*

References
1 Hanks, S.K. et al. (1988) Science 241, 42–52.
2 Heidecker, G. et al. (1992) Adv. Cancer Res. 58, 53–73.
3 Schultz, A.M. et al. (1988) Oncogene 2, 187–193.
4 MacNicol, A.M. et al. (1993) Cell 73, 571–583.
5 Morrison, D.K. et al. (1989) Cell 58, 649–657.
6 Baccarini, M. et al. (1990) EMBO J. 9, 3649–3657.
7 Kovacina, K.S. et al. (1990) J. Biol. Chem. 265, 12115–12118.
8 Blackshear, P.J. et al. (1990) J. Biol. Chem. 265, 12131–12134.
9 App, H. et al. (1991) Mol. Cell. Biol. 11, 913–919.
10 Kolch, W. et al. (1993) Nature 364, 249–252.
11 Warne, P.H. et al. (1993) Nature 364, 352–355.
12 Zhang, X. et al. (1993) Nature 364, 308–313.
13 Hallberg et al. (1994). J. Biol. Chem. 269, 3913–3916.
14 Turner, B. et al. (1991) Proc. Natl Acad. Sci. USA 88, 1227–1231.
15 Maslinski, W. et al. (1992) J. Biol. Chem. 267, 15281–15284.

16 Carroll, M.P. et al. (1991) J. Biol. Chem. 266, 14964–14969.
17 Thompson, P.A. et al. (1991) Cell Growth Differ. 2, 609–617.
18 Siegel, J.N. et al. (1990) J. Biol. Chem. 265, 18472–18480.
19 Kyriakis, J.M. et al. (1993) J. Biol. Chem. 268, 16009–16019.
20 Dent, P. et al. (1992) Science 257, 1404–1407.
21 Howe, L.R. et al. (1992) Cell 71, 335–342.
22 Muslin, A.J. et al. (1993) Mol. Cell. Biol. 13, 4197–4202.
23 Huang, W. et al. (1993) Proc. Natl Acad. Sci. USA 90, 10947–10951.
24 Wasylyk, C. et al. (1989) Mol. Cell. Biol. 9, 2247–2250.
25 Bruder, J.T. et al. (1994) Nucl. Acids Res. 21, 5229–5234.
26 Li, S. and Sedivy, J.M. (1993) Proc. Natl Acad. Sci. USA 90, 9247–9251.
27 Kaibuchi, K. et al. (1989) J. Biol. Chem. 264, 20855–20858.
28 Jamal, S. and Ziff, E., (1990) Nature 344, 463–466.
29 Qureshi, S.A. et al. (1991) J. Biol. Chem. 266, 20594–20597.
30 Rim, M. et al. (1992) Oncogene 7, 2065–2068.
31 Cornwell, M.M. and Smith, D.E. (1993) J. Biol. Chem. 268, 15347–15350.
32 Noda, M. et al. (1983) Proc. Natl Acad. Sci. USA 80, 5602–5606.
33 Rapp, U.R. (1991) Oncogene 6, 495–500.
34 Kolch, W. et al. (1991) Nature 349, 426–428.
35 Troppmair, J. et al. (1992) Oncogene 7, 1867–1873.
36 Sozeri, O. et al. (1992) Oncogene 7, 2259–2262.
37 Kolch, W. et al. (1993) Oncogene 8, 361–370.
38 Shimizu, K. et al. (1985) Proc. Natl Acad. Sci. USA 82, 5641–5645.
39 Kasid, U. et al. (1987) Science 237, 1039–1041.
40 Stanton, V.P. and Cooper, G.M. (1987) Mol. Cell. Biol. 7, 1171–1179.
41 Fukui, M. et al. (1985) Proc. Natl Acad. Sci. USA 82, 5954–5958.
42 Graziano, S.L. et al. (1987) Cancer Res. 48, 2148–2155.
43 Hajj, C. et al. (1990) Cancer 66, 733–739.
44 Keski-Oja, A. et al. (1982) J. Cell. Biochem. 20, 139–148.
45 Klinken, S.P. et al. (1989) J. Virol. 63, 1489–1492.
46 Huleihel, M. et al. (1986) Mol. Cell. Biol. 6, 2655–2662.
47 Beck, T.W. et al. (1990) Mol. Cell. Biol. 10, 3325–3333.
48 Bonner, T.I. et al. (1985) Mol. Cell. Biol. 5, 1400–1407.
49 Heidecker, G. et al. (1990) Mol. Cell. Biol. 10, 2503–2512.
50 Ishikawa, F. et al. (1988) Oncogene 3, 635–658.
51 McGrew, B.R. et al. (1992) Oncogene 7, 33–42.
52 Fabian, J.R. et al. (1993) Mol. Cell. Biol. 13, 7170–7179.
53 Ishikawa, F. et al. (1987) Mol. Cell. Biol. 7, 1226–1232.
54 Schultz, A.M. et al. (1985) Virol. 146, 78–89.
55 Bonner, T.I. et al. (1986) Nucl. Acids Res. 14, 1009–1015.
56 Beck, T.W. et al. (1987) Nucl. Acids Res. 15, 595–609.
57 Ikawa, S. et al. (1988) Mol. Cell. Biol. 8, 2651–2654.
58 Sithanandam, G. et al. (1990) Oncogene 5, 1775–1780.
59 Eychene, A. et al. (1992) Oncogene 7, 1657–1660.
60 Stephens, R.M. et al. (1992) Mol. Cell. Biol. 12, 3733–3742.

RAS

IDENTIFICATION

There are three forms of *Ras*: *Hras* (the oncogene of Harvey murine sarcoma virus, Ha-MuSV), *Kras* (oncogene of Kirsten murine sarcoma virus, Ki-MuSV) and *Nras* (detected in tumours but not in retroviruses). Ha-MuSV and Ki-MuSV were first isolated by inoculating rats with the corresponding mouse leukaemia viruses (Mo-MuLV and Ki-MuLV): following the induction of leukaemia, plasma from these animals was injected into BALB/c mice which rapidly developed solid tumours (*rat sarcomas*) from the effects of v-*ras*^{H} or v-*ras*^{K}. BALB-MuSV, AF-1 and Rasheed-MuSV are additional murine sarcoma viruses in which acquired cellular *Ras* genes have been identified. The human homologues are *HRAS1*, *KRAS2* and *NRAS*: *HRAS2* and *KRAS1* are inactive pseudogenes.

RELATED GENES

The *Ras* superfamily comprises nearly 50 currently known *Ras* related genes encoding GTP-binding proteins (G proteins). These include *NRASL1*, *NRASL2* and *NRASL3*, *RRAS*, *RhoA*, *RhoB* and *RhoC*, *Rac1* and *Rac2*, *Ral*, *Rap1A* (also called *Krev-1* or *Smg-p21A*), *RAB2*, yeast *YPT1*, human and mouse *MEL*, the *Drosophila Dras* genes, *Caenorhabditis elegans let-60* and *Saccharomyces cerevisiae RAS1* and *RAS2*. The elongation factor EF-Tu in *E.coli* has four regions that are homologous with regions in the RAS family.

	NRAS	HRAS1	KRAS2
Nucleotides (kb)	32	4.5	50
Chromosome	1p13	11p15.5	12p12.1
Mass (kDa): expressed	21	21	21

Cellular location

Inner surface of the plasma membrane.

Tissue distribution

Ubiquitous (6.8×10^4 molecules per cell in NIH 3T3 cells and 6.8×10^5 molecules per cell in v-*Hras*-transformed 3T3 cells [1,2])

PROTEIN FUNCTION

RAS proteins are membrane-bound GTPases. Normal p21^{ras} (RAS) hydrolyses GTP at rates comparable with those reached by purified G proteins and exists in an equilibrium between an active (GTP.RAS) and an inactive (GDP.RAS) state. The rates of GDP release and GTP hydrolysis are increased by the actions of two classes of regulatory proteins: guanine nucleotide release proteins (GNRPs) that catalyse the release of bound GDP [3] and GTPase-activating proteins (GAPs) that increase the rate of hydrolysis of GTP [4-7].

Normal RAS proteins are involved in the control of cell growth and differentiation but any one of many single amino acid mutations can give rise to highly oncogenic proteins. The action of a variety of growth factors increases the concentration of GTP.RAS in normal cells and the conformational change induced by GTP binding activates RAS, enabling it to interact with cellular target ("effector") proteins. The mammalian effector of RAS activates a cascade of serine/threonine protein kinases that includes RAF1, MAP kinase kinase (MAPKK) and extracellular signal-regulated kinases (ERKs or MAP kinases) [8,9].

Oncogenic *Ras* stimulates the activity of protein kinase C and the Na$^+$/H$^+$ exchange protein, phospholipid metabolism and in various types of cell has been reported to activate transcription of many genes, including ornithine decarboxylase (*ODC1*), *FOS*, *JUN*, *JUNB*, *MDR1*, *MYC*, transin, p9Ka/42A, *TGFα* and *TGFβ* and to repress transcription of the *MYOD1*, *MYOH*, myogenin, PDGF receptor and fibronectin genes [10].

The yeast *RAS1* and *RAS2* genes encode proteins with GTPase activity that have strong homology with human RAS proteins. The yeast proteins activate adenylate cyclase in a manner analogous to the action of G_s in mammalian plasma membranes. However, there is no evidence that RAS proteins regulate adenylate cyclase in vertebrate cells, although they can substitute for RAS1 and RAS2 in yeast [11].

Regulation of RAS by GAPs

Most cells express two GAPs, type I p120^{GAP} and NF1/GAP (see **Tumour Suppressor Genes: NF1**), with similar activities. p120^{GAP} acts catalytically on normal, but not transforming, RAS proteins to stimulate their relatively weak hydrolytic activity for bound GTP by 100-fold [12]. In general, GAP appears to function as an upstream regulator of normal RAS, maintaining it in an inactive, GDP-bound state. However, GAP may also be involved in coupling RAS to downstream effector proteins. Thus, mutant forms of RAS lacking effector function still associate with GAP but remain bound to GTP, although such complexes are not oncogenic [13] and either RAS or GAP proteins inhibit the coupling of muscarinic receptors to atrial potassium channels [14]. p120^{GAP} possesses SRC homology domains SH2 and SH3 through which it can associate with tyrosine phosphorylated proteins, whereas NF1/GAP does not, indicating that different activated RAS complexes may have distinct cellular targets [15]. Three point mutations in

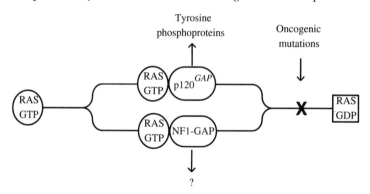

the SH2 domain of GAP have been detected in human basal cell carcinomas: mutations in this region may therefore play a role in tumorigenesis [16].

Conserved RAS signalling pathways

Homologues of RAS act as crucial signal transducing elements in all eukaryotic organisms that have been examined. Homologous components of pathways that couple to RAS in *C. elegans*, *Drosophila* and mammals are shown below. In mammals phosphorylated tyrosine residues on activated tyrosine kinase receptors associate with the SH2 domain of growth factor receptor-bound protein 2 (GRB2). GRB2 binds to SOS1 via its SH3 domains. SOS1 is thus recruited to the plasma membrane where it activates RAS [17–23].

C. elegans	*Drosophila*	Mammalian	
LET-23	SEVENLESS	PDGFR EGFR	(Receptor tyrosine kinases)
↓	↓	↓	
SEM-5	DRK [E(sev)2B]	GRB2	(Adaptor proteins) {SH3/SH2/SH3}
↓	↓	↓	
?	SOS	mSOS1,2	(Guanine nucleotide release proteins)
↓	↓	↓	
GTP-RAS↑	GTP-RAS↑	GTP-RAS↑	
↓	↓	↓	
Vulval induction, etc.	Eye development, etc.	Cell growth, etc.	

RAS in cell proliferation

The evidence indicates that, except for oncoproteins located in the cytosol (e.g. MOS), the stimulation of proliferation involves RAS. Thus, insulin, together with bombesin, PDGF or EGF form potent co-mitogenic combinations for quiescent cells *in vitro*. PDGF or EGF cause activation of RAS (i.e. increase the cellular GTP.RAS concentration) and the tyrosine phosphorylation of GAP. PDGF causes ~10% of total cellular GAP to associate with the PDGFR [24,25], together with PLCγ, PtdIns 3-kinase and RAF1. Ligand-activated association of GAP with receptors may thus be a mechanism for switching on the mitogenic pathway. However, in CHO cells, PtdIns 3-kinase appears to function upstream of both RAF1 and RAS. Thus, insulin stimulation of the serum response element (SRE) of the *Fos* promoter is inhibited by expression of dominant negative *Ras*- or *Raf*-encoding plasmids [25]. Furthermore, PDGF receptors mutated in the PtdIns 3 kinase-binding sites are unable to stimulate RAS, whereas GAP-binding site mutants do so, suggesting an important role for PtdIns 3-kinase or a protein binding to the same site in PDGF-stimulated RAS activation [27].

Neither insulin nor bombesin elevate the GTP.RAS concentration in normal cells, although insulin causes tyrosine phosphorylation of the SRC tyrosine kinase substrate SHC which then binds to GRB2/SOS. Furthermore, in Swiss 3T3 fibroblasts, microinjection of anti-RAS antibody inhibits DNA synthesis stimulated by PDGF or EGF and also by insulin and bombesin, suggesting that RAS is involved in the insulin/bombesin-stimulated pathway.

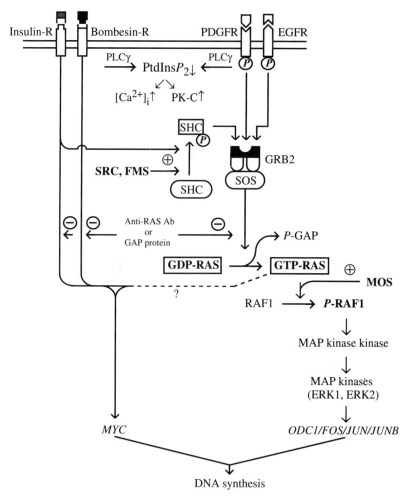

PtdInsP$_2$: phosphatidylinositol 4,5-bisphosphate; PLCγ: phospholipase Cγ; PK-C: protein kinase C; [Ca^{2+}]$_i$: intracellular free Ca^{2+} concentration.

Cancer

Activating mutations in *RAS* oncogenes occur in a wide variety of human tumours. The overall incidence is only between 10% and 15% but is as high as 95% in pancreatic carcinomas [28–30]. Individual *RAS* genes are commonly associated with specific tumours, for example, *KRAS2* with cancers of the lung [31], colon or pancreas, *NRAS* with acute myelogenous leukaemia (AML). However, there is no specificity in thyroid tumours and in thyroid adenomas and carcinomas mutations in all three genes (*HRAS, KRAS2* and *NRAS*) may occur within one tumour. Simultaneous mutations in *KRAS2* and *NRAS* have also been detected in multiple myeloma [32]. The highly polymorphic *HRAS1* minisatellite locus (unstable repetitive DNA sequences), just downstream from the *HRAS1* gene, consists of four common progenitor alleles and several dozen rare alleles, which apparently derive from mutations of the progenitors. Mutant alleles of the HRAS1 minisatellite locus represent a major risk factor for common types of cancer (~10% of breast, colorectum, and bladder cancers) [33]. In non-small cell lung cancer hypomethylation of CCGG sites in the 3' region and allelic loss of *HRAS* can occur, even in the absence mutations at codons 12, 13 or 61 [34].

These observations indicate the probable importance of *RAS* oncogenes in neoplasia, although there is as yet no discernible pattern to the expression of activated *RAS* genes and they occur in benign as well as malignant tumours.

Transgenic animals

The expression of *Nras*, v-*Hras* or human *HRAS1* causes non-neoplastic proliferation and malignant tumours in a tissue-specific manner. Co-expression of v-*Hras* and *Myc* causes a synergistic increase in the initiation of tumours, indicating that the expression of an activated *Ras* gene alone is not sufficient to transform differentiated cells *in vivo* [35–37].

In animals

In tumours induced chemically (e.g. by nitrosomethylurea (NMU), dimethylbenzanthracene (DMBA) or *N*-methyl-*N*'-nitro-*N*-nitrosoguanidine (MNNG)) or physically (e.g. by X-ray treatment) induced in rodents the frequency of *Ras* mutations is usually ~70%, commonly arising from point mutations at codons 12 or 61 [38,39]. The expression of oncogenic *Hras in vivo* can rapidly confer metastatic potential on benign rat mammary cells [40].

In vitro

Normal fibroblasts are not transformed either by cellular or retroviral *Ras* oncogenes [41,42] and mutant *RAS* from human tumours only transforms transfected primary fibroblasts when supplemented with immortalizing oncogenes such as *Myc* [43], v-*myc*, *Nmyc* [44], adenovirus E1A [45] mutant *P53* or polyoma large T antigen. E1B or polyoma middle T antigen can replace *Ras*. However, NIH 3T3 fibroblasts are transformed by overexpression of normal RAS proteins [46–48]. Transformation of NIH 3T3 cells by *Hras* is greatly enhanced by the expression of *Raf-1* and RAF-1 kinase appears to be rate-limiting for *Ras* transformation [49]. It is inhibited by the expression of normal p105^{RB1} [50]. *Ras* oncogenes efficiently transform erythroid [51], myeloid [52] and murine mast cells [53].

Rap1A/Krev-1 is a *Ras*-related protein that suppresses the activity of v-*Kras-2* and causes transformed NIH 3T3 cells to revert to a normal phenotype [54]. RAP1 has a higher affinity for GAP than RAS and may also interact specifically with effector molecules. Reversion of the transformed phenotype has also been demonstrated on expression of tropomyosin 1 [55] or of a mutated form of gelsolin, the actin regulatory protein, which may inhibit PtdInsP_2 hydrolysis [56].

The evidence from cellular studies of *Ras* is consistent with the pathology and epidemiology of spontaneously arising cancer in humans, suggesting that transformation is at least a two-stage process and that one oncogene may be needed for immortalization and another for transformation. However, massive overexpression of a single gene (e.g. v-*myc* or *Ras*) can probably override this distinction.

Transformation by either *Kras* or *Hras* oncogenes of a variety of rodent cells increases TGFα and TGFβ secretion. TGFα may function as an autocrine growth factor for *Ras*-transformed malignant cells and TGFβ may promote metastasis [57].

NRAS gene structure

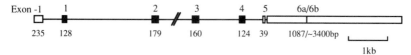

Exons 1–4 encode 37, 60, 53 and 39 amino acids, respectively. The sizes of the corresponding exons in *HRAS* are 110, 230, 160 and 117 bp and in *KRAS2* 122, 179, 160 and 124 bp, respectively. *NRAS* contains two 3' non-coding exons (5 and 6) not present in *HRAS1* or *KRAS2*. *KRAS2* has alternative fourth exons (4A and 4B) separated by ~5600 bp that encode 39 and 38 amino acids, respectively. Codons 12 and 13 of wild-type *Hras* constitute a strong pause site for *in vitro* DNA synthesis catalysed by DNA polymerase α [58]. Pausing at these codons is abolished by mutation to an activated oncogene.

TRANSCRIPTIONAL REGULATION

The promoter regions of *RAS* genes do not contain TATA or CAT boxes but have multiple GC boxes and utilize more than one transcription start site [59]. The human *NRAS* promoter contains consensus binding sites for CREB/ATF, AP-1, AP-2, MYB, E4TF1, SP1 and MLTF/MYC [60].

PROTEIN STRUCTURE

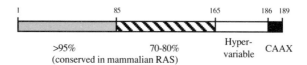

Several different wild-type and oncogenic RAS complexes have been crystallized to provide the first atomic descriptions of proto-oncogenes and oncogenes. RAS comprises a central, six-stranded β sheet and five helices, two of which (α2 and α3) lie below the plane defined by the β sheet. Of the 10 loops in the protein, L1 contains Gly12 (the most frequent site of mutation in human tumours), L2 includes the residues believed to interact with the effector and L4 contains Gln61 [61].

The sequence of Ha-MuSV HRAS differs from human HRAS1 only at positions 12 (lysine for glycine) and 143 (lysine for glutamate): that of

Ki-MuSV KRAS differs from human KRAS 2A in five positions (Gly12→Ser, Glu37→Gln, Ala59→Thr, Asp132→Glu, Ile187→Val).

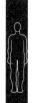

SEQUENCE OF NRAS

```
  1 MTEYKLVVVG AGGVGKSALT IQLIQNHFVD EYDPTIEDSY RKQVVIDGET
 51 CLLDILDTAG QEEYSAMRDQ YMRTGEGFLC VFAINNSKSF ADINLYREQI
101 KRVKDSDDVP MVLVGNKCDL PTRTVDTKQA HELAKSYGIP FIETSAKTRQ
151 GVEDAFYTLV REIRQYRMKK LNSSDDGTQG CMGLPCVVM (189)
```

SEQUENCE OF HRAS1

```
  1 MTEYKLVVVG AGGVGKSALT IQLIQNHFVD EYDPTIEDSY RKQVVIDGET
 51 CLLDILDTAG QEEYSAMRDQ YMRTGEGFLC VFAINNTKSF EDIHQYREQI
101 KRVKDSDDVP MVLVGNKCDL AARTVESRQA QDLARSYGIP YIETSAKTRQ
151 GVEDAFYTLV REIRQHKLRK LNPPDESGPG CMSCKCVLS (189)
```

Underlined residues differ from NRAS.

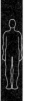

SEQUENCE OF KRAS2A

```
  1 MTEYKLVVVG AGGVGKSALT IQLIQNHFVD EYDPTIEDSY RKQVVIDGET
 51 CLLDILDTAG QEEYSAMRDQ YMRTGEGFLC VFAINNTKSF EDIHHYREQI
101 KRVKDSEDVP MVLVGNKCDL PSRTVDTKQA QDLARSYGIP FIETSAKTRQ
151 RVEDAFYTLV REIRQYRLKK ISKEEKTPGC VKIKKCIIM (189)
```

Underlined residues differ from NRAS.

SEQUENCE OF KRAS2B

```
  1 MTEYKLVVVG AGGVGKSALT IQLIQNHFVD EYDPTIEDSY RKQVVIDGET
 51 CLLDILDTAG QEEYSAMRDQ YMRTGEGFLC VFAINNTKSF EDIHHYREQI
101 KRVKDSEDVP MVLVGNKCDL PSRTVDTKQA QDLARSYGIP FIETSAKTRQ
151 GVDDAFYTLV REIRKHKEKM SKDGKKKKKK SKTKCVIM (188)
```

Underlined residues differ from KRAS 2A; 175–180 is a polybasic region involved in plasma membrane targeting.

Domain structures

5–63, 77–92, 109–123, 139–165 and 186–189	Non-contiguous domains essential for RAS transforming activity
10–16, 57–62 and 116–119	Highly conserved nucleotide binding regions

32–40	"Effector domain": substitutions in this region reduce the biological effect of RAS proteins in both mammalian and yeast cells but do <u>not</u> affect GTP binding or hydrolysis. Essential for stimulation of GTPase activity by GAP. Mutations in this region reduce the direct interaction that occurs between RAS and RAF1 [62,63]
61–65	Confer RAS/GAP sensitivity on RAS protein
165–184	Hypervariable region
186–189	CAAX box: Cys186 essential for transforming activity
12, 13, 59, 61	Sites of naturally occurring activating point mutations that inhibit GTP hydrolysis. Oncogenic mutations therefore enable the GTP.RAS complex to remain in an active form that is presumed to stimulate a growth-promoting event
63, 116, 117, 119 and 146	Activating point mutations created by *in vitro* mutagenesis
164	Mutagenesis causes loss of GTP binding
177	HRAS1 serine phosphorylation site
186	Farnesyl alkylation of NRAS, KRAS2A, HRAS1: palmitoylation of Cys residues (HRAS1 Cys184) in the hypervariable region
185	Farnesyl alkylation of KRAS 2B. Inhibition of farnesyltransferase activity selectively blocks *Ras*-dependent transformation *in vitro* [64,65].

DATABASE ACCESSION NUMBERS

	PIR	SWISSPROT	EMBL/GENBANK	REFERENCES
Human *NRAS*	A01359	P01111	X02751	66
	A21700		X00642 to X00645	67
			L00040 to L00043	68
			M10055, K03211	69,70
Human *KRAS2A*	A01364	P01116	L00045 to L00049	71
Human *KRAS2B*	A01367	P01118	K01519, K01520,	
			X01669	72–74
			X02825, K03209,	
			K03210	75–77
Human *HRAS1*	A01360	P01112	V00574	78–81

References
1 Hand, P.H. et al. (1987) Biochim. Biophys. Acta 908, 131–142.
2 Miller, A.C. et al. (1993) Mol. Cell. Biol. 13, 4416–4422.
3 Schweighoffer, F. et al. (1993) Oncogene 8, 1477–1485.
4 **Bourne, H.R. et al. (1990) Nature 348, 125–132.**

5 **Downward, J. (1992) BioEssays 14, 177–184.**
6 **Boguski, M.S. and McCormick, F. (1993) Nature 366, 643–654.**
7 **Santos, E. and Nebreda, A.R. (1989) FASEB J. 3, 2151–2163.**
8 De Vries-Smits, A.M.M. et al. (1992) Nature 357, 602–604.
9 Cook, S.J. et al. (1993) EMBO J. 12, 3475–3485.
10 Sistonen, L. et al. (1989) EMBO J. 8, 815–822.
11 **Broach, J.R. and Deschenes, R.J. (1990) Adv. Cancer Res. 54, 79–139.**
12 Marshall, M.S. et al. (1989) EMBO J. 8, 1105–1110.
13 Krengel, U. (1990) Cell 62, 539–548.
14 Yatani, A. et al. (1990) Cell 61, 769–776.
15 McCormick, F. et al. (1992) Phil. Trans. R. Soc. Lond. B 336, 43–48.
16 Friedman, E. et al. (1993) Nature Genetics 5, 242–247.
17 Lowenstein, E.J. et al. (1992) Cell 70, 431–442.
18 Gale, N.W. et al. (1993) Nature 363, 88–92.
19 Rozakis-Adcock, M. et al. (1993) Nature 363, 83–88.
20 Liu, B.X. et al. (1993) Oncogene 8, 3081–3084.
21 Burgering, B.M.Th. et al. (1993) EMBO J. 12, 4211–4220.
22 Egan, S.E. et al. (1993) Nature 363, 45–51.
23 Skolnik, E.Y. et al. (1993) EMBO J. 12, 1929–1936.
24 Molloy, C.J. et al. (1989) Nature 342, 711–714.
25 Kazlauskas, A. et al. (1990) Science 247, 1578–1581.
26 Yamauchi, K. et al. (1993) J. Biol. Chem. 268, 14597–14600.
27 Satoh, T. et al. (1993) Mol. Cell. Biol. 13, 3706–3713.
28 **Bos, J.L. (1988) Mutat. Res. 195, 255–271.**
29 Almoguera, C. et al. (1988) Cell 53, 549–554.
30 Rochlitz, C.F. et al. (1989) Cancer Res. 49, 357–360.
31 Rodenhuis, S. and Slebos, R.J.C. (1992) Cancer Res. 52, 2665s–2669s.
32 Portier, M. et al. (1992) Oncogene 7, 2539–2543.
33 Krontiris, T.G. et al. (1993) N. Engl. J. Med. 329, 517–523.
34 Vachtenheim, J. et al. (1994) Cancer Res. 54, 1145–1148.
35 Sinn, E. et al. (1987) Cell 49, 465–475.
36 Andres, A.-C. et al. (1987) Proc. Natl Acad. Sci. USA 84, 1299–1303.
37 Mangues, R. et al. (1992) Oncogene 7, 2073–2076.
38 **Barbacid, M. (1987) Annu. Rev. Biochem. 56, 779–827.**
39 Nakazawa, H. et al. (1992) Oncogene 7, 2295–2301.
40 Nicolson, G.L. et al. (1992) Oncogene 7, 1127–1135.
41 Newbold, R.F. and Overell, R.W. (1983) Nature 304, 648–651.
42 Sager, R. et al. (1983) Proc. Natl Acad. Sci. USA 87, 7601–7605.
43 Land, H. et al. (1983) Nature 304, 596–602.
44 Schwab, M. et al. (1985) Nature 316, 160–162.
45 Ruley, H.E. (1983) Nature 304, 602–606.
46 Ricketts, M.H. and Levinson, A.D. (1988) Mol. Cell. Biol. 8, 1460–1468.
47 Reynolds, V.L. et al. (1987) Oncogene 1, 323–330.
48 Doppler, W. et al. (1987) Gene, 54, 147–153.
49 Cuadrado, A. et al. (1993) Oncogene 8, 2443–2448.
50 Kivinen, L. et al. (1993) Oncogene 8, 2703–2711.
51 Hankins, W.D. and Scolnick, E.M. (1981) Cell 26, 91–97.
52 Pierce, J.H. and Aaronson, S.A. (1985) Mol. Cell. Biol. 5, 667–674.
53 Rein, A. et al. (1985) Mol. Cell. Biol. 5, 2257–2264.

54 Beranger, F. et al. (1991) Proc. Natl Acad. Sci. USA 88, 1606–1610.

55 Prasad, G.L. et al. (1993) Proc. Natl Acad. Sci. USA 90, 7039–7043.

56 Mullauer, L. et al. (1993) Oncogene 8, 2531–2536.

57 Colletta, G. et al. (1991) Oncogene 6, 583–587.

58 Hoffmann, J.-S. et al. (1993) Cancer Res. 53, 2895–2900.

59 Hoffman, E.K. et al. (1987) Mol. Cell. Biol. 7, 2592–2596.

60 Thorn, J.T. et al. (1991) Oncogene 6, 1843–1850.

61 Wittinghofer, F. (1992) Semin. Cancer Biol. 3, 189–198.

62 Warne, P.H. et al. (1993) Nature 364, 352–355.

63 Zhang, X. et al. (1993) Nature 364, 308–313.

64 Kohl, N.E. et al. (1993) Science 260, 1934–1937.

65 James, G.L. et al. (1993) Science 260, 1937–1942.

66 Taparowsky, E. et al. (1983) Cell 34, 581–586.

67 Brown, R. et al. (1984) EMBO J. 3, 1321–1326.

68 Yuasa, Y. et al. (1984) Proc. Natl Acad. Sci. USA 81, 3670–3674

69 Gambke, C. et al. (1985) Proc. Natl Acad. Sci. USA. 82, 879–882.

70 Hall, A. and Brown, R. (1985) Nucl. Acids Res. 13, 5255–5268.

71 McGrath, J.P. et al. (1983) Nature 304, 501–506.

72 Shimizu, K. et al. (1983) Nature 304, 497–500.

73 Capon, D.J. et al. (1983) Nature 304, 507–513.

74 McCoy, M.S. et al. (1984) Mol. Cell. Biol. 4, 1577–1582.

75 Nakano, H. et al. (1984) Proc. Natl Acad. Sci. USA. 81, 71–75.

76 Hirai, H. et al. (1985) Biochem. Biophys. Res. Commun. 127, 68–174.

77 Yamamoto, F. and Perucho, M. (1988) Oncogene Res. 3, 123–138.

78 Capon, D.J. et al. (1983) Nature 302, 33–37.

79 Reddy, E.P. (1983) Science 220, 1061–1063.

80 Tabin, C.J. et al. (1982) Nature 300, 143–149.

81 Sekiya, T. et al. (1984) Proc. Natl Acad. Sci. USA 81, 4771–4775.

IDENTIFICATION

v-*rel* is the oncogene of avian reticuloendotheliosis virus strain T (REV-T), originally isolated from turkeys that had contracted lymphoid leukosis. *REL* was detected by screening DNA with v-*rel* probes.

RELATED GENES

REL genes are members of the nuclear factor κB (NF-κB) transcription factor family [1, 2]. Human *REL* encodes HIVEN86A, a κB site-binding transcription factor. v-REL is unrelated to any other known oncoprotein [3]. These proteins have an N-terminal conserved REL homology domain of ~300–350 amino acids that includes sequences important for DNA binding, dimerization and nuclear localization.

Other members of the REL family include NF-κB1 (human κ binding factor, formerly KBF1, p110 or EBP-1: an early response gene expressed as a homodimer in T cells [4,5]), NF-κB2 (formerly p49, p50B, H2TF1 or LYT10) [6], murine REL-B, I-REL (the human homologue of REL-B which may function as an inhibitor of REL proteins), and the *dorsal* gene product of *Drosophila melanogaster*.

NF-κB is a complex of the REL family proteins p50 (*NFKB1*) and p65 (*RELA*). p50 is synthesized as a precursor protein (p105) that is proteolytically cleaved to release the p50 DNA binding protein, comprised mainly of the REL homology domain. p65 is not processed and has a strong C-terminal transcription activation domain. NF-κB occurs in an active form in the nucleus of mature B cells, differentiated monocytes and some T cell lines. It is generally inactive in the cytoplasm of other cells where it is complexed with I-κB which, when underphosphorylated, acts via p65 to prevent translocation to the nucleus. I-κB is directly phosphorylated by protein kinase C. Following cell activation by mitogens, cytokines phorbol esters and some viruses, NF-κB is released from I-κB and translocated to the nucleus where it binds to the Ig κ enhancer and to the H-2K^b palindrome and activates genes involved in the immune, inflammatory and acute phase responses.

NF-κB p65 also has N-terminal sequence homology with REL and a C-terminal transcription activation domain [7]. NF-κB p65 is a powerful *trans*-activating factor when transiently expressed in Jurkat T cells: its action is completely suppressed by v-REL.

	REL/Rel	v-*rel*
Nucleotides (kb)	>24 (chicken, turkey)	1.4 (REV-T)
Chromosome	2p13–p12	
Mass (kDa): predicted	65	56
expressed	68	pp59$^{v\text{-}rel}$

Cellular location

REL is cytoplasmic in chick embryo fibroblasts (CEFs). v-REL is nuclear in non-transformed CEFs [8]. v-REL and REL are primarily cytoplasmic in transformed avian and murine cells and exist in a complex with REL, p115, I-κB and NF-κB [9-11]. However, v-REL with an added SV40 T antigen nuclear localization signal also transforms these cells, when the protein is nuclear. In transformed lymphoid cells the majority of v-REL (90%) is cytoplasmic and complexed with I-κB, the minority is nuclear and associated with p115 and NF-κB. In the human lymphoblastoid cell line Jurkat, p40 is exclusively cytoplasmic and is not present in nuclear complexes of REL and NF-κB p105 [12].

Tissue distribution

In humans high concentrations of *REL* mRNA occur in relatively mature lymphocytes [13]. In chickens *Rel* mRNA is mainly in haematopioetic cells [14] but there is ubiquitous, low level embryonic expression [15]. *Rel* mRNA expression is depressed in immature thymocytes and may therefore play a role in lymphocyte differentiation, in contrast to the evidence for *Myb* and *Ets* [13].

PROTEIN FUNCTION

REL and v-REL are transcription factors that interact to form homodimers or heterodimers with NF-κB or its precursor p105 and bind to NF-κB motifs (NGGNN^A/$_T$TTCC) [4,11,16-18]. Immunoprecipitates of v-REL have an associated serine/threonine protein kinase activity [19,20].

REL homodimers and heterodimers show distinct DNA binding specificities and affinities for various κB motifs [21]. Human REL and NF-κB p105 protein synthesis is induced by the action of cytokines, mitogenic lectins, phorbol esters and viral gene products and both proteins are tyrosine kinase substrates [12]. REL is tyrosine phosphorylated in T cells following PHA or TPA treatment and in neutrophils in response to granulocyte colony stimulating factor (G-CSF) [22].

REL homodimers activate transcription of IL6, IL2 receptor, IFNβ, IFNγ and NF-κB [23-26] and the heterodimer of REL/NF-kB subunit p65 binds to the phorbol ester (TPA) responsive sequence 5'-GGGAAAGTAC-3' in the 5' flanking region of the human urokinase gene [27]. REL proteins also modulate gene expression by acting via the HIV LTR NF-κB sites [28] and induce κB-site dependent stimulation of polyoma virus replication [29]. Mutant NF-κB (p50) that is unable to bind to DNA but can form homo- or heterodimers prevents transcriptional activation via the HIV LTR or the MHC class I H-2K^b promoter [30].

In most cells v-REL represses gene expression, including that of *Myc* [28,31,32] but in some cells (e.g. undifferentiated F9 cells, rat fibroblasts, chicken cells) it acts as a κB-specific transcriptional activator rather than as a repressor [33] and can stimulate transcription of the MHC class I gene cluster and of high mobility group protein 14b [34]. In P19 embryonal carcinoma cells either REL or v-REL induce differentiation[35].

The activation regions of both REL and v-REL proteins interact with the TATA binding protein (TBP) and transcription factor IIB (TFIIB), suggesting that the transcription regulating activites of REL proteins may be mediated by interaction with basal transcription factors [36]. v-REL appears to compete with endogenous proteins of the *REL* family, the expression and activity of which is cell specific. v-REL probably transforms cells by acting as a dominant negative version of REL [3].

Cancer

Rearrangement or amplification of the *REL* locus occurs in some lymphomas. A B cell lymphoma-associated chromosomal translocation, t(10;14)(q24;q32), translocates the immunoglobulin $C\alpha_1$ locus into that of *NF-KB2*: the fusion gene product includes the REL homology domain and binds κB sequences *in vitro* [37]. A cell line derived from a diffuse large cell lymphoma expresses a *REL* fusion mRNA (*NRG*, non-rel gene) [38].

In animals

In REV-T infection p59[v-rel] causes acute neoplasia in birds that is rapidly fatal [14, 39].

In vitro

Overexpression of REL transforms primary avian fibroblasts but in bone marrow cells induces programmed cell death [15]. v-rel primarily transforms lymphoid cells but may also transform erythroid and myeloid cells and only partially transforms CEFs [39, 40]. Chicken spleen cells transformed *in vitro* by REV-T are tumorigenic on transplantation [41].

GENE STRUCTURE

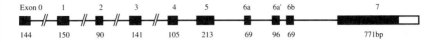

Exon 6a′ is not present in turkey *Rel*, from which v-*rel* was transduced, and is a portion of an inverted *Alu* repeat [42].

TRANSCRIPTIONAL REGULATION

The promoter region of the normal chicken *Rel* gene is GC-rich, contains an NF-κB consensus binding sequence and lacks a TATA box. *In vitro* v-rel expression suppresses transcription from the *Rel* promoter by a mechanism that does not involve the NF-κB site [43].

PROTEIN STRUCTURE OF V-REL, REL, P50 AND P65

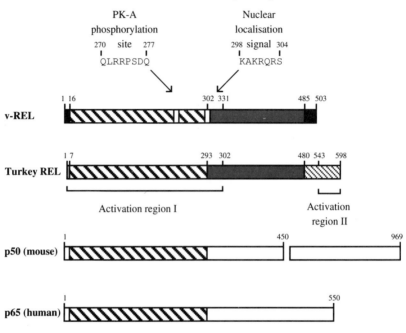

Within the REL homology domain (dark cross-hatch) all REL proteins have a nuclear localization signal, although transformation of spleen cells appears independent of whether v-REL is nuclear or cytoplasmic [8]. REL (and *dorsal*) contain C-terminal sequences that are important for cytoplasmic retention and transcriptional activation that are deleted in v-REL [31,43]. p50 contains a unique ~40 amino acid insert in the REL domain. The p50 precursor is cleaved to release the REL domain, containing the DNA binding subunit, and a C-terminal region containing around six ankyrin repeats, that has I-κB activity [4,45,46].

SEQUENCE OF REL

```
  1    MASGAYNPYI  EIIEQPRQRG  MRFRYKCEGR  SAGSIPGEHS  TDNNRTYPSI
 51    NIMNYYGKGK  VRITLVTKND  PYKPHPHDLV  GKDCRDGYYE  AEFGNERRPL
101    FFQNLGIQCV  KKKEVKEAII  TRIKAGINPF  NVPEKQLNDI  EDCDLNVVRL
151    CFQVFLPDEH  GNLTTALPPV  VSNPIYDNRA  PNTAELRICR  VNKNCGSVRG
201    GDEIFLLCDK  VQKDDIEVRF  VLNDWEAKGI  FSQADVHRQV  AIVFKTPPYC
251    KAITEPVTVK  MQLRRPSDQE  VSESMDFRYL  PDEKDTYGNK  AKKQKTTLIF
301    QKLCQDHVET  GFRHVDQDGL  ELLTSGDPPT  LASQSAGITV  NFPERPRPGL
351    LGSIGEGRYF  KKEPNLFSHD  AVVREMPTGV  GVQAESYYPS  PGPISSGLSH
401    HASMAPLPSS  SWSSVAHPTP  RSGNTNPLSS  FSTRTLPSNS  QGIPPFLRIP
451    VGNDLNASNA  CIYNNADDIV  GMEASSMPSA  DLYGISDPNM  LSNCSVNMMT
501    TSSDSMGETD  NPRLLSMNLE  NPSCNSVLDP  RDLRQLHQMS  SSSMSAGANS
551    NTTVFVSQSD  AFEGSDFSCA  DNSMINESGP  SNSTNPNSHG  FVQDSQYSGI
601    GSMQNEQLSD  SFPYEFFQV  (619)
```

Domain structure

1–300	REL homology domain
19–27	DNA binding motif (RXXRXRXXC) conserved in all REL proteins (underlined)
264–267	Putative cAMP-dependent protein kinase phosphorylation site (underlined)
290–296	Nuclear localization signal (underlined)
308–340	*Alu* sequence encoded by exon 6a' (italics)

v-*rel* has transduced the turkey *Rel* sequence encoding the first 478 amino acids of REL. In v-REL this is flanked by 11 N-terminal amino acids and 18 C-terminal amino acids derived from *env* [47,48]. The percentage homology (identical plus conserved residues) between turkey and human REL is 87–100% (exons 0–6a), 70% (exon 6b) and 49% (exon 7).

DATABASE ACCESSION NUMBERS

	PIR	SWISSPROT	EMBL/GENBANK	REFERENCES
Human *REL*			M11595	42
Turkey *Rel*	A01377	P01125	X03508	47
			X03616 to X03623	
			K02447	

References

1 Rushlow, C. and Warrior, R. (1992) BioEssays 14, 89–95.
2 Hannink, M. and Temin, H.M. (1991) Crit. Rev. Oncogenes 2, 293–309.
3 Gilmore, T.D. (1992) Cancer Surveys 15, 69–87.
4 Kieran, M. et al. (1990) Cell 62, 1007–1018.
5 Bours, V. et al. (1990) Nature 348, 76–80.
6 Nabel, G.J. and Verma, I.M. (1993) Genes Devel. 7, 2063.
7 Nolan, G.P. et al. (1991) Cell 64, 961–969.
8 Gilmore, T.D. and Temin, H.M. (1988) J. Virol. 62, 703–714.
9 Simek, S. and Rice, N.R. (1988) J. Virol. 62, 4730–4736.
10 Davis, N. et al. (1991) Science 253, 1268–1271.
11 Capobianco, A.J. et al. (1992) J. Virol. 66, 3758–3767.
12 Neumann, M. et al. (1992) Oncogene 7, 2095–2104.
13 Brownell, E. et al. (1987) Mol. Cell. Biol. 7, 1304–1309.
14 Moore, B.E. and Bose, H.R. Jr. (1989) Oncogene 4, 845–852.
15 Abbadie, C. et al. (1993) Cell 75, 899–912.
16 Kamens, J. and Brent, R. (1991) New Biol. 3, 1005–1013.
17 Kochel, T. and Rice, N.R. (1992) Oncogene 7, 567–572.
18 Kunsch, C. et al. (1992) Mol. Cell. Biol. 12, 4412–4421.
19 Rice, N.R. et al. (1986) Virology 149, 217–229.
20 Walro, D.S. et al. (1987) Virology 160, 433–444.
21 Nakayama, K. et al. (1992) Mol. Cell. Biol. 12, 1736–1746.
22 Druker, B.J. et al. (1994) J. Biol. Chem. 269, 5387–5390.
23 Muchardt, C. et al. (1992) J. Virol. 66, 244–250.
24 Tan, T.-H. et al. (1992) Mol. Cell. Biol. 12, 4067–4075.

25 Sica, A. et al. (1992) Proc. Natl Acad. Sci. USA 89, 1740–1744.

26 Cogswell, P.C. et al. (1993) J. Immunol. 150, 2794–2804.

27 Hansen, S.K. et al. (1992) EMBO J. 11, 205–213.

28 McDonnell, P.C. et al. (1992) Oncogene 7, 163–170.

29 Ishikawa, H. et al. (1993) Oncogene 8, 2889–2896.

30 Logeat, F. et al. (1991) EMBO J. 10, 1827–1832.

31 Richardson, P.M. and Gilmore, T.D. (1991) J. Virol. 65, 3122–3130.

32 Ballard, D.W. et al. (1992) Proc. Natl Acad.Sci. USA 89, 1875–1879.

33 Walker, W.H. et al. (1992) J. Virol. 66, 5018–5029.

34 Boehmelt, G. et al. (1992) EMBO J. 11, 4641–4652.

35 Inuzuka, M. et al. (1994) Oncogene 9, 133–140.

36 Xu, X. et al. (1993) Mol. Cell. Biol. 13, 6733–6741.

37 Neri, A. et al. (1991) Cell 67, 1075–1087.

38 Lu, D. et al. (1991) Oncogene 6, 1235–1241.

39 Moore, B.E. and Bose, H.R. (1988) Virology 162, 377–387.

40 Morrison, L.E. et al. (1991) Oncogene 6, 1657–1666.

41 Lewis, R.B. et al. (1981) Cell 25, 421–431.

42 Brownell, E. et al. (1989) Oncogene 4, 935–942.

43 Capobianco, A.J. and Gilmore, T.D. (1991) Oncogene 6, 2203–2210.

44 Kamens, J. et al. (1990) Mol. Cell Biol. 10, 2840–2847.

45 Ghosh, S. et al. (1990) Cell 62, 1019–1029.

46 Inoue, J.-I. et al. (1992) Cell 68, 1109–1120.

47 Wilhelmsen, K.C. et al. (1984) J. Virol. 52, 172–182.

48 Capobianco, A.J. et al. (1990) Oncogene 5, 257–265.

RET

IDENTIFICATION

RET is a human transforming gene with no homology with known viral oncogenes orginally detected by NIH 3T3 fibroblast transfection with DNA from a T cell lymphoma.

RELATED GENES

RET has homology with *Tek* receptor tyrosine kinase and the Ca^{2+}-binding sites of cadherins [1]. RET^{TPC} and RET^{PTC} (papillary thyroid carcinoma) are synonymous notations for the oncoprotein.

Nucleotides (kb)	30
Chromosome	10q11.2
Mass (kDa): predicted	91 (RET)
	57–60 (RET/PTC1)
expressed	gp150/gp170
	p96/p100 (in *RET*-transformed cells)
	p57$^{RET/PTC1}$/p64$^{RET/PTC1}$
	p76$^{RET/PTC2}$/p81$^{RET/PTC2}$

Cellular location

Plasma membrane. p96 and oncoproteins: cytoplasm.

Tissue distribution

Expressed in the developing central and peripheral nervous systems and the excretory systems of mice. Undetectable or low in adult rat or mouse normal tissues but present in the rat placenta during the mid-term of gestation [2].

The proto-oncogene form of *RET* is expressed in human medullary thyroid carcinomas (MTCs) and pheochromocytomas and in neuroblastoma cells after induction of differentiation [3,4].

PROTEIN FUNCTION

RET encodes two forms of receptor tyrosine kinases not phosphorylated on tyrosine. Ligand unknown. *RET* may be involved in neuronal differentiation [4,5]. The dominant oncogenic forms of RET (RET/PTC1, RET/PTC2 and RET/PTC3) are constitutively phosphorylated on tyrosine and have autophosphorylation activity [6,7]. p76$^{RET-PTC2}$ and p81$^{RET-PTC2}$ form homo- and heterodimers with each other [8].

Cancer

An activated form of *RET* (*RET-PTC1*) has been found with high frequency (11–33%) in papillary thyroid carcinomas [9,10] and in the TPC-1 human

241

papillary thyroid carcinoma cell line [11]. There is one report of RET–PTC1 activation in follicular adenomas and adenomatous goitres [12]. A second type of RET oncogenic rearrangement, RET–PTC2, occurs with lower frequency in papillary thyroid carcinomas [8]. These tumours are usually sporadic. Germline point mutations in RET also occur in familial medullary thyroid carcinoma (FMTC) [13], multiple endocrine neoplasia (MEN) types 2A [14] and 2B [15] and Hirschsprung's disease [16,17].

Transgenic animals

Mice carrying the metallothionein/Ret (MT/Ret) fusion gene develop melanosis and melanocytic tumours [18]. In MMTV/Ret transgenic mice mammary and salivary gland adenocarcinomas develop in a stochastic manner [19]. Mice homozygous for the deletion of Ret die soon after birth and reveal that Ret is essential for renal organogenesis and enteric neurogenesis [20].

GENE STRUCTURE

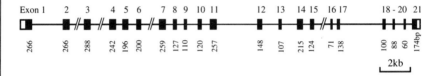

TRANSCRIPTIONAL REGULATION

The promoter region of proto-RET contains a GC-rich region without a TATA box. Putative binding motifs for SP1, AP-2, epidermal growth factor receptor-specific transcription factor (ETF) and the transcription suppressor GC factor (GCF) occur in this repeated GC region [21,22].

PROTEIN STRUCTURE

The RET transforming gene isolated by Takahashi et al. [23] had been activated in vitro during the transfection assay in a rearragement that juxtaposed two unlinked human DNA segments, the RET proto-oncogene and the putative zinc finger-containing RFP gene (ret finger protein) [24].

RET/PTC1 is a different fusion protein of a 5′ non-RET region (D10S170) and the kinase domain encoded by RET. This is a somatic, tumour-specific event, in contrast to the recombination between RET and RFP. Alternative splicing of proto-RET gives rise to differing C-termini and corresponding PTC cDNAs have been isolated.

A second rearrangement (RET/PTC2) has been detected in papillary thyroid carcinoma in which the C-terminus of normal RET, including the tyrosine kinase domain, is fused with part of the RIα regulatory subunit of protein kinase A [7,8].

A third rearrangement (*RET/PTC3*) has also been detected in papillary thyroid carcinomas in which the C-terminal 360 amino acids of RET are linked to 238 N-terminal residues of RFG (*R*ET *f*used *g*ene) [25].

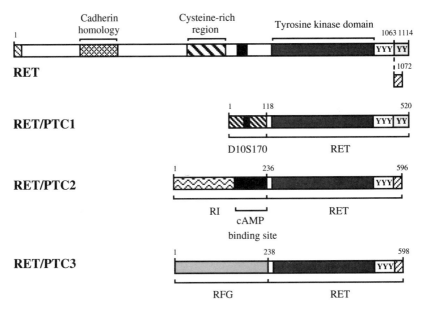

SEQUENCE OF RET

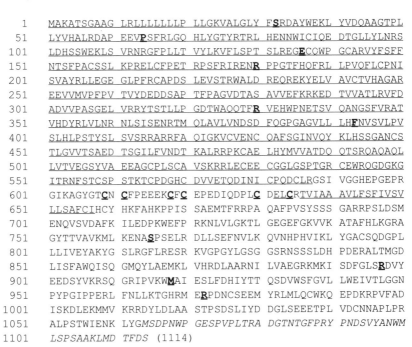

```
   1   MAKATSGAAG LRLLLLLLLP LLGKVALGLY FSRDAYWEKL YVDQAAGTPL
  51   LYVHALRDAP EEVPSFRLGQ HLYGTYRTRL HENNWICIQE DTGLLYLNRS
 101   LDHSSWEKLS VRNRGFPLLT VYLKVFLSPT SLREGECQWP GCARVYFSFF
 151   NTSFPACSSL KPRELCFPET RPSFRIRENR PPGTFHQFRL LPVQFLCPNI
 201   SVAYRLLEGE GLPFRCAPDS LEVSTRWALD REQREKYELV AVCTVHAGAR
 251   EEVVMVPFPV TVYDEDDSAP TFPAGVDTAS AVVEFKRKED TVVATLRVFD
 301   ADVVPASGEL VRRYTSTLLP GDTWAQQTFR VEHWPNETSV QANGSFVRAT
 351   VHDYRLVLNR NLSISENRTM QLAVLVNDSD FQGPGAGVLL LHFNVSVLPV
 401   SLHLPSTYSL SVSRRARRFA QIGKVCVENC QAFSGINVQY KLHSSGANCS
 451   TLGVVTSAED TSGILFVNDT KALRRPKCAE LHYMVVATDQ QTSRQAQAQL
 501   LVTVEGSYVA EEAGCPLSCA VSKRRLECEE CGGLGSPTGR CEWRQGDGKG
 551   ITRNFSTCSP STKTCPDGHC DVVETQDINI CPQDCLRGSI VGGHEPGEPR
 601   GIKAGYGTCN CFPEEEKCFC EPEDIQDPLC DELCRTVIAA AVLFSFIVSV
 651   LLSAFCIHCY HKFAHKPPIS SAEMTFRRPA QAFPVSYSSS GARRPSLDSM
 701   ENQVSVDAFK ILEDPKWEFP RKNLVLGKTL GEGEFGKVVK ATAFHLKGRA
 751   GYTTVAVKML KENASPSELR DLLSEFNVLK QVNHPHVIKL YGACSQDGPL
 801   LLIVEYAKYG SLRGFLRESR KVGPGYLGSG GSRNSSSLDH PDERALTMGD
 851   LISFAWQISQ GMQYLAEMKL VHRDLAARNI LVAEGRKMKI SDFGLSRDVY
 901   EEDSYVKRSQ GRIPVKWMAI ESLFDHIYTT QSDVWSFGVL LWEIVTLGGN
 951   PYPGIPPERL FNLLKTGHRM ERPDNCSEEM YRLMLQCWKQ EPDKRPVFAD
1001   ISKDLEKMMV KRRDYLDLAA STPSDSLIYD DGLSEEETPL VDCNNAPLPR
1051   ALPSTWIENK LYGMSDPNWP GESPVPLTRA DGTNTGFPRY PNDSVYANWM
1101   LSPSAAKLMD TFDS (1114)
```

Domain structure

1–587	RET sequence replaced by RFP in the chimeric protein generated *in vitro* (underlined)
1–712	RET sequence replaced by D10S170 sequence in the PTC1 fusion protein
636–657	Transmembrane region (underlined)
722–999	Tyrosine protein kinase domain
730–738 and 758	ATP binding site
874	Active site
1064–1114	51 C-terminal amino acids of one isoform of RET (italics). The alternative 9 amino acid terminus is shown in the RET/PTC2 sequence below [26].

Mutations detected (underlined, bold): MEN 2A: Cys609→mis-sense, Cys618→Gly, Arg or Ser, Cys620→Arg, Tyr, Cys634→Arg, Gly, Tyr, Ser or Phe; MEN2B: Met918→Thr; FMTC: Cys611→Trp, Cys618→Ser or Tyr, Cys620→Arg. Hirschsprung's disease: deletions, truncation, Ser32→Leu, Pro64→Leu, Glu136→STOP, Arg180→STOP, Arg330→Gln, Phe393→Leu, Ser765→Pro, Arg897→Gln, Arg972→Gly. Sporadic MTC: Cys630→deletion [27].

SEQUENCE OF RET/PTC2

```
  1  MQSGSTAASQ QARSLRQCQL YVEKHNIEAL LKDSIVQLCT ARPERPMAFL
 51  REYFERLEKE EAKQIQNLQK AGTRTDSRED EISPPPPNPV VKGRRRRGAI
101  SAEVYTEEDA ASYVRKVIPK DYKTMAALAK AIEKNVLFSH LDDNERSDIF
151  DAMFSVSFIA GETVIQQGDE GDNFYVIDQG ETDVYNNEW ATSVGEGGSF
```
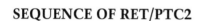
```
                                       RIα/RET
201  GELALIYGTP RAATVKAKTN VKLWGIDRDS YRRILMEDPK WEFPRKNLVL
251  GKTLGEGEFG KVVKATAFHL KGRAGYTTVA VKMLKENASP SELRDLLSEF
301  NVLKQVNHPH VIKLYGACSQ DGPLLLIVEY AKYGSLRGFL RESRKVGPGY
351  LGSGGSRNSS SLDHPDERAL TMGDLISFAW QISQGMQYLA EMKLVHRDLA
401  ARNILVAEGR KMKISDFGLS RDVYEEDPYV KRSQGRIPVK WMAIESLFDH
451  IYTTQSDVWS FGVLLWEIVT LGGNPYPGIP PERLFNLLKT GHRMERPDNC
501  SEEMYRLMLQ CWKQEPDKRP VFADISKDLE KMMVKRRDYL DLAASTPSDS
551  LIYDDGLSEE ETPLVDCNNA PLPRALPSTW IENKLYGRIS HAFTRF (596)
```

Domain structure

1–236	Sequence of RIα (underlined)
236/237	RIα/RET fusion point (the same as in D10S170-RET)
588–596	Nine amino acid form of C-terminus (italics)

DATABASE ACCESSION NUMBERS

	PIR	SWISSPROT	EMBL/GENBANK	REFERENCES
Human *RET*	A27203	P07949	M16029	5
			X12949, X15262	28
Human *RET/PTC2*			L03357	8
Human *RET/PTC3*			M31213	25

References
1 Iwamoto, T. et al. (1993) Oncogene 8, 1087–1091.
2 Szentirmay, Z. et al. (1990) Oncogene 5, 701–705.
3 Santoro, M. et al. (1990) Oncogene 5, 1595–1598.
4 Tahira, T. et al. (1991) Oncogene 6, 2333–2338.
5 Takahashi, M. and Cooper, G.M. (1987) Mol. Cell. Biol. 7, 1378–1385.
6 Ishizaka, Y. et al. (1992) Oncogene 7, 1441–1444.
7 Lanzi, C. et al. (1992) Oncogene 7, 2189–2194.
8 Bongarzone, I. et al. (1993) Mol. Cell. Biol. 13, 358–366.
9 Jhiang, S.M. et al. (1992) Oncogene 7, 1331–1337.
10 Santoro, M. et al. (1992) J. Clin. Invest. 89, 1517–1522.
11 Ishizaka, Y. et al. (1990) Biochem. Biophys. Res. Commun. 168, 402–408.
12 Ishizaka, Y. et al. (1991) Oncogene 6, 1667–1672.
13 Donis-Keller, H. et al. (1993) Hum. Molec. Genet. 2, 851–856.
14 Mulligan, L. et al. (1993) Nature 363, 458–460.
15 Hofstra, R.M.W. et al. (1994) Nature 367, 375–376.
16 Edery, P. et al. (1994) Nature 367, 378–380.
17 Romeo, G. et al. (1994) Nature 367, 377–378.
18 Taniguchi, M. et al. (1992) Oncogene 7, 1491–1496.
19 Iwamoto, T. et al. (1990) Oncogene 5, 535–542.
20 Schuchardt, A. et al. (1994) Nature 367, 380–383.
21 Itoh, F. et al. (1992) Oncogene 7, 1201–1205.
22 Kwok, J.B.J. et al. (1993) Oncogene 8, 2575–2582.
23 Takahashi, M. et al. (1985) Cell 42, 581–588.
24 Takahashi, M. et al (1988) Mol. Cell. Biol. 8, 1853–1856.
25 Santoro, M. et al. (1994) Oncogene 9, 509–516.
26 Tahira, T. et al. (1990) Oncogene 5, 97–102.
27 Carlson, K.M. et al. (1994) Proc. Natl Acad. Sci. USA 91, 1579–1583.
28 Takahashi, M. et al. (1989) Oncogene 4, 805–806.

ROS1

IDENTIFICATION

v-*ros* is the oncogene of the acutely transforming avian sarcoma virus UR2 (University of Rochester), so designated because it is unrelated to any other ASV gene. *MCF3* is an activated form of *ROS1* detected by transfection of cDNA derived from a human mammary carcinoma cell line (MCF-7) into NIH 3T3 cells and injection of these cells into nude mice. The *MCF3* gene was expressed in some of the tumours generated. *ROS1* was detected by screening cDNA with an *MCF3* probe.

RELATED GENES

ROS1 has homology with SRC tyrosine kinases and with receptor-type tyrosine kinases including the insulin and EGF receptors. Close similarity in overall structure and sequence exists between vertebrate ROS and *Drosophila sevenless*.

	ROS1	v-*ros*
Nucleotides	32 kb	1273 bp
Chromosome	6q21–q22	
Mass (kDa): predicted	256	61
expressed	gp260	P68*gag-ros*

Cellular location

Plasma membrane.

Tissue distribution

Ros-1 mRNA expression in the mouse occurs transiently during the development of the kidney, intestine and lung and coincides with major morphogenetic and differentiation events [1]. Chicken *Ros-1* is significantly expressed in the kidney and intestine with low expression in the gonads, thymus, bursa and brain [2].

PROTEIN FUNCTION

ROS1 is a receptor-like tyrosine kinase with autophosphorylation capacity. p68*gag-ros* co-precipitates with PtdIns kinase and in UR2-transformed cells the levels of PtdIns4*P*, PtdIns(4,5)P_2 and Ins(1,4,5)P_3 are increased [3]. The pattern of expression during the differentiation of normal tissues is unusual for a tyrosine kinase receptor and indicates a specific role for *Ros-1* during developmen [1].

Cancer

ROS1 expression is elevated in cell lines derived from human glioblastomas [5] but not in primary human glioblastomas [6].

In animals

Injected UR2 induces tumours in chickens. UR2-transformed rat cells induce fatal fibrosarcomas on injection into rats [7]. *MCF3*-transformed NIH 3T3 cells form tumours in nude mice [8].

In vitro

Infected cells from chicken tumours transform chick embryo fibroblasts and infected CEFs transform rat-1 cell lines.

GENE STRUCTURE

The genomic structure of *ROS1* has not been completely characterized.

PROTEIN STRUCTURE OF ROS

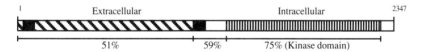

The figures indicate percentage identity with chicken ROS1. v-ROS is an N-terminally truncated version of chicken ROS1 with an alternative 12 amino acid C-terminus. Rat ROS1 is related to *Drosophila sev* protein and both have a unique insert in the tyrosine kinase domain. ROS proteins contain a 20 residue hydrophobic sequence 50 amino acids downstream of the initiating Met residue and may form a loop structure from the plasma membrane. In MCF3, an activated form of ROS1, all but eight amino acids of the ROS1 extracellular domain are replaced by sequences of unknown origin.

SEQUENCE OF ROS1

```
  1 MKNIYCLIPK LVNFATLGCL WISVVQCTVL NSCLKSCVTN LGQQLDLGTP
 51 HNLSEPCIQG CHFWNSVDQK NCALKCRESC EVGCSSAEGA YEEEVLENAD
101 LPTAPFASSI GSHNMTLRWK SANFSGVKYI IQWKYAQLLG SWTYTKTVSR
151 PSYVVKPLHP FTEYIFRVVW IFTAQLQLYS PPSPSYRTHP HGVPETAPLI
201 RNIESSSPDT VEVSWDPPQF PGGPILGYNL RLISKNQKLD AGTQRTSFQF
251 YSTLPNTIYR FSIAAVNEVG EGPEAESSIT TSSSAVQQEE QWLFLSRKTS
301 LRKRSLKHLV DEAHCLRLDA IYHNITGISV DVHQQIVYFS EGTLIWAKKA
351 ANMSDVSDLR IFYRGSGLIS SISIDWLYQR MYFIMDELVC VCDLENCSNI
```

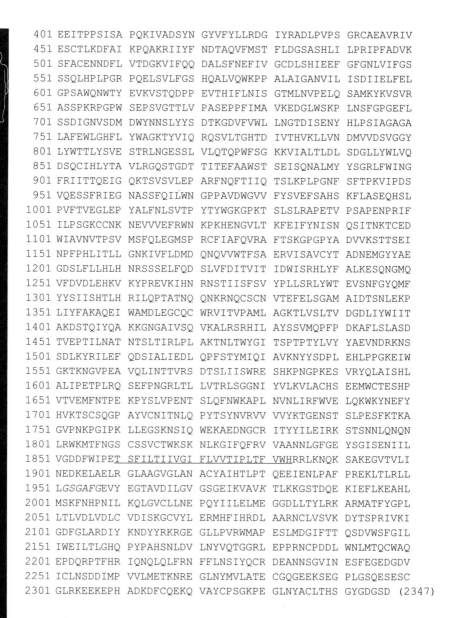

```
 401 EEITPPSISA PQKIVADSYN GYVFYLLRDG IYRADLPVPS GRCAEAVRIV
 451 ESCTLKDFAI KPQAKRIIYF NDTAQVFMST FLDGSASHLI LPRIPFADVK
 501 SFACENNDFL VTDGKVIFQQ DALSFNEFIV GCDLSHIEEF GFGNLVIFGS
 551 SSQLHPLPGR PQELSVLFGS HQALVQWKPP ALAIGANVIL ISDIIELFEL
 601 GPSAWQNWTY EVKVSTQDPP EVTHIFLNIS GTMLNVPELQ SAMKYKVSVR
 651 ASSPKRPGPW SEPSVGTTLV PASEPPFIMA VKEDGLWSKP LNSFGPGEFL
 701 SSDIGNVSDM DWYNNSLYYS DTKGDVFVWL LNGTDISENY HLPSIAGAGA
 751 LAFEWLGHFL YWAGKTYVIQ RQSVLTGHTD IVTHVKLLVN DMVVDSVGGY
 801 LYWTTLYSVE STRLNGESSL VLQTQPWFSG KKVIALTLDL SDGLLYWLVQ
 851 DSQCIHLYTA VLRGQSTGDT TITEFAAWST SEISQNALMY YSGRLFWING
 901 FRIITTQEIG QKTSVSVLEP ARFNQFTIIQ TSLKPLPGNF SFTPKVIPDS
 951 VQESSFRIEG NASSFQILWN GPPAVDWGVV FYSVEFSAHS KFLASEQHSL
1001 PVFTVEGLEP YALFNLSVTP YTYWGKGPKT SLSLRAPETV PSAPENPRIF
1051 ILPSGKCCNK NEVVVEFRWN KPKHENGVLT KFEIFYNISN QSITNKTCED
1101 WIAVNVTPSV MSFQLEGMSP RCFIAFQVRA FTSKGPGPYA DVVKSTTSEI
1151 NPFPHLITLL GNKIVFLDMD QNQVVWTFSA ERVISAVCYT ADNEMGYYAE
1201 GDSLFLLHLH NRSSSELFQD SLVFDITVIT IDWISRHLYF ALKESQNGMQ
1251 VFDVDLEHKV KYPREVKIHN RNSTIISFSV YPLLSRLYWT EVSNFGYQMF
1301 YYSIISHTLH RILQPTATNQ QNKRNQCSCN VTEFELSGAM AIDTSNLEKP
1351 LIYFAKAQEI WAMDLEGCQC WRVITVPAML AGKTLVSLTV DGDLIYWIIT
1401 AKDSTQIYQA KKGNGAIVSQ VKALRSRHIL AYSSVMQPFP DKAFLSLASD
1451 TVEPTILNAT NTSLTIRLPL AKTNLTWYGI TSPTPTYLVY YAEVNDRKNS
1501 SDLKYRILEF QDSIALIEDL QPFSTYMIQI AVKNYYSDPL EHLPPGKEIW
1551 GKTKNGVPEA VQLINTTVRS DTSLIISWRE SHKPNGPKES VRYQLAISHL
1601 ALIPETPLRQ SEFPNGRLTL LVTRLSGGNI YVLKVLACHS EEMWCTESHP
1651 VTVEMFNTPE KPYSLVPENT SLQFNWKAPL NVNLIRFWVE LQKWKYNEFY
1701 HVKTSCSQGP AYVCNITNLQ PYTSYNVRVV VVYKTGENST SLPESFKTKA
1751 GVPNKPGIPK LLEGSKNSIQ WEKAEDNGCR ITYYILEIRK STSNNLQNQN
1801 LRWKMTFNGS CSSVCTWKSK NLKGIFQFRV VAANNLGFGE YSGISENIIL
1851 VGDDFWIPET SFILTIIVGI FLVVTIPLTF VWHRRLKNQK SAKEGVTVLI
1901 NEDKELAELR GLAAGVGLAN ACYAIHTLPT QEEIENLPAF PREKLTLRLL
1951 LGSGAFGEVY EGTAVDILGV GSGEIKVAVK TLKKGSTDQE KIEFLKEAHL
2001 MSKFNHPNIL KQLGVCLLNE PQYIILELME GGDLLTYLRK ARMATFYGPL
2051 LTLVDLVDLC VDISKGCVYL ERMHFIHRDL AARNCLVSVK DYTSPRIVKI
2101 GDFGLARDIY KNDYYRKRGE GLLPVRWMAP ESLMDGIFTT QSDVWSFGIL
2151 IWEILTLGHQ PYPAHSNLDV LNYVQTGGRL EPPRNCPDDL WNLMTQCWAQ
2201 EPDQRPTFHR IQNQLQLFRN FFLNSIYQCR DEANNSGVIN ESFEGEDGDV
2251 ICLNSDDIMP VVLMETKNRE GLNYMVLATE CGQGEEKSEG PLGSQESESC
2301 GLRKEEKEPH ADKDFCQEKQ VAYCPSGKPE GLNYACLTHS GYGDGSD (2347)
```

Domain structure

11–42 and 1860–1883   Hydrophobic regions (underlined)
  1952–1957 and 1980   ATP binding site (italics)

DATABASE ACCESSION NUMBERS

	PIR	SWISSPROT	EMBL/GENBANK	REFERENCE
Human *ROS1*			M34353	9

References

1 Sonnenberg, E. et al. (1991) EMBO J. 10, 3693–3702.
2 Neckameyer, W.S. et al. (1986) Mol. Cell. Biol. 6, 1478–1486.
3 Macara, I.G. et al. (1984) Proc. Natl Acad. Sci. USA 81, 2728–2732.
4 Chen, J. et al. (1994) Oncogene 9, 773–780.
5 Sharma, S. et al. (1989) Oncogene Res. 5, 91–100.
6 Wu, J.K. and Chikaraishi, D.M. (1990) Cancer Res. 50, 3032–3035.
7 Neckameyer, W.S. and Wang, L.-H. (1985) J. Virol. 53, 879–884.
8 Birchmeier, C. et al. (1986) Mol. Cell. Biol. 6, 3109–3116.
9 Birchmeier, C. et al. (1990) Proc. Natl Acad. Sci. USA 87, 4799–4803.

IDENTIFICATION

v-*sea* (*s*arcoma, *e*rythroblastosis and *a*naemia) is the oncogene of the acutely transforming virus AEV-S13. Chicken *Sea* was detected by low stringency hybridization screening of cDNA with a v-*src* probe.

RELATED GENES

SEA is a member of the tyrosine protein kinase family with strong homology to the insulin receptor family and MET.

	SEA	*v-sea*
Nucleotides (kb)	Not fully mapped	8.5 (S13)
Chromosome	11q13	
Mass (kDa): predicted	190	42 (v-SEA)
expressed		gp155$^{env-sea}$
		gp85^{env}/gp70$^{env-sea}$

Cellular location

SEA: Plasma membrane. v-SEA: Plasma membrane.

Tissue distribution

Chicken *Sea* is expressed in most tissues with highest levels in peripheral white blood cells and the intestine [1]. *Sea* mRNA is elevated fivefold in chicken embryo cells transformed by v-*src*.

PROTEIN FUNCTION

SEA is a growth factor receptor tyrosine protein kinase. Transformation by *env–sea* correlates with tyrosine phosphorylation of SHC proteins [2].

Cancer

Expressed at low frequency (~1%) in breast carcinomas together with *BCL1*, *HSTF1* and *INT2* [3].

In animals

Injection of AEV S13 into young chickens causes sarcomas, erythroblastosis and anaemias [4]. Fibroblasts transformed by v-*sea* are only weakly oncogenic when injected into chicks: cells expressing a retrovirus carrying both v-*sea* and v-*ski* are highly malignant [5].

In vitro

v-*sea* transforms fibroblasts and erythroblasts [6] but does not transform avian myeloid cells [7]. v-*sea* induces the synthesis of chicken myeloid growth factor (cMGF) and causes autocrine growth in myeloid cells transformed by v-*myb* or v-*myc* [8]. The differentiation of v-*sea*-transformed erythroid cells into erythrocytes is blocked by the expression of v-*ski* [5]. This effect of v-*ski* is similar to that of v-*erbA* but is associated with different effects on gene expression.

GENE STRUCTURE

The *env* sequence is 96% homologous with that of the RAV2 strain of ALV. The ~1085 bp insert between *env* and the viral 3' non-coding region encodes the *sea* ORF. A single base deletion 14 bp upstream of the normal *env* termination codon permits read-through into the *sea* gene. The termination codon lies within the 3' viral non-coding region.

The S13 virus encodes normal *gag* and *gag–pol* proteins and an abnormal *env* glycoprotein (gp155) that is cleaved to gp85^{env} and gp70$^{env-sea}$. gp155$^{env-sea}$ retains the entire extracellular and transmembrane domains of *env*. Replacement of the entire *env* sequence by the myristylation target signal of pp60^{v-src} does not affect the capacity of v-*sea* to transform fibroblasts [6]. The uncleaved but fully glycosylated gp155$^{env-sea}$ retains the capacity to transform chicken embryo fibroblasts [9].

PROTEIN STRUCTURE

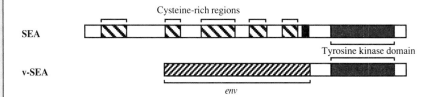

The extracellular and transmembrane regions of v-SEA are derived from the viral *env* gene.

SEQUENCE OF CHICKEN SEA

```
   1 MGPRCLVCLL LLLAPSLLQA GAWQCRRIPF SSTRNFSVPY TLPSLDAGSP
  51 VQNIAVFPDP PTVFVAVRNR ILVVDPELRL RSVLVTGPTG SAPCEICRLC
 101 PAAVDAPGPE DVDNVLLLLD PVEPWLYSCG TARRGLCYLH QLDVRGSEVT
 151 IASTRCLYSA AANSPVNCPD CVASPLGSTA TVVADRYTAS FYLGSTVNSS
 201 VAARYSPRSV SVRRLKGTRD GFADPFHSLT VLPHYQDVYP IHYVHSFTDG
 251 DHVYLVTVQP EFPGSSTFHT RLVRLSAHEP ELRRYREIVL DCRYESKRRR
 301 RRRGAEEETE RDVAYNVLQA AHAARPGARL ARDLGIDGTE TVLFGAFAES
 351 HPESRAPQHN SAVCAFPLRL LNQAIREGMD KCCGTGTQTL KRGLAFFQPQ
 401 QYCPHSVNLS APVTNTSCWD QPTLVPAASH KVDLFNGRLS GTLLTSIFVT
 451 VLQNVTVAHL GTAQGRVLQM VLQRSSSYVV ALTNFSLGEP GLVQHATGLQ
 501 GHSLLFAAGT KVWRVNVTGP GCRHFSTCDR CLRAERFMGC GWCGNGCTRH
 551 HECAGPWVQD SCPPVLTDFH PRSAPLRGQT RVTLCGMTFH SPPDPTAHHS
 601 LPGPYRVAVG GRSCTVLLDE SESYRPLPTF RRKDFVDVLV CVLEPGEPAV
 651 AAGPADVVLN VTESAGTSRF RVQGSSTLSG FVFVEPHIST LHPSFGPQGG
 701 GTLMSLYGTH LSAGSSWRVT INGSECLLDG QPSEGDGEIR CTAPAATSLG
 751 AAPVALWIDG EEFLAPLPFE YRPDPSVLTV VPNCSYGGST LTLIGTHLDS
 801 VYRAKIQFQG GGGGKTEATE CEGPQSPNWL LCRSPAFPIE IKPVPGNLSV
 851 LLDGAADRWL FRLRYFPQPQ MFSFGQQGER YQLKPGDNEI KVNQLGLDSV
 901 AGCMNITMTV GGRDCHPNVL KNEVTCRVPR DVDLTPAGAP VQICVNGDCQ
 951 ALGLVLPASS LDMAASLALG TGVTFLVCCV LAAVLLRWRW RKRRGLENLE
1001 LLVHPPRIEH PITIQRPNVD YREVQVLPVA DSPGLARPHA HFASAGADAA
1051 GGGSPVPLLR TTSCCLEDLR PELLEEVKDI LIPEERLITH RSRVIGRGHF
1101 GSVYHGTYMD PLLGNLHCAV KSLHRITDLE EVEEFLREGI LMKSFHHPQV
1151 LSLLGVCLPR HGLPLVVLPY MRHGDLRHFI RAQERSPTVK ELIGFGLQVA
1201 LGMEYLAQKK FVHRDLAARN CMLDETLTVK VADFGLARDV FGKEYYSIRQ
1251 HRHAKLPVKW MALESLQTQK FTTKSDVWSF GVLMWELLTR GASPYPEVDP
1301 YDMARYLLRG RRLPQPQPCP DTLYGVMLSC WAPTPEERPS FSGLVCELER
1351 VLASLEGERY VNLAVTYVNL ESGPPFPPAP RGQLPDSEDE EDEEDEEDED
1401 AAVR (1404)
```

Domain structure

1–22	Signal sequence (italics)
297–303	Proteolytic processing site
964–986	Transmembrane domain (underlined)
1096–1357	Tyrosine kinase domain
1118–1121	ATP binding site
35, 408, 415, 454, 484, 516, 660, 722, 847, 905	Potential *N*-linked glycosylation sites

DATABASE ACCESSION NUMBERS

	PIR	*SWISSPROT*	*EMBL/GENBANK*	*REFERENCES*
Chicken *Sea*			L12024	*1*

References

1 Huff, J.L. et al. (1993) Proc. Natl Acad. Sci. USA 90, 6140–6144.
2 Crowe, A.J. et al. (1994) Oncogene 9, 537–544.
3 Theillet, C. et al. (1990) Oncogene 5, 147–149.
4 Stubbs, E.L. and Furth, J. (1935) J. Exp. Med. 61, 593–616.
5 Larsen, J. et al. (1992) Oncogene 7, 1903–1911.
6 Crowe, A.J. and Hayman, M.J. (1991) J. Virol. 65, 2533–2538.
7 Beug, H. and Graf, T. (1989) Eur. J. Clin. Invest. 19, 491–502.
8 Adkins, B. et al. (1984) Cell 39, 439–445.
9 Crowe, A.J. and Hayman, M.J. (1993) Oncogene 8, 181–189.

SKI

IDENTIFICATION

v-*ski* is the common oncogene of Sloan–Kettering viruses (SKVs), a group of acutely transforming chicken retroviruses. It was first detected in chick embryo fibroblasts infected with an originally non-transforming ALV strain, from which three isolates (SKV770, SKV780, SKV790) were prepared. SKI was detected by screening cDNA with a v-*ski* probe.

RELATED GENES

SNOA, *SNOI* and *SNON* (*S*KI-related *no*vel) are produced by alternative splicing of the same gene (giving different C-termini) and *SNOI* utilizes an alternative third exon [1,2]. *SKI* and *SNO* are closely related but show no marked sequence homology to other oncogenes. SKI proteins contain an extensive C-terminal helical domain that has homology with domains present in myosin, intermediate filaments and lamins.

	SKI/Ski	*v-ski*
Nucleotides (kb)	>70 (chicken)	3.0–8.9 (SKV-derived genomes)
Chromosome	1q22–q24	
Mass (kDa): predicted	80	p49$^{v\text{-}ski}$
expressed (chicken)	p90 (7 exons) p50 (lacking exon 7), p60 (lacking exon 6)	p125$^{\Delta gag\text{-}ski}$; p110$^{\Delta gag\text{-}ski\text{-}pol}$; p45$^{\Delta gag\text{-}ski}$

Cellular location

SKI: Nucleus. v-SKI: Nucleus.

Tissue distribution

Detectable at low levels in all chicken and quail tissues [3]. *Xenopus Ski* RNA accumulates in developing oocytes: following fertilization, the level declines during the mid-blastula transition. In *Xenopus* adult tissues *Ski* expression is high in the lungs and ovaries [4].

PROTEIN FUNCTION

Unknown. v-*ski* induces MyoD and myogenin expression and myogenesis in non-muscle cells [5]. These genes are also induced by a transformation-defective v-*ski* mutant that does not induce myotube formation. However, in *Ski* transgenic mice the levels of MyoD and myogenin are not affected [6].

The effect of wild-type v-*ski* is the opposite to that of v-*jun* which inhibits myogenic differentiation.

The combination of v-*ski* and v-*sea* is highly malignant, indicating that v-*ski* can cooperate with a tyrosine kinase oncogene as does v-*erbA* with v-*erbB* [7].

The C-terminal helical domain, deleted in v-SKI, may permit the formation of homodimers or interaction with other proteins. Phosphorylation in the C-terminal region of normal SKI may release the protein to function via its N-terminus as a regulator of transcription [4].

Cancer

The chromosomal region 1q22–q24, to which *SKI* maps, is a common site of breakage in carcinomas and haematopoietic tumours [8].

Transgenic animals

Transgenic mice expressing a region of chicken *Ski* have distinctive muscle growth caused by selective hypertrophy of fast skeletal muscle fibres [6,9].

In animals

In chickens, injection of SKV-CEFs causes non-metastasizing squamous cell carcinomas in 50% of animals [3,10]. v-*ski* enhances the leukaemogenic potential of v-*sea* [7].

In vitro

v-*ski* or overexpressed *Ski* transforms CEFs and induces myogenic differentiation of quail embryo cells [11,12]. v-*ski* transforms chicken bone marrow cells but requires co-expression of v-*sea* for the initiation of transformation [13]. v-*ski* also transforms bone marrow cells *in vitro* in the presence of the KIT ligand SCF.

PARTIAL STRUCTURE OF THE CHICKEN SKI GENE

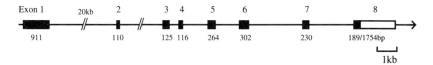

The region between exons 2 and 3 has not been fully mapped. The open box indicates the untranslated region of exon 8 and the arrow indicates that the 3' end has not been defined [14].

PROTEIN STRUCTURE

v-SKI is highly homologous (91%) with human SKI except for a 37 amino acid insertion in v-SKI (280–316) that corresponds to exon 2 of chicken *Ski* from which it is derived and a 15 amino acid insertion in SKI (55–69).

SEQUENCE OF SKI

```
  1  MEAAAGGRGC FQPHPGLQKT LEQFHLSSMS SLGGPAAFSA RWAQEAYKKE
 51  SAKEAGAAAV PAPVPAATEP PPVLHLPAIQ PPPPVLPGPF FMPSDRSTER
101  CETVLEGETI SCFVVGGEKR LCLPQILNSV LRDFSLQQIN AVCDELHIYC
151  SRCTADQLEI LKVMGILPFS APSCGLITKT DAERLCNALL YGGAYPPPCK
201  KELAASLALG LELSERSVRV YHECFGKCKG LLVPELYSSP SAACIQCLDC
251  RLMYPPHKFV VHSHKALENR TCHWGFDSAN WRAYILLSQD YTGKEEQARL
301  GRCLDDVKEK FDYGNKYKRR VPRVSSEPPA SIRPKTDDTS SQSPAPSEKD
351  KPSSWLRTLA GSSNKSLGCV HPRQRLSAFR PWSPAVSASE KELSPHLPAL
401  IRDSFYSYKS FETAVAPNVA LAPPAQQKVV SSPPCAAAVS RAPEPLATCT
451  QPRKRKLTVD TPGAPETLAP VAAPEEDKDS EAEVEVESRE EFTSSLSSLS
501  SPSFTSSSSA KDLGSPGARA LPSAVPDAAA PADAPSGLEA ELEHLRQALE
551  GGLDTKEAKE KFLHEVVKMR VKQEEKLSAA LQAKRSLHQE LEFLRVAKKE
601  KLREATEAKR NLRKEIERLR AENEKKMKEA NESRLRLKRE LEQARQARVC
651  DKGCEAGRLR AKYSAQIEDL QVKLQHAEAD REQLRADLLR EREAREHLEK
701  VVKELQEQLW PRARPEAAGS EGAAELEP (728)
```

Domain structure

112, 122, 143, 150, 153, 174, 187, 224, 228, 244, 247, 250 and 272	13 cysteine residues conserved among all known SKI/SNO proteins (italics, underlined)
538–561, 562–586, 587–611, 612–636	Four major contiguous 25-mer repeated elements defined by the regular position of five hydrophobic, one acidic and two basic residues (underlined) [4]

DATABASE ACCESSION NUMBERS

	PIR	SWISSPROT	EMBL/GENBANK	REFERENCES
Human *SKI*	S06053	P12755	X15218	[1]
Human *SNOA*		P12756	S06054, X15217	[2]
Human *SNON*		P12757	X15219, S06052	[1,2]
Human *SNOI*			Z19588	[2]

References

[1] Nomura, N. et al. (1989) Nucl. Acids Res. 17, 5489–5500.
[2] Pearson-White, S. et al. (1993) Nucl. Acids Res. 21, 4632–4638.
[3] Stavnezer, E. et al. (1989) Mol. Cell. Biol. 9, 4038–4045.
[4] Sleeman, J.P. and Laskey, R.A. (1993) Oncogene 8, 67–77.

5   Colmenares, C. et al. (1991) Mol. Cell. Biol. 11, 1167–1170.
6   Sutrave, P. et al. (1992) In Neuromuscular Development and Disease, Molecular and Cellular Biology, Kelly, A.M. and Blau, H.M., eds, vol. 2, Raven Press, New York, pp. 107–114
7   Larsen, J. et al. (1992) Oncogene 7, 1903–1911.
8   Koduru, P.R.K. et al. (1987) Blood 69, 97–102.
9   Sutrave, P. et al. (1990) Genes Devel. 4, 1462–1473.
10 **Sutrave, P. and Hughes, S.H. (1991) Oncogene 6, 353–356.**
11 Colmenares, C. and Stavnezer, E. (1989) Cell 59, 293–303.
12 Colmenares, C. et al. (1991) J. Virol. 65, 4929–4935.
13 Larsen, J. et al. (1993) Oncogene 8, 3221–3228.
14 Grimes, H.L. et al. (1992) Nucl. Acids Res. 20, 1511–1516.

SRC

IDENTIFICATION

v-*src* is the transforming gene of the chicken Rous *sarc*oma virus (RSV). *SRC* was identified by screening human genomic DNA with a v-*src* probe.

RELATED GENES

SRC-like genes have been found in all species that have been examined. They are members of the superfamily of kinases [1].

In vertebrates eight genes of the *SRC* family have been identified (*SRC*, *Blk*, *FGR* (*SRC-2*), *FYN*, *HCK*, *LCK/Tkl*, *LYN*, *YES*) of which *SRC*, *FGR* and *YES* have viral homologues. All the proteins contain Gly2 that becomes myristylated and contributes to membrane anchoring of the proteins; all share sequences throughout the SRC homology domains 1 (the tyrosine kinase catalytic region), 2 and 3 (SH1, SH2, SH3) [2] and all have the capacity to be regulated by phosphorylation of a common C-terminal tyrosine residue.

SH2 and/or SH3 domains also occur in the ABL/ARG family of non-receptor tyrosine kinases, the FPS/FES family, the growth factor receptor coupling proteins (SHCs and GRBs), v-AKT, the PTP1 and PTP2 tyrosine phosphatases, ATK, HTK-16, ITK, SYK, TEC, TYK and ZAP-70 tyrosine kinases, RAS–GAP, p47$^{gag\text{-}crk}$, NCK, the transcription factor ISGF3α, phospholipase Cγ$_1$, PtdIns 3-kinase, ASH, yeast actin binding protein ABP1p, myosin-I, tensin and α-spectrin.

	SRC	v-src
Nucleotides (kb)	~60	7–9 (RSVs)
Chromosome	20q13.3	
Mass (kDa): predicted	60	59
expressed	60 (pp60^{SRC})	pp60$^{v\text{-}src}$

Cellular location

Plasma membrane associated [3].

Tissue distribution

SRC (pp60^{SRC}) is expressed in most avian and mammalian cells although it is barely detectable in lymphocytes. The highest concentrations of protein and tyrosine kinase activity occur in neuronal tissues [4] and in platelets where SRC comprises 0.2–0.4% of total protein.

PROTEIN FUNCTION

SRC is the prototype of the SRC family of membrane-associated protein tyrosine kinases [5]. The activity of v-SRC greatly exceeds that of SRC which is normally inhibited *in vivo* by nearly stoichiometric phosphorylation of Tyr527.

SRC and/or other members of the SRC family (e.g. YES and FYN) are rapidly activated by the stimulation of a variety of transmembrane signalling receptors [6], including the PDGFR with which phosphorylated SRC associates [7]. Activation of the PDGFR subsequently leads to the release of activated SRC from the plasma membrane caused by cAMP-dependent phosphorylation of the SRC N-terminus [8]. SRC is also phosphorylated during mitosis by p34^{CDC2}. Phosphorylation may therefore sensitize SRC Tyr527 to phosphatase action or de-sensitize it to a kinase and there is evidence that sustained expression of protein tyrosine phosphatase PTPα causes SRC activation, cell transformation and tumorigenesis [9-11].

SRC forms complexes with polyoma middle T antigen in polyoma-transformed cells. This augments many-fold the tyrosine kinase activity of SRC and is necessary but not sufficient for transformation by polyoma virus. Activation of SRC is partly caused by the enzyme being locked in a conformation that prevents its being negatively regulated by Tyr527 phosphorylation [12-15].

v-SRC induces the cell-type specific activation of MAP kinase kinase [16] and the sustained transcription of the *Egr-1*, *Junb*, *TIS10* and *CEF-4/9E3* genes that are transiently activated by exposure of fibroblasts to serum [17,18]. v-SRC does not activate *Fos* transcription in murine fibroblasts, although it causes detectable activation in chick embryo fibroblasts [19]. Transformation of fibroblasts by v-SRC also activates S6 kinase II, although it is not a substrate for v-SRC *in vitro* [20, 21]. v-SRC, but not SRC, associates with the 90 kDa heat shock protein (HSP90) during or immediately after synthesis. This interaction decreases v-SRC kinase activity during transfer to the plasma membrane and modulates its specificity [22].

v-SRC causes multiple alterations in the metabolism of phosphatidylinositol and its derivatives, stimulating PtdInsP_2 hydrolysis and the accumulation of inositoltrisphosphate, enhancing the activity of Ins(1,4,5)P_3 3-kinase and activating PtdIns 3-kinase [23, 24].

SH2 domains regulate protein interactions by binding directly to tyrosine phosphorylated proteins and the SH2 and SH3 domains of SRC regulate substrate specificity in a host-dependent manner and are thus important for transformation. PtdIns 3-kinase, which possesses two SH2 domains, binds to v-SRC and also to SRC in cells transformed by polyoma virus. v-SRC causes tyrosine phosphorylation of the SH2-containing SHC proteins and promotes their association with the GRB2 SH2 domain: GRB2 can in turn can couple via SOS to RAS activation. RAS–GAP binds to the SH2 domain of SRC but is tyrosine phosphorylated only in complexes with v-SRC from transformed cells [25].

SRC substrates

The only known function of SRC is as a tyrosine kinase and it is generally believed that the loss of anchorage dependence and growth control, together with the changes in metabolite transport and organization of the cytoskeleton that occur in v-SRC-transformed cells derive from the phosphorylation of specific target proteins [26]. The activation of SRC correlates with the phosphorylation on tyrosine residues of a wide range of substrates, many of which are similarly phosphorylated during the mitogenesis of normal cells and in transformed cells. However, in intact cells essential targets of SRC involved in regulating cell proliferation have not been identified, although the activation by phosphorylation of focal adhesion kinase (p125^{FAK}), a possible mediator of integrin signalling that contains a high-affinity binding site for the SRC SH2 domain [27], may represent a common point of convergence of growth factor- and SRC-activated pathways.

Proteins phosphorylated by SRC

p42, p50, p75, p80/85^{EMS1} [28], p130 [29], p120 [30], gp130
Calmodulin
Catenin
CD3-ζ
Clathrin
Connexin 43
Enolase
Lactate dehydrogenase
NCK
p34^{CDC2}
Phosphoglycerate mutase, G$_\alpha$ subunits [31]
Platelet fibrinogen receptor (gpIIb/gpIIIa)
RAS-GAP
Synaptophysin
Cytoskeletal proteins p110 (actin filament-associated protein
     (AFAP-110) [29]
Annexin II (p36, calpactin I or lipocortin II) [32]
α-Fodrin
α- and β-Tubulin
MAP2
Tau
Integrin
Talin
Paxillin [33]
Vinculin
p125^{FAK} [34]

Regulation of SRC tyrosine kinase activity

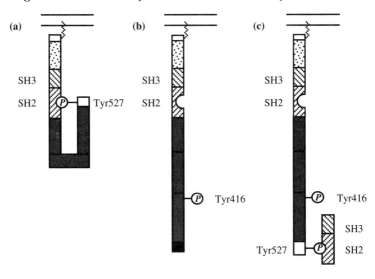

(a) In normal, unstimulated cells SRC Tyr527 is phosphorylated and its interaction with the SH2 domain results in very low kinase activity [35]. Treatment with phosphatase or an antibody directed against the C-terminal region of SRC generates a kinase activity comparable to that of v-SRC [36]. The substitution of Tyr527 by Phe produces an oncogenic mutant that has high kinase activity throughout the cell cycle [37–40].

(b) v-SRC in which the absence of Tyr527 permits constitutive activation of the kinase.

(c) Hypothetical model for the activation of SRC by a cellular SH2 domain protein associating with Tyr527.

Cancer

SRC protein kinase activity is enhanced in some human colon cancers [41,42], skin tumours [43] and breast carcinomas. Association of SRC with EGFR and HER2 has been detected in human breast carcinoma cell lines [44]. SRC expression and kinase activity are increased in some human neuroblastoma-derived cell lines.

Transgenic animals

Mice homozygous for a null mutation in *Src* have impaired osteoclast function, are deficient in bone remodelling and develop osteopetrosis [45,46]. Rapidly metastasizing tumours arising in transgenic mice expressing polyomavirus middle T antigen are rarely detected when *Src* is inactivated [47]. Transgenic mice expressing high levels of v-SRC kinase activity die by mid-gestation with the formation of twin or multiple embryos [48].

In animals

The original RSV strain is tumorigenic in only a few strains of chicken: later variants are tumorigenic in a range of avian species. Some *src* variants induce cellular anti-tumour immunity [49].

In vitro

Infection with RSV transforms many types of cell. Expression of v-SRC is sufficient to initiate and maintain cellular transformation of chicken or mammalian fibroblasts. SRC is non-transforming, even when expressed at high levels [50–52].

GENE STRUCTURE

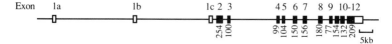

An additional fourth 5' non-coding exon is present in chicken *Src*. Multiple mRNAs are generated by the differential splicing of the human or chicken non-coding exons and by the use of distinct initiation sites: all have the potential to encode SRC, as their 5' exons are all eventually joined to exon 2.

An alternative splicing mechanism occurs in normal avian and rodent neurons and in some human neuroblastomas that yields a variant (p60^{src+}) with 6, 11 or 17 additional amino acids [53].

TRANSCRIPTIONAL REGULATION

The human *SRC* promoter has a high GC content and several SP1 and AP-2 sites but no TATA or CAAT boxes [54].

PROTEIN STRUCTURE

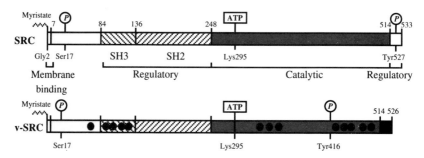

Human and chicken SRC (shown above) are 94.6% identical. v-*src* is derived from chicken *Src*: dots indicate point mutations scattered through v-SRC. The C-terminal regions (12 amino acids in v-SRC and 19 in SRC) are unrelated in sequence.

SRC can be converted to a transforming protein by various amino acid substitutions [55,56], by replacement or truncation of the C-terminus [40,57] or by dephosphorylation of Tyr527 [12]. Mutations of Lys295 or in the vicinity of the consensus sequence block kinase activity and transformation [58,59]. The site of SRC *trans*-phosphorylation, Tyr416, is highly conserved in tyrosine kinases and is the major phosphorylation site in v-SRC (Tyr527 is deleted). All transforming SRC mutants have increased kinase activity that correlates with Tyr416 *trans*-phosphorylation [60, 61].

The three-dimensional structures of SRC SH2 and SH3 domains have been determined [62, 63].

SEQUENCE OF SRC

```
  1   MGSNKSKPKD  ASQRRRSLEP  AENVHGAGGG  AFPASQTPSK  PASADGHRGP
 51   SAAFAPAAAE  PKLFGGFNSS  DTVTSPQRAG  PLAGGVTTFV  ALYDYESRTE
101   TDLSFKKGER  LQIVNNTEGD  WWLAHSLSTG  QTGYIPSNYV  APSDSIQAEE
151   WYFGKITRRE  SERLLLNAEN  PRGTFLVRES  ETTKGAYCLS  VSDFDNAKGL
201   NVKHYKIRKL  DSGGFYITSR  TQFNSLQQLV  AYYSKHADGL  CHRLTTVCPT
251   SKPQTQGLAK  DAWEIPRESL  RLEVKLGQGC  FGEVWMGTWN  GTTRVAIKTL
301   KPGTMSPEAF  LQEAQVMKKL  RHEKLVQLYA  VVSEEPIYIV  TEYMSKGSLL
351   DFLKGETGKY  LRLPQLVDMA  AQIASGMAYV  ERMNYVHRDL  RAANILVGEN
401   LVCKVADFGL  ARLIEDNEYT  ARQGAKFPIK  WTAPEAALYG  RFTIKSDVWS
451   FGILLTELTT  KGRVPYPGMV  NREVLDQVER  GYRMPCPPEC  PESLHDLMCQ
501   CWRKEPEERP  TFEYLQAFLE  DYFTSTEPQY  QPGENL (536)
```

Underlined: differences between human and chicken SRC.

Domain structure

1–7	Myristylation domain [64]
2	Myristate attachment site
8–87	Unique domain
276–284 and 298	ATP binding
389	Active site
420	Autophosphorylation site
530	Phosphorylation site
84–145	SH3 domain
151–248	SH2 domain (italics)
249–517	Catalytic domain
518–536	Regulatory domain
93, 95, 134, 139 and 152	Potential tyrosine phosphorylation sites: the phosphorylation of each of these amino acids does not directly affect kinase activity although, as the total kinase activity is dependent on the overall phosphorylation state of this region, it presumably influences the structure of SRC [65].

Percentage sequence identity with SRC in domains of the SRC family proteins

	Myristylation and unique domains	SH2 and SH3 domains	Catalytic domain
YES	22	74	89
FYN	20	67	81
FGR	11	57	78
LCK	4	50	67
HCK	17	56	69
LYN	11	52	66
BLK	18	53	67

DATABASE ACCESSION NUMBERS

	PIR	SWISSPROT	EMBL/GENBANK	REFERENCES
Human *SRC1*	A26891	P12931	M16243 to M16245	66
			K03212 to K03218	67
			X03995 to X04000	68
RSV (Prague C) v-*src*	A00632	P00526	V01197	69
				70
RSV v-*src*	A00631	P00524	X13745	71
			V01169	72,73

References

1 Hanks, S.K. et al. (1988) Science 241, 42–52.
2 Pawson, T. and Gish, G.D. (1992) Cell 71, 359–362.
3 Anand, R. et al. (1993) Oncogene 8, 3013–3020.
4 Brugge, J. et al. (1987) Genes Devel. 1, 287–296.
5 Jove, R. and Hanafusa, H. (1987) Annu. Rev. Cell Biol. 3, 31–56.
6 Eiseman, E. and Bolen, J.B. (1990) Cancer Cells 2, 303–310.
7 Twamley-Stein, G.M. et al. (1993) Proc. Natl Acad. Sci. USA 90, 7696–7700.
8 Walker, F. et al. (1993) J. Biol. Chem. 268, 19552–19558.
9 Zheng, X.M. et al. (1992) Nature 359, 336–339.
10 den Hertog, J. et al. (1993) EMBO J. 12, 3789–3798.
11 Cobb, B.S. and Parsons, J.T. (1993) Oncogene 8, 2897–2903.
12 Courtneidge, S.A. (1985) EMBO J. 4, 1471–1477.
13 Bolen, J.B. et al. (1984) Cell 38, 767–777.
14 Cartwright, C.A. et al. (1985) Mol. Cell. Biol. 5, 2647–2652.
15 Cooper, J.A. and Howell, B. (1993) Cell 73, 1051–1054.
16 Gardner, A.M. et al. (1993) J. Biol. Chem. 268, 17896–17901.
17 Dehbi, M. et al. (1992) Mol. Cell. Biol. 12, 1490–1499.
18 Apel, I. et al. (1992) Mol. Cell. Biol. 12, 3356–3364.
19 Catling, A.D. et al. (1993) Oncogene 8, 1875–1886.
20 Sweet, L.J. et al. (1990) Mol. Cell. Biol. 10, 2413–2417.

21 Chung, J. et al. (1991) Mol. Cell. Biol. 11, 1868–1874.
22 Xu, Y. and Lindquist, S. (1993) Proc. Natl Acad. Sci. USA 90, 7074–7078.
23 Fukui, Y. et al. (1991) Oncogene 6, 407–411.
24 Ruggiero, M. et al. (1991) FEBS Letts 291, 203–207.
25 Brott, B.K. et al. (1991) Proc. Natl Acad. Sci. USA 88, 755–759.
26 **Kellie, S. et al. (1991) J. Cell Sci. 99 (2), 207–211.**
27 Schaller, M.D. et al. (1994) Mol. Cell. Biol. 14, 1680–1688.
28 Schuuring, E. et al. (1993) Mol. Cell. Biol. 13, 2891–2898.
29 Flynn, D.C. et al. (1993) Mol. Cell. Biol. 13, 7892–7900.
30 Reynolds, A.B. et al. (1992) Oncogene 7, 2439–2445.
31 Hausdorff, W.P. et al. (1992) Proc. Natl Acad. Sci. USA 89, 5720–5724.
32 Ozaki, T. and Sakiyama, S. (1993) Oncogene 8, 1707–1710.
33 Weng, Z. et al.(1993) J. Biol. Chem. 268, 14956–14963.
34 Cobb, B.S. et al. (1994) Mol. Cell. Biol. 14, 147–155.
35 Liu, X. et al. (1993) Oncogene 8, 1119–1126.
36 Cooper, J.A. and King, C.S. (1986) Mol. Cell. Biol. 6, 4467–4477.
37 Cartwright, C.A. et al. (1987) Cell 49, 83–91.
38 Kmiecik, T.E. and Shalloway, D. (1987) Cell 49, 65–73.
39 Piwnica–Worms, H. et al. (1987) Cell 49, 75–82.
40 Reynolds, A.B. et al. (1987) EMBO J. 6, 2359–2364.
41 Garcia, R. et al. (1991) Oncogene 6, 1983–1989.
42 Cartwright, C.A. et al. (1990) Proc. Natl Acad. Sci. USA 87, 558–562.
43 Barnekow, A. et al. (1987) Cancer Res. 47, 235–240.
44 Luttrell, D.K. et al. (1994) Proc. Natl Acad. Sci. USA 91, 83–87.
45 Soriano, P. et al. (1991) Cell 64, 693–702.
46 Lowe, C. et al. (1993) Proc. Natl Acad. Sci. USA 90, 4485–4489.
47 Guy, C.T. et al. (1994) Genes Devel. 8, 23–32.
48 Boulter, C.A. et al. (1991) Development 111, 357–366.
49 Gelman, I.H. et al. (1993) Oncogene 8, 2995–3004.
50 Iba, H. et al. (1984) Proc. Natl Acad. Sci. USA 81, 4424–4428.
51 Parker, R.C. et al. (1984) Cell 37, 131–139.
52 Shalloway, D. et al. (1984) Proc. Natl Acad. Sci. USA 81, 7071–7075.
53 Wiestler, O.D. and Walter, G. (1988) Mol. Cell. Biol. 8, 502–504.
54 Bonham, K. and Fujita, D.J. (1993) Oncogene 8, 1973–1981.
55 Kato, J.-Y. et al. (1986) Mol. Cell. Biol. 6, 4155–4160.
56 Levy, J.B.et al. (1986) Proc. Natl Acad. Sci. USA 83, 4228–4232.
57 Yaciuk, P. et al. (1989) Mol. Cell. Biol. 9, 2453–2463.
58 Kamps, M.P. and Sefton, B.M. (1986) Mol. Cell. Biol. 6, 751–757.
59 DeClue, J.E. and Martin, G.S. (1989) J. Virol. 63, 542–554.
60 Jove, R. et al. (1989) Oncogene Res. 5, 49–60.
61 Sato, M. et al. (1989) J. Virol. 63, 683–688.
62 Waksman, G. et al. (1993) Cell 72, 779–790.
63 Yu, H. et al. (1992) Science 258, 1665–1668.
64 **Resh, M.D. (1994) Cell 76, 411–413.**
65 Espino, P.C. et al. (1990) Oncogene 5, 283–93.
66 Anderson, S.K. et al. (1985) Mol. Cell. Biol. 5, 1112–1129.
67 Tanaka, A. et al. (1987) Mol. Cell. Biol. 7, 1978–1983.
68 Parker, R.C. et al. (1985) Mol. Cell. Biol. 5, 831–838.

69 Schwartz, D.E. et al. (1983) Cell 32, 853–869.

70 Neil, J.C. et al. (1981) Nature 291, 675–677.

71 Barnier, J.V. et al. (1989) Nucl. Acids Res. 17, 1252.

72 Czernilofsky, A.P. et al. (1983) Nature 301, 736–738.

73 Takeya, T. and Hanafusa, H. (1983) Cell 32, 881–890 (and correction: Cell 34, 319, 1983).

TAL1

IDENTIFICATION

TAL1 (*T* cell *a*cute *l*eukaemia *1*, also called *SCL* (*s*tem *c*ell *l*eukaemia) or *TCL5*) was identified in a chromosome translocation in a stem cell leukaemia.

RELATED GENES

Member of the basic helix–loop–helix (bHLH) family closely related to TAL2 and LYL1.

Nucleotides (kb)	16
Chromosome	1p32
Mass (kDa): predicted	34
expressed	22/42

Cellular location

Nucleus.

Tissue distribution

Expressed in developing brain, normal bone marrow and mast cells, mast cell lines, leukaemic T cells megakaryocytic and erythroleukaemic cell lines [1] and in endothelial cells [2] but not in normal T cells.

PROTEIN FUNCTION

TAL1 is a transcription factor that forms heterodimers with any of the known class A bHLH proteins (E12, E47, E2-2 and HEB) that bind to the E box (CANNTG) eukaryotic enhancer element, as does MyoD [3]. *TAL1* expression is necessary for erythroid cell differentiation and is regulated by the erythroid transcription factor GATA1 [4]. In the early myeloid cell line 416B, GATA1 but not TAL1 induces differentiation into megakaryocytes[5]. *TAL1* may be involved in neural and endothelial cell differentiation [1,2].

Cancer

In 3% of T cell acute lymphoblastic leukaemias (T-ALLs) the translocation (1;14)(p32;q11) transposes *TAL1* into the T cell receptor (TCR) δ gene resulting in elevated expression of *TAL1* mRNA.

In 25% of T-ALL there is a 90 kb deletion (*tal*d or *tal*d1) upstream from one allele of the *TAL1* locus, probably due to aberrant Ig recombinase activity [6,7]. A second specific deletion (*tal*d2) occurs in 6% of T-ALLs. The t(1;14) translocations and both *tal*d deletions disrupt the 5′ end of the *TAL1* gene so that its expression is controlled by the regulatory elements of the TCRδ or *SIL* genes that are both normally expressed in T cell ontogeny [8].

In ~20% of T-ALL *SIL* (*S*CL *i*nterrupting *l*ocus, chromosome 1p33), a highly conserved mammalian gene, fuses with *TAL1*, even though neither encodes TCR genes that normally rearrange during T cell ontogeny and are common sites for chromosomal translocation in T cell leukaemias. The rearrangement is similar in effect to the t(1;14)(p32;q11) translocation. There is also one example in which recombination with TCRδ affects the 3' side of *TAL1*, transcription being initiated from a promoter in the fourth exon [9] and one in which the gene is not disrupted, the breakpoint occurring 25 kb downstream of *TAL1* [10].

In animals

TAL1 cooperates with v-ABL in promoting tumorigenesis when *TAL1* is expressed from a synthetic retrovirus in v-*abl*-transformed T cells injected into mice [11].

GENE STRUCTURE OF SIL AND TAL1

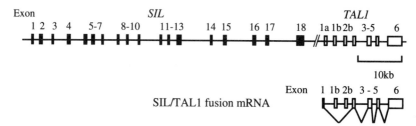

TAL1 type A (exons 1a-4-5/6); type B (exons 1b-2-3-4-5/6). Alternative splicing can link exon 1a to 2 or 1b to 4 or utilize an alternative intron to split exons 5 and 6. In *SIL–TAL1* an interstitial deletion removes most of the *SIL* gene, splicing *SIL* exon 1 to *TAL1* exon 3 and the 3' *TAL1* exons (4, 5 and 6).

SEQUENCE OF TAL

```
  1  MTERPPSEAA RSDPQLEGRD AAEASMAPPH LVLLNGVAKE TSRAAAAEPP
 51  VIELGARGGP GGGPAGGGGA ARDLKGRDAA TAEARHRVPT TELCRPPGPA
101  PAPAPASVTA ELPGDGRMVQ LSPPALAAPA APGRALLYSL SQPLASLGSS
151  FFGEPDAFPM FTTNNRVKRR PSPYEMEITD GPHTKVVRRI FTNSRERWRQ
201  QNVNGAFAEL RKLIPTHPPD KKLSKNEILR LAMKYINFLA KLLNDQEEEG
251  TQRAKTGKDP VVGAGGGGGG GGGGAPPDDL LQDVLSPNSS CGSSLDGAAS
301  PDSYTEEPAP KHTARSLHPA MLPAADGAGP R (331)
```

Domain structure

122	MAP kinase phosphorylation site
176–331	Sequence of p22^{*TAL1*}
188–239	Helix–loop–helix motif (underlined)
263–274	Poly-glycine
122	Ser122 is phosphorylated *in vitro* by ERK1 protein kinase and in intact cells after stimulation by EGF[12].

DATABASE ACCESSION NUMBERS

	PIR	SWISSPROT	EMBL/GENBANK	REFERENCES
Human *TAL1*	A34519	P17542	M29038	6
	A36358		M61103 to M61105	
			M63572, M63576,	
			M63584, M63589	

References

1 Green, A.R. et al. (1992) Oncogene 7, 653–660.
2 Hwang, L.-Y. et al. (1993) Oncogene 8, 3043–3046.
3 Hsu, H.-L. et al. (1994) Mol. Cell. Biol. 14, 1256–1265.
4 Aplan, P.D. et al. (1992) EMBO J. 11, 4073–4081.
5 Visvader, J.E. et al. (1992) EMBO J. 11, 4557–4564.
6 Aplan, P.D. et al. (1990) Mol. Cell. Biol. 10, 6426–6435.
7 Brown, L. et al. (1990) EMBO J. 9, 3343–3351.
8 Bernard, O. et al. (1991) Oncogene 6, 1477–1488.
9 Bernard, O. et al. (1992) J. Exp. Med. 176, 919–925.
10 Xia, Y. et al. (1992) Genes, Chromosomes & Cancer 4, 211–216.
11 Elwood, N.J. et al. (1993) Oncogene 8, 3093–3101.
12 Cheng, J.-T. et al. (1993) Mol. Cell. Biol. 13, 801–808.

THR/ErbA

IDENTIFICATION

v-*erbA* and v-*erbB* are the oncogenes carried by the AEV-ES4 strain of avian *ery*thro*b*lastosis virus, detected by hybridization with cDNA probes directed against AEV DNA.

THRA1/ErbA-1 encodes thyroid hormone receptor α. *THRB/ErbA-2* encodes thyroid hormone receptor β. Both are receptors for triiodothyronine (T_3), detected by screening cDNA libraries with a v-*erbA* probe.

RELATED GENES

THRA1 and *THRB* are members of a superfamily numbering nearly 30 that includes the receptors for steroids, retinoic acid and vitamin D_3. The subfamily of thyroid hormone receptors (THRs) and retinoic acid receptors (RARs) comprises three RARs (α, β and γ), three retinoid X receptors (RXRα, β, γ), two THRs (α and β) and several "orphan receptors" for which ligands have yet to be identified.

Other *THRA1*-related genes are *EAR2* (*erbA*-related/*ERBAL2*), *EAR3* (*ERBAL3*) and *EAR3* (or chicken ovalbumin upstream promoter, COUP) which is closely similar to *Drosophila seven-up*.

	THRA	THRB	v-*erbA*
Nucleotides (kb)	27	60	5.7 (AEV-ES4)
Chromosome	17q11.2–q12	3p24.1–p22	
Mass (kDa): predicted	47 (THRA1)/55 (THRA2)	52	72
expressed	48/55	52/55	P75*gag-erbA*

Cellular location

Nucleus.

Tissue distribution

THRA1 ubiquitous. *THRB* restricted. Rat THRB is strongly expressed in the liver, thyroid, adrenal and anterior and posterior pituitary glands [1]. In chick brain ontogenesis *ErbA-1* is expressed from the early embryonic stages, *ErbA-2* is rapidly induced after embryonic day 19 and is substantially expressed in brain, lung, kidney, eye and yolk sac but is undetectable in haematopoietic tissues [2].

PROTEIN FUNCTION

THRA1 and THRB are transcription factors possessing zinc finger domains. Human THRA1 and THRB are the high-affinity receptors (K_d = 0.2 nM) for T_3. THRA1 binds to a palindromic response element, repressing transcription: T_3 binding to THRA1 activates transcription[3]. THRA2 does not bind T_3 and has been proposed to act as a dominant negative regulator of thyroid hormone receptors. There is a second functional form of human THRB (*THRB2/ErbA-2*).

Overexpression of THRB1 in murine muscle cells indicates that it is involved in triggering muscle terminal differentiation [4]. Thus, it blocks the activity of the myogenesis inhibitor AP-1, increases T_3-induced *MyoD* expression and causes T_3 to stimulate growth arrest and terminal differentiation in the presence of serum factors acting, like SKI, as a positive regulator of muscle differentiation.

v-ERBA does not bind hormone or *trans*-activate and it acts as a constitutive repressor and an antagonist of thyroid hormone and retinoic acid receptors [5]. Thus v-ERBA blocks apoptosis of normal early erythrocyte progenitor cells induced by T_3 or retinoic acid in the absence of differentiation-inducing agents [6]. v-erbA cooperates with v-erbB and related sarcoma-inducing oncogenes (and with *Hras*) to block erythroid cell differentiation (into erythrocytes) and to promote transformation. v-ERBA suppresses transcription of avian erythrocyte anion transport (band III), carbonic anhydrase II and β-globin genes. The capacity of v-erbA to block differentiation correlates with transcriptional arrest of erythrocyte-specific genes [7].

Rous sarcoma virus LTR contains a unique hormone responsive element (RSV-T3RE) that mediates strong activation by THRA or v-ERBA homodimers or by THRA/RXR heterodimers, but not THRB, in the absence of T_3 and activation is reversed by T_3 [8].

Cancer

Loss of heterozygosity at the *THRA1* locus has been detected in sporadic breast cancers and in a breast cancer cell line (BT474) *THRA1* undergoes fusion to *BTR*, the truncated form of *THRA1* resembling v-erbA. In some colon carcinomas expression of the larger transcript (6 kb) of *THRB* is suppressed: expression of *THRA1* and *THRA2* is unaffected [9,10].

In animals

v-erbA alone is not tumorigenic but cooperates with v-ets to cause avian erythroleukaemia [11].

In vitro

v-erbA alone can transform erythrocytic progenitor cells and stimulate CEF growth, although it does not cause tumours. However, v-erbA enhances the tumorigenicity of v-erbB-transformed CEFs [12]. v-erbA affects transformed erythroblasts in two ways: (i) it increases the pH range within which the cells will grow and (ii) it blocks the differentiation of erythroblasts into erythrocytes. The potent repressor function of v-ERBA requires the formation of heterodimeric complexes with retinoid X receptor (RXR-α) and C-terminal mutations in v-ERBA that abolish heterodimer formation also block v-ERBA repressor function [13]. Despite being a constitutive repressor in animal cells, v-ERBA is a hormone-activated transcriptional activator in yeast. The functional domains of the protein required for activation of gene expression in yeast and for transformation of avian cells are closely similar [14].

STRUCTURE OF THE HUMAN *THRA1* GENE

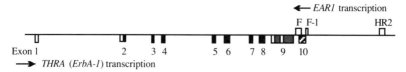

Boxes below the line represent *THRA1* (exons 1-9): open boxes above the line represent the exons of the *THRA*-related *EAR1* gene (F: final, F-1: adjacent to final, HR2: homologue of rat exon 2) that is transcribed in the reverse direction [15]. The use of an alternative splice site in *THRA1* exon 9 generates THRA2 (exons 1–10).

TRANSCRIPTIONAL REGULATION

The human *THRA* promoter lacks TATA elements but is very GC-rich and contains many Sp1 sites as well as hormone-responsive elements [16].

PROTEIN STRUCTURE

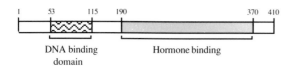

Human THRA1 differs from chicken ERBA1, from which v-ERBA is derived, in having two additional amino acids in the N-terminal region and 41 scattered substitutions. P75$^{v-gag-erbA}$ is a highly mutated version of ERBA-1 with two point mutations in the DNA binding domain and 11 others in the hormone binding domain, a 9 amino acid C-terminal deletion in the hormone binding domain and an N-terminal third encoded by *gag*. These changes result in the loss of T$_3$ binding capacity (although the hormone binding region is retained) but the retention of sequence-specific DNA binding. v-ERBA acts as a constitutive repressor of T$_3$-regulated genes. In the AEV-ES4 viral genome both the *ErbA* and *ErbB* genes are inserted between *gag* and *env* and are independently expressed, remaining colinear with the coding domains of their cellular progenitors.

SEQUENCE OF THRA1

```
  1  MEQKPSKVEC  GSDPEENSAR  SPDGKRKRKN  GQCSLKTSMS  GYIPSYLDKD
 51  EQCVVCGDKA  TGYHYRCITC  EGCKGFFRRT  IQKNLHPTYS  CKYDSCCVID
101  KITRNQCQLC  RFKKCIAVGM  AMDLVLDDSK  RVAKRKLIEQ  NRERRRKEEM
151  IRSLQQRPEP  TPEEWDLIHI  ATEAHRSTNA  QGSHWKQRRK  FLPDDIGQSP
201  IVSMPDGDKV  DLEAFSEFTK  IITPAITRVV  DFAKKLPMFS  ELPCEDQIIL
251  LKGCCMEIMS  LRAAVRYDPE  SDTLTLSGEM  AVKREQLKNG  GLGVVSDAIF
301  ELGKSLSAFN  LDDTEVALLQ  AVLLMSTDRS  GLLCVDKIEK  SQEAYLLAFE
351  HYVNHRKHNI  PHFWPKLLMK  VTDLRMIGAC  HASRFLHMKV  ECPTELFPPL
401  FLEVFEDQEV  (410)
```

Domain structure

1–52	Modulating domain
53–73 and 91–115	Two C4-type zinc fingers
158–179	Putative *trans*-repression domain (underlined). Mutation of Pro160 (or of the corresponding v-ERBA residue), between the DNA and hormone-binding domains, abolishes the capacity to suppress basal transcription but does not prevent hormone-induced *trans*-activation by THRA1 [17]. v-ERBA may therefore function by *trans*-repression, rather than as a dominant negative inhibitor of THR or RAR activation
190–370	Hormone binding
371–410	C-terminal region (underlined) that differs from THRA2 (THRA1 and THRA2 are identical up to amino acid 370)

C-TERMINUS OF THRA2

```
371  EREVQSSILY  KGAAAEGRPG  GSLGVHPEGQ  QLLGMHVVQG  PQVRQLEQQL
421  GEAGSLQGPV  LQHQSPKSPQ  QRLLELLHRS  GILHARAVCG  EDDSSEADSP
471  SSSEEEPEVC  EDLAGNAASP  (490)
```

SEQUENCE OF THRB

```
  1  MTENGLTAWD  KPKHCPDREH  DWKLVGMSEA  CLHRKSHSER  RSTLKNEQSS
 51  PHLIQTTWTS  SIFHLDHDDV  NDQSVSSAQT  FQTEEKKCKG  YIPSYLDKDE
101  LCVVCGDKAT  GYHYRCITCE  GCKGFFRRTI  QKNLHPSYSC  KYEGKCVIDK
151  VTRNQCQECR  FKKCIYVGMA  TDLVLDDSKR  LAKRKLIEEN  REKRRREELQ
201  KSIGHKPEPT  DEEWELIKTV  TEAHVATNAQ  GSHWKQKPKF  LPEDIGQAPI
251  VNAPEGGKVD  LEAFSHFTKI  ITPAITRVVD  FAKKLPMFCE  LPCEDQIILL
301  KGCCMEIMSL  RAAVRYDPES  ETLTLNGEMA  VIRGQLKNGG  LGVVSDAIFD
351  LGMSLSSFNL  DDTEVALLQA  VLLMSSDRPG  LACVERIEKY  QDSFLLAFEH
401  YINYRKHHVT  HFWPKLLMKV  TDLRMIGACH  ASRFLHMKVE  CPTELLPPLF
451  LEVFED  (456)
```

Domain structure

1–101	Modulating domain
102–122 and 140–164	Two C4-type zinc fingers
239–456	Hormone binding

DATABASE ACCESSION NUMBERS

	PIR	SWISSPROT	EMBL/GENBANK	REFERENCES
Human *THRA1*	A30893; A40917	P21205	X55004 to X55005	18
	S06247; B32286		X55068 to X55074	
			Y00479	
Human *THRA2*	A30893; S06247	P10827	J03239; X55004	19
	B32286		X55066; X55069	13
			X55071 to X55074	20
Human*THRB*	A25237	P10828	X04707	21, 22

References

1 Macchia, E. et al. (1990) Endocrinology 126, 3232–3239.
2 Forrest, D. et al. (1991) EMBO J. 10, 269–275.
3 Damm, K. et al. (1989) Nature 339, 593–597.
4 Carnac, G. et al. (1993) Oncogene 8, 3103–3110.
5 Sande, S. et al. (1993) J. Virol. 67, 1067–1074.
6 Gandrillon, O. et al. (1994) Oncogene 9, 749–758.
7 Zenke, M. et al. (1988) Cell 52, 107–119.
8 Saatcioglu, F. et al. (1994) Cell 75, 1095–1105.
9 Futreal, P.A. et al. (1994) Cancer Res. 54, 1791–1794.
10 Markowitz, S. et al. (1989) J. Clin. Invest. 84, 1683–1687.
11 Metz, T. and Graf, T. (1992) Oncogene 7, 597–605.
12 Zenke, M. et al. (1990) Cell 61, 1035–1049.
13 Yen, P.M. et al. (1994) J. Biol. Chem. 269, 903–909.
14 Smit-McBride, Z. and Privalsky, M.L. (1993) Oncogene 8, 1465–1475.
15 Miyajima, N. et al. (1989) Cell 57, 31–39.
16 Laudet, V. et al. (1993) Oncogene 8, 975–982.
17 Damm, K. and Evans, R.M. (1993) Proc. Natl Acad. Sci. USA 90, 10668–10672.
18 Nakai, A. et al. (1988) Proc. Natl Acad. Sci. USA 85, 2781–2785.
19 Pfahl, M. and Benbrook, D. (1987) Nucl. Acids Res. 15, 9613.
20 Laudet, V. et al. (1991) Nucleic Acids Res. 19, 1105–1112.
21 Weinberger, C. et al. (1986) Nature 324, 641–646.
22 Sakurai, A. et al. (1990) Mol. Cell. Endocrinol. 71, 83–91.

IDENTIFICATION

TRK (*t*ropomyosin-*r*eceptor-*k*inase) is a human transforming gene that has no homology with known viral oncogenes, originally detected by NIH 3T3 fibroblast transfection with genomic DNA from a colon carcinoma. Additional *TRK* oncogenes have been isolated from thyroid tumours and over 40 *TRK* oncogenes have been generated *in vitro*.

RELATED GENES

The extracellular regions of TRK proteins contain three leucine-rich motifs (LRMs) flanked by conserved cysteine residues, a characteristic of the LRM super-family that includes human platelet von Willebrand factor receptor, ribonuclease/angiogenin inhibitor, cell adhesion proteins and extracellular matrix proteins. The extracellular domains also contain two C_2 Ig-like loops similar to those present in neural cell adhesion molecules and in the receptors for fibroblast growth factors, PDGF and CSF1, in KIT and in *Drosophila Dtrk* and *toll*. TRK also has homology with the receptor tyrosine kinase domains of EGFR, the insulin receptor family and the SRC family and with ROR1 and ROR2 and *Drosophila Dror*. A muscle-specific receptor in *Torpedo californica* contains a TRK-related kinase domain but also has a kringle domain close to the transmembrane region [1].

	TRK	TRKB	TRKC
Nucleotides (kb)	20	>100	Not fully mapped
Chromosome	1q23–1q24 (*NTRK1*)	1q23–q31 (*NTRK2*)	1q23–q31 (*NTRK3*)
Mass (kDa): predicted	87 70 (TRK1)/49 (TRK2)	95	90
expressed	gp140^{trk} 70^{trk} (tropomyosin-TRK) 55 (TRK-T1)	gp95^{trkB}/gp145^{trkB}	gp145^{trkC} K1 gp145^{trkC} K2 gp145^{trkC} K3

Cellular location

Plasma membrane.

Tissue distribution

TRK, *TRKB* and *TRKC* are primarily expressed in the nervous system. In humans and rats the *TRKAII* isoform occurs in neuronal tissues and *TRKAI* is expressed mainly in non-neuronal tissues [2]. *TRKE* is the first member of the family found widely and abundantly expressed in human tissues (brain, placenta, lung, skeletal muscle, kidney, pancreas but not liver) [3].

PROTEIN FUNCTION

TRK genes (*TRK* (or *TRKA*), *TRKB*, *TRKC* and *TRKE*) encode trans-membrane tyrosine kinases that are receptors for the nerve growth factor (NGF) family of neurotrophins (NGF, brain-derived neurotrophic factor (BDNF), NT-3, NT-4 or NT-5) and probably mediate specific cell adhesion events during neuronal cell development. Some of the multiple *TRKB* and *TRKC* transcripts encode truncated, non-catalytic receptors [4,5]. TRK oncoproteins bind to SHC proteins that are phosphorylated on tyrosine and bound to GRB2 and the activation of TRKA by NGF induces SHC phosphorylation and GRB2 binding.

gp140trkA: High-affinity receptor for NGF also activated by NT-5 [6–8].
NGF binding stimulates the tyrosine kinase activity and rapid tyrosine phosphorylation of gp140trkA [9]. The activation of chimeric receptors comprised of the EGFR extracellular ligand-binding domain and TRK transmembrane and intracellular sequences promotes association of phosphorylated PLCγ, RAS.GTP, SHC and the non-catalytic subunit of PtdIns 3-kinase (p85) with TRK [10]. In PC-12 cells the activation of gp140trkA by NGF stimulates RAF1 and MAP kinases and results in differentiation into neuronal-type cells [11]. In transfected NIH 3T3 fibroblasts expressing gp140trkA NGF causes *Fos* transcription, DNA synthesis and morphological transformation [12] and in *Xenopus* oocytes expressing gp140trkA NGF induces meiotic maturation [13]. Monoamine-activated α2-macroglobulin inhibits NGF-stimulated neurite outgrowth by binding to gp140trkA [14].

gp145trkB: Receptor for BDNF, NT-4 and NT-5. *TrkB* mediates the survival and proliferation of NIH 3T3 cells in response to BDNF and the co-expression of gp145trkB and either BDNF or NT-4 transforms these cells. BDNF or NT-4 induce PC12 cells expressing gp145trkB to differentiate [15–18].

gp95trkB: Function unknown but the differential pattern of expression with respect to gp145trkB suggests that this non-catalytic form may transport gp145trkB ligands within or to the brain.

gp145trkC: All three isoforms are high-affinity receptors for NT-3 and, when expressed in NIH 3T3 fibroblasts, undergo rapid tyrosine phosphorylation in response to NT-3. Activated gp145trkC K1 phosphorylates PLCγ1 and PtdIns 3-kinase but gp145trkC K2 and gp145trkC K3 do not [4,5,19].

TRKE: Probable ligand: NGF.

Cancer

Transforming *TRK* (*NTRK1*) alleles are found in human colon carcinomas and with high frequency in thyroid papillary carcinomas [20,21]. *TRKA* expression is high in many early-stage neuroblastomas but undetectable in most advanced tumours and appears to correlate inversely with amplification of *MYCN*. *TRKB* and its ligand BDNF are expressed in the *MYCN* amplified cell line SMS-KCN [22].

Transgenic animals

Mice carrying a germline mutation that eliminates *Trk* have severe sensory and sympathetic neuropathies and most die within one month of birth [23]. Most of the tissues known to express *Trk* in both the peripheral and central nervous systems are affected, in contrast to the effects of *TrkB* or *TrkC* disruption in which only a limited subset of expressing cells are affected. Mice lacking *TrkB* have multiple central and peripheral nervous system deficiencies and die soon after birth [24]. Mice defective in *TrkC* lack Ia muscle afferent projections to spinal motor neurons and display abnormal movements and postures [25]. Thus NGF signalling via *Trk* appears essential for the development of both the peripheral and central nervous systems.

In vitro

NIH 3T3 fibroblasts are transformed by NGF, the ligand for TRKA, or by co-transfection of plasmids expressing *TrkB* and BDNF or NT-3 or by co-expression of *TrkC* and NT-3 [12,26,27]. The human oncogene *TRK-T1* transforms NIH 3T3 cells [28].

PROTEIN STRUCTURE

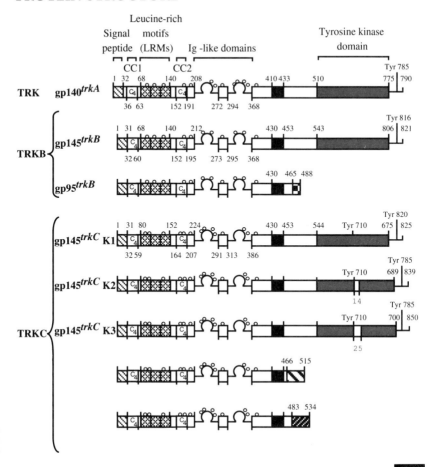

The N-terminal region of the extracellular domains contains a signal peptide, two cysteine clusters (C_4) each including four of the 12 cysteine residues conserved in all known TRK proteins, three tandem LRM repeats and two C_2 Ig-like domains. Circles (o) denote conserved potential N-glycosylation sites [29]. gp145*trkC* K2 contains an insert of 14 amino acids in the sequence of gp145*trkC* K1 and gp145*trkC* K3 has a 25 amino acid insert. Two putative non-catalytic isoforms have also been identified.

TRK oncoproteins

The *TRK* oncogene first isolated from a colon carcinoma was generated by rearrangement of a non-muscle tropomyosin gene and *TRK* [20]. Tropomyosin has 27 residues deleted at the C-terminus and the N-terminal 360 amino acids of TRK are truncated but the transmembrane region and the tyrosine kinase domain are unmodified ((b) below). Thus activation of *TRK* to an oncogene is the result of fusion of the tropomyosin sequences.

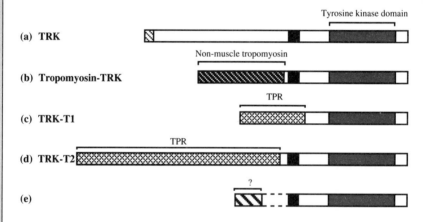

The tropomyosin-activated *TRK* oncogene has also been isolated from human thyroid papillary carcinomas but other chimeric *TRK* oncogenes have been isolated from these tumours that contain different activating sequences [21,28]. TRK-T1 (c), TRK-T2 (d) and TRK-T3 (not shown) contain TPR sequences. A further isolate contains uncharacterized sequences ((e) above).

Activation of *TRK* can also occur by recombination *in vitro* and over 40 such *TRK* oncogenes have been detected [3,30]. The products of these *TRK* oncogenes retain the parental tyrosine kinase activity and have an intact C-terminus. However, the N-termini acquired may generate non-glycosylated cytoplasmic molecules or transmembrane glycoproteins.

SEQUENCE OF TRKAI

```
  1  MLRGGRRGQL GWHSWAAGPG SLLAWLILAS AGAAPCPDAC CPHGSSGLRC
 51  TRDGALDSLH HLPGAENLTE LYIENQQHLQ HLELRDLRGL GELRNLTIVK
101  SGLRFVAPDA FHFTPRLSRL NLSFNALESL SWKTVQGLSL QELVLSGNPL
151  HCSCALRWLQ RWEEEGLGGV PEQKLQCHGQ GPLAHMPNAS CGVPTLKVQV
201  PNASVDVGDD VLLRCQVEGR GLEQAGWILT ELEQSATVMK SGGLPSLGLT
251  LANVTSDLNR KNLTCWAEND VGRAEVSVQV NVSFPASVQL HTAVEMHHWS
301  IPFSVDGQPA PSLRWLFNGS VLNETSFIFT EFLEPAANET VRHGCLRLNQ
351  PTHVNNGNYT LLAANPFGQA SASIMAAFMD NPFEFNPEDP IPDTNSTSGD
401  PVEKKDETPF GVSVAVGLAV FACLFLSTLL LVLNKCGRRN KFGINRPAVL
451  APEDGLAMSL HFMTLGGSSL SPTEGKGSGL QGHIIENPQY FSDACVHHIK
501  RRDIVLKWEL GEGAFGKVFL AECHNLLPEQ DKMLVAVKAL KEASESARQD
551  FQREAELLTM LQHQHIVRFF GVCTEGRPLL MVFEYMRHGD LNRFLRSHGP
601  DAKLLAGGED VAPGPLGLGQ LLAVASQVAA GMVYLAGLHF VHRDLATRNC
651  LVGQGLVVKI GDFGMSRDIY STDYYRVGGR TMLPIRWMPP ESILYRKFTT
701  ESDVWSFGVV LWEIFTYGKQ PWYQLSNTEA IDCITQGREL ERPRACPPEV
751  YAIMRGCWQR EPQQRHSIKD VHARLQALAQ APPVYLDVLG (790)
```

Domain structure

1–32	Signal sequence (italics)
36–63 and 152–191	Conserved cysteine domains 1 and 2
68–92, 93–116 and 117–140	LRM domains
208–272 and 294–268	Ig-like domains
33–409	Extracellular domain
418–433	Transmembrane domain (underlined)
434–790	Cytoplasmic domain
510–518 and 538	ATP binding site
644	Active site
674	Autophosphorylation site
394	Translocation breakpoint for tropomyosin/TRK oncoprotein formation
510–775	Tyrosine kinase domain
490	SHC binding site (Tyr490)
785	Phospholipase Cγ binding site (Tyr785)
751	PtdIns 3-kinase (p85) binding site (Tyr751) [32]
67, 95, 121, 188, 202, 253, 262, 281, 318, 323, 338, 358 and 395	Potential carbohydrate attachment sites

The human TRK sequence shown is for the TRKAI isoform; human and rat TRKAII contain a six amino acid insert (VSFSPV) after Pro392 (human) [2]. TRK (human), TRKB (mouse) and TRKC (pig) share 67% overall amino acid homology. The catalytic domain of TRKE is 41% identical to that of TRKA (extracellular region 16%).

DATABASE ACCESSION NUMBERS

	PIR	*SWISSPROT*	*EMBL/GENBANK*	*REFERENCES*
Human *TRK*	A30124	P04629	M23102	*19, 33*
Human *TRKE*			X74979	*3*
Mouse *TrkB*		P15209	X17647	*34*
Pig *TrkC*		P24786	M80800	*27*

References
1 Jennings, C.G.B. et al. (1993) Proc. Natl Acad. Sci. USA 90, 2895–2899.
2 Barker, P.A. et al. (1993) J. Biol. Chem. 268, 15150–15157.
3 Di Marco, E. et al. (1993) J. Biol. Chem. 268, 24290–24295.
4 **Barbacid, M. et al. (1993) Oncogene 8, 2033–2042.**
5 **Barbacid, M. et al. (1993) In Molecular Genetics of Nervous System Tumors, Wiley-Liss, New York, pp. 123–135.**
6 Klein, R. et al. (1991) Cell 65, 189–197.
7 Berkemeier, L.R. et al. (1991) Neuron 7, 857–866.
8 Kaplan, D.R. et al. (1991) Science 252, 554–558.
9 Kaplan, D.R. et al. (1991) Nature 350, 158–160.
10 Obermeier, A. et al. (1993) J. Biol. Chem. 268, 22963–22966.
11 Ohmichi, M. et al. (1992) J. Biol. Chem. 267, 14604–14610.
12 Cordon-Cardo, C. et al. (1991) Cell 66, 173–183.
13 Nebreda, A.R. et al. (1991) Science 252, 558–561.
14 Koo, P.H. and Qiu, W.-S. (1994) J. Biol. Chem. 269, 5369–5376.
15 Klein, R. et al. (1992) Neuron 8, 947–956.
16 Soppet, D. et al. (1991) Cell 65, 895–903.
17 Squinto, S.P. et al. (1991) Cell 65, 886–893.
18 Ip, N.Y. et al. (1993). Neuron 10, 137–149.
19 Lamballe, F. et al. (1993) EMBO J. 12, 3083–3094.
20 Martin-Zanca, D. et al. (1986) Nature 319, 743–748.
21 Bongarzone, I. et al. (1989) Oncogene 4, 1457–1462.
22 Nakagawara, A. et al. (1994) Mol. Cell. Biol. 14, 759–767.
23 Klein, R. et al. (1994) Nature 368, 246–249.
24 Klein, R. et al. (1993) Cell 75, 113–122.
25 Smeyne, R.J. et al. (1994) Nature 368, 249–251.
26 Klein, R. et al. (1991) Cell 66, 395–403.
27 Lamballe, F. et al. (1991) Cell 66, 967–979.
28 Greco, A. et al. (1992) Oncogene 7, 237–242.
29 Schneider, R. and Schweiger, M. (1991) Oncogene 6, 1807–1811.
30 Kozma, S.C. et al. (1988) EMBO J. 7, 147–154.
31 Oskam, R. et al. (1988) Proc. Natl Acad. Sci. USA 85, 2964–2968.
32 Obermeier, A. et al. (1993) EMBO J. 12, 933–941.
33 Martin-Zanca, D. et al. (1989) Mol. Cell. Biol. 9, 24–33.
34 Klein, R. et al. (1989) EMBO J. 8, 3701–3709.

VAV

IDENTIFICATION

VAV (sixth letter of the Hebrew alphabet) was first identified by *in vitro* replacement of 67 N-terminal proto-VAV amino acids by 19 Tn5 transposase residues.

RELATED GENES

The central domain (198–434) shares homology with DBL, BCR, murine CDC25MM, CDC24 and CDC25 and (see *ABL*).

Nucleotides (kb)	>35 kb
Chromosome	19p13.2
Mass (kDa): predicted	96
expressed	p95 (oncogenic form ~p85)

Cellular location

Cytoplasm and nucleus.

Tissue distribution

Normal human *VAV* appears to be specifically expressed in cells of haematopoietic origin (erythroid, lymphoid, myeloid) regardless of their differentiation lineage.

PROTEIN FUNCTION

Probable exchange factor for a small RAS-like GTP binding protein. VAV undergoes rapid and transient tyrosine phosphorylation following activation of the T cell receptor or IgM antigen receptors on B cells [1] or in response to EGF or PDGF in transfected NIH 3T3 cells [2, 3] and in human haematopoietic cells after stimulation by IFNα [4] or stem cell factor (see *KIT*) [5]. In activated B cells VAV rapidly and transiently associates via its SH2 domain with a 70 kDa tyrosine-phosphorylated protein, VAP1. VAV may therefore participate in proliferation-associated signalling processes.

Cancer

The region of chromosome 19 to which VAV maps is involved in karyotypic abnormalities in a variety of malignancies including melanomas and leukaemias.

In vitro

VAV is a weak NIH 3T3 cell-transforming agent; transformation is greatly enhanced by truncation of the N-terminal helix–loop–helix/leucine zipper region [6].

PROTEIN STRUCTURE

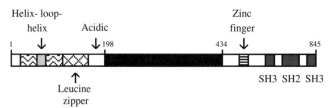

The C-terminal region of VAV contains one SH2 domain and two SH3 domains (see **DBL**). Point mutations in the SH2 domain inhibit the transforming potential of oncogenic VAV but do not activate that of normal VAV [7]. VAV proteins also contain a cysteine-rich domain that includes two putative metal-binding regions, $Cys-X_2-Cys-X_{13}-Cys-X_2-Cys$ and $His-X_2-Cys-X_6-Cys-X_2-His$. Mutations in these regions can completely abolish transforming activity [8].

SEQUENCE OF VAV (see also *DBL*)

```
  1  MELWRQCTHW  LIQCRVLPPS  HRVTWDGAQV  CELAQALRDG  VLLCQLLNNL
 51  LPHAINLREV  NLRPQMSQFL  CLKNIRTFLS  TCCEKFGLKR  SELFEAFDLF
101  DVQDFGKVIY  TLSALSWTPI  AQNRGIMPFP  TEEESVGDED  IYSGLSDQID
151  DTVEEDEDLY  DCVENEEAEG  DEIYEDLMRS  EPVSMPPKMT  EYDKRCCCLR
201  EIQQTEEKYT  DTLGSIQQHF  LKPLQRFLKP  QDIEIIFINI  EDLLRVHTHF
250  LKEMKEALGT  PGAPNLYQVF  IKYKERFLVY  GRYCSQVESA  SKHLDRVAAA
301  REDVQMKLEE  CSQRANNGRF  TARPADGAYA  ASSQISPPSP  GAGETHAGGD
351  GARKLRLALD  AMRDLAQCVN  EVKRDNETLR  QITNFQLSIE  NLDQSLAHYG
401  RPKIDGELKI  TSVERRSKMD  RYAFLLDKAL  LICKRRGDSY  DLKDFVNLHS
451  FQVRDDSSGD  RDNKKWSHMF  LLIEDQGAQG  YELFF*KTREL* *KKK*WMEQFEM
501  AISNIYPENA  TANGHDFQMF  SFEETTS<u>CKA</u> <u>CQMLLRGTFY</u> <u>QGYRCHRCRA</u>
551  SA<u>HKECLGRV</u> <u>PPCGRH</u>GQDF  PGTM*KKDKLH* *RR*AQDKKRNE  LGLPKMEVFQ
601  EYYGLPPPPG  AIGPFLRLNP  GDIVELTKAE  AEQNWWEGRN  TSTNEIGWFP
651  CNRVKPYVHG  PPQDLSVHLW  YAGPMERAGA  ESILANRSDG  TFLVRQRVKD
701  AAEFAISIKY  NVEVKHTVKI  MTAEGLYRIT  EKKAFRGLTE  LVEFYQQNSL
751  KDCFKSLDTT  LQFPFKEPEK  RTISRPAVGS  TKYFGTAKAR  YDFCARDRSE
801  LSLKEGDIIK  ILNKKGQQGW  WRGEIYGRVG  WFPANYVEED  YSEYC (845)
```

Domain structure

515–563	Phorbol ester and diacylglycerol binding
671–761	SH2. The VAV SH2 domain has Thr at the βD5 position and recognizes phosphopeptides with the general motif *P*-Tyr-Met-Glu-Pro [9]
782–842	SH3
486–493 and 575–582	Putative nuclear localization signals (italics)
541–548 and 553–566	Zinc finger domains (underlined)

DATABASE ACCESSION NUMBERS

	PIR	SWISSPROT	EMBL/GENBANK	REFERENCES
Human *VAV*	S05382	P15498	X16316, M59834	6,10

References
1 Bustelo, X.R. and Barbacid, M. (1992) Science 256, 1196–1199.
2 Bustelo, X.R. et al. (1992) Nature 356, 68–71.
3 Margolis, B. et al. (1992) Nature 356, 71–74.
4 Platanias, L.C. and Sweet, M.E. (1994) J. Biol. Chem. 269, 3143–3146.
5 Alai, M. et al. (1992) J. Biol. Chem. 267, 18021–18025.
6 Katzav, S. et al. (1991) Mol. Cell. Biol. 11, 1912–1920.
7 Katzav, S. (1993) Oncogene 8, 1757–1763.
8 Coppola, J. et al. (1991) Cell Growth Differ. 2, 95–105.
9 Songyang, Z. et al. (1994) Mol. Cell. Biol. 14, 2777–2785.
10 Katzav, S. et al. (1989) EMBO J. 8, 2283–2290.

WNT1, WNT2, WNT3

IDENTIFICATION

Wnt-1/Int-1 was originally identified as a frequent target for MMTV insertion in mammary carcinomas [1]. *Wnt-3* is related to *Wnt-1* and is also activated by proviral insertion. *WNT1* and *WNT3* were detected by screening genomic DNA with mouse *Int-1* and *Wnt-3* probes. *WNT2* was detected by isolation of a methylation-free CpG island from a human lung cDNA library.

RELATED GENES

There are at least 10 genes in the mouse *Wnt-1/Int-1* family [2]. On the basis of their similarity to the *Drosophila melanogaster wingless* gene product, *Int-1* and related genes have been reclassified as *Wnt* (wingless-type MMTV integration site). At least 12 *Xenopus laevis Xwnt* genes have been detected and there are *Caenorhabditis elegans* homologues of *Wnt-1*, *Wnt-2* and *Wnt-5B*.

	WNT1 (INT1)	*WNT2* (IRP)	*WNT3* (INT4)
Nucleotides (kb)	30	Not fully mapped	>50
Chromosome	12q13	7q31	17q21–q22
Mass (kDa): predicted	41	38	40
expressed	gp40/gp42	gp35	

Cellular location

WNT1 and WNT2: Secreted. Tightly associated with extracellular matrix and cell surface [3,4]. WNT3: unknown.

Tissue distribution

Murine *Wnt* genes are expressed in a variety of embryonic and adult tissues, particularly in brain and lung. *Wnt-1* is also expressed in the adult testis [5] and *Wnt-2* during the ductal phase of mouse mammary gland development [6]. *WNT2* is expressed in human fetal lung fibroblast cell lines [7]. *Xwnt-3A* may participate in patterning the central nervous system during early *Xenopus* development [8].

PROTEIN FUNCTION

WNT1 is probably a growth factor but its receptor is unknown. Normal function is in embryogenesis: in the mouse it is required for development of the mid-brain and anterior hindbrain. Secretion of WNT1 is inefficient and substantial amounts are present in the endoplasmic reticulum associated with Bip [9,10]. Expression of *Wnt-1* in embryos can reproduce the effects of lithium treatment, suggesting that WNT1 may modulate the way cells respond to inducing agents by suppressing the concentration of phosphoinositides available to generate second messenger signals [11,12]. In PC12 cells *Wnt-1* expression enhances cell–cell adhesion and correlates with increased expression of E-cadherin and plakoglobulin and decreased expression of N-CAM.

These observations are generally consistent with the evidence that *Drosophila* and *Xenopus* wnt genes are involved in the generation of the central nervous system [13].

Cancer

WNT1 is amplified in some primary retinoblastoma tumours [14]. Amplification of *Wnt-2* has been detected in mouse mammary tumours [15]. No amplification or rearrangement of *WNT3* has been detected in human breast tumours [16].

Transgenic animals

Wnt-1 causes hyperplasia in the mammary glands of male and female mice which can progress to mammary and salivary adenocarcinomas [17,18]. Bi-transgenic mice carrying both *Wnt-1* and *Int-2* transgenes regulated by the MMTV LTR develop mammary carcinomas more rapidly and with higher frequency than occurs when either gene is expressed alone [19]. This indicates that *Wnt-1* and *Int-2* cooperate in mammary tumorigenesis, although amplification or rearrangement of *WNT1* has not been detected in human breast carcinomas.

In animals

Wnt-1 and *Int-2* are the most frequent targets in MMTV-induced tumours. Either *Wnt-1* or *Int-2* or both may be activated [20] and insertion at each site has been detected in both pre-malignant lesions and in malignant tumours [21]. The frequency with which the *Wnt-1* and *Int-2* loci are rearranged by MMTV insertional mutagenesis is a function of the host genetic background [22–24], indicating that strains inbred for a high incidence of mammary tumours have acquired host mutations that complement the activity of specific *Wnt/Int* genes.

In vitro

Wnt-1 transforms fibroblasts with very low efficiency but expression of the gene by fibroblasts causes morphological transformation of co-cultured mammary epithelial cells [25]. Thus WNT1 protein may participate in a paracrine mechanism.

Wnt-1 partially transforms the C57 mammary epithelial cell line [26] and renders the RAC mammary cell line tumorigenic [27]. WNT2 transforms epithelial cells.

GENE STRUCTURE OF *WNT1*

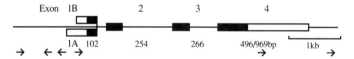

The sequence and organization of the *WNT1* gene is highly conserved in organisms ranging from man to *Drosophila*. The conservation between human *WNT1* and mouse *Wnt-1* includes extensive intronic regions as well as 5′ and 3′ non-translated regions [28].

Arrows indicate integration sites and orientations in *Wnt-1* of MMTV proviruses in a variety tumours, the majority being orientated away from *Wnt-1*. For *Wnt-1*, *Int-2*, *Hst-1* and *Wnt-4* proviral integration of MMTV does not perturb the DNA encoding these genes [29, 30].

The structure of *Wnt-3* is similar to that of *Wnt-1*. All introns are at homologous positions compared with *Wnt-1* except for a unique intron before a fifth exon that is completely non-coding [29].

TRANSCRIPTIONAL REGULATION

The 5′ exon has two forms (1A and 1B) with identical 3′ ends but different 5′ ends [31]. There are two TATA boxes upstream of the 1B start site at –35 and –25. The region upstream of 1A contains no TATA boxes but is very GC-rich and includes at least two SP1 binding sites.

PROTEIN STRUCTURE

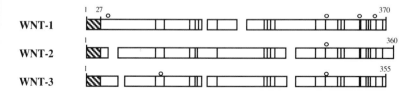

The vertical bars represent the 22 cysteine residues conserved throughout the WNT family. Circles indicate potential *N*-glycosylation sites. The cross-hatched box indicates the signal sequence.

SEQUENCE OF WNT1 (INT1)

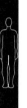

```
  1  MGLWALLPGW VSATLLLALA ALPAALAANS SGRWWGIVNV ASSTNLLTDS
 51  KSLQLVLEPS LQLLSRKQRR LIRQNPGILH SVSGGLQSAV RECKWQFRNR
101  RWNCPTAPGP HLFGKIVNRG CRETAFIFAI TSAGVTHSVA RSCSEGSIES
151  CTCDYRRRGP GGPDWHWGGC SDNIDFGRLF GREFVDSGEK GRDLRFLMNL
201  HNNEAGRTTV FSEMRQECKC HGMSGSCTVR TCWMRLPTLR AVGDVLRDRF
251  DGASRVLYGN RGSNRASRAE LLRLEPEDPA HKPPSPHDLV YFEKSPNFCT
301  YSGRLGTAGT AGRACNSSSP ALDGCELLCC GRGHRTRTQR VTERCNCTFH
351  WCCHVSCRNC THTRVLHECL (370)
```

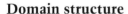

Domain structure

1–27	Signal sequence (italics)
29, 316, 346, 359	Potential carbohydrate attachment sites

SEQUENCE OF WNT2

```
  1  MNAPLGGIWL WLPLLLTWLT PEVNSSWWYM RATGGSSRVM CDNVPGLVSS
 51  QRQLCHRHPD VMRAISQGVA EWTAECQHQF RQHRWNCNTL DRDHSLFGRV
101  LLRSSRESAF VYAISSAGVV FAITRACSQG EVKSCSCDPK KMGSAKDSKG
151  IFDWGGCSDN IDYGIKFARA FVDAKERKGK DARALMNLHN NRAGRKAVKR
201  FLKQECKCHG VSGSCTLRTC WLAMADFRKT GDYLWRKYNG AIQVVMNQDG
251  TGFTVANERF KKPTKNDLVY FENSPDYCIR DREAGSLGTA GRVCNLTSRG
301  MDSCEVMCCG RGYDTSHVTR MTKCGCKFHW CCAVRCQDCL EALDVHTCKA
351  PKNADWTTAT (360)
```

Domain structure

1–21 or 25	Signal sequence
24, 295	Potential carbohydrate attachment sites

SEQUENCE OF MOUSE WNT3

```
  1  MEPHLLGLLL GLLLSGTRVL AGYPIWWSLA LGQQYTSLAS QPLLCGSIPG
 51  LVPKQLRFCR NYIEIMPSVA EGVKLGIQEC QHQFRGRRWN CTTIDDSLAI
101  FGPVLDKATR ESAFVHAIAS AGVAFAVTRS CAEGTSTICG CDSHHKGPPG
151  EGWKWGGCSE DADFGVLVSR EFADARENRP DARSAMNKHN NEAGRTTILD
201  HMHLKCKCHG LSGSCEVKTC WWAQPDFRAI GDFLKDKYDS ASEMVVEKHR
251  ESRGWVETLR AKYALFKPPT ERDLVYYENS PNFCEPNPET GSFGTRDRTC
301  NVTSHGIDGC DLLCCGRGHN TRTEKRKEKC HCVFHWCCYV SCQECIRIYD
351  VHTCK (355)
```

Domain structure

1–27	Signal sequence (italics)
90, 301	Potential carbohydrate attachment sites

DATABASE ACCESSION NUMBERS

	PIR	SWISSPROT	EMBL/GENBANK	REFERENCES
Human *WNT1 (INT1)*	A24674	P04628	X03072	*28, 31*
Human *WNT2*	S00834	P09544	X07876	*32*
Mouse *Wnt-3*	A35503	P17553	M32502	*29*

References
1 **Peters, G. (1991) Semin. Virol. 2, 319–328.**
2 **Nusse, R. and Varmus, H.E. (1992) Cell 69, 1073–1087.**
3 Papkoff, J. (1994) Oncogene 9, 313–317.
4 Parkin, N.T. et al. (1993) Genes Devel. 7, 2181–2193.
5 Jakobovits, A. et al. (1986) Proc. Natl Acad. Sci. USA 83, 7806–7810.
6 Buhler, T. A. et al. (1993) Devel. Biol. 155, 87–96.
7 Levay-Young, B. K. and Navre, M. (1992) Am. J. Physiol. 262, L672–683.
8 Wolda, S. L. et al. (1993) Devel. Biol. 155, 46–57.
9 van Ooyen, A. and Nusse, R. (1984) Cell 39, 233–240.
10 Kitajewski, J. et al. (1992) Mol. Cell. Biol. 12, 784–790.
11 Sokol, S. et al. (1991) Cell 67, 741–752.
12 Olson, D.J. et al. (1991) Science 252, 1173–1176.
13 Christian, J.L. et al. (1991) Devel. Biol. 143, 230–234.
14 Arheden, K. et al. (1988) Cytogen. Cell Genet. 48, 174–177.
15 Roelink, H. et al. (1992) Oncogene 7, 487–492.
16 Roelink, H. J. et al. (1993) Genomics 17, 790–792.
17 Tsukamoto, A.S. et al. (1988) Cell 55, 619–625.
18 Edwards, P.A.W. et al. (1992) Oncogene 7, 2041–2051.
19 Kwan, H. et al. (1992) Mol. Cell. Biol. 12, 147–154.
20 Gray, D.A. et al. (1986) Virology 154, 271–278.
21 Morris, D.W. et al. (1990) J. Virol. 64, 1794–1802.
22 Escot, C. et al. (1986) J. Virol. 58, 619–625.
23 Etkind, P., (1989) J. Virol. 63, 4972–4975.
24 Marchetti., A. et al. (1991) J. Virol. 65, 4550–4554.
25 Jue, S.F. et al. (1992) Mol. Cell. Biol. 12, 321–328.
26 Blasband, A. et al. (1992) Oncogene 7, 153–161.
27 Rijsewijk, F. et al. (1987) EMBO J. 6, 127–131.
28 van Ooyen, A. et al. (1985) EMBO J. 4, 2905–2909.
29 Roelink, H. et al. (1990) Proc. Natl Acad. Sci. USA 87, 4519–4523.
30 Peters, G. et al. (1989) Proc. Natl Acad. Sci. USA 86, 5678–5682.
31 Nusse, R. et al. (1990) Mol. Cell. Biol. 10, 4170–4179.
32 Wainwright, B.J. et al. (1988) EMBO J. 7, 1743–1748.

YES1

IDENTIFICATION

v-*yes* (originally *yas*) is the oncogene of two avian sarcoma viruses, Y73 and Esh sarcoma virus (ESV). Y73 *a*vian *s*arcoma virus was isolated from a transplantable tumour arising in a chicken of the same strain on a farm in Yamaguchi Prefecture. Esh was isolated from a tumour arising in a White leghorn owned by Mr Esh of Pennsylvania. *YES* was detected by screening DNA with a v-*yes* probe.

RELATED GENES

Member of the *SRC* tyrosine kinase family (*Blk, FGR, FYN, HCK, LCK/Tkl, LYN, SRC, YES*). Chicken *YRK* (*Y*es-*r*elated *k*inase) is 72.4% identical to chicken YES [1]. *YESP/YES2* is a human pseudogene.

	YES1	v-yes
Nucleotides	>30 kb	3718 bp (Y73)
Chromosome	18q21.3	
Mass (kDa): predicted	61	
expressed	62	P90*gag-yes* (Y73)
		P80*gag-yes* (ESV)

Cellular location

YES1: Plasma membrane and attached to the cytoskeleton. v-YES: More diffusely distributed but concentrated in cell junction and adhesion plaques, similar to SRC.

Tissue distribution

YES mRNA is widely distributed. In humans expression is high in the brain and kidney and low in spleen, muscle and thymus [2–4]. YES kinase activity is high in platelets, peripheral blood T cells and natural killer cells but low in monocytes and B lymphocytes [5, 6]. Expression is stimulated during lymphocyte mitogenesis [3].

PROTEIN FUNCTION

YES genes encode membrane-associated protein tyrosine kinases, functionally related to SRC. As for SRC, there is evidence implicating YES in the tyrosine phosphorylation of multiple substrates and in the modulation of PtdIns metabolism that occurs during the activation of many normal cell types and in transformed cells.

In normal quiescent fibroblasts stimulated by PDGF a small proportion of YES associates with the PDGF receptor and PtdIns kinase [7]. This complex formation is correlated with a transient increase in the activity of the YES kinase. For transforming mutants of polyomavirus middle T antigen the extent of association of middle T antigen with YES and PtdIns kinase correlates with transforming capacity [8].

In a variety of cell types, activated YES associates with stimulated plasma membrane signalling receptors. Other SRC family kinases (FYN, LYN, SRC) may be simultaneously or alternatively activated, indicating that the SRC family kinases are involved in a cell-specific manner in generating the patterns of protein tyrosine phosphorylation that occur after cell stimulation [9,10]. In keratinocytes and other types of cell YES is in-activated by a Ca^{2+}-dependent association with proteins that overrides its activation by tyrosine dephosphorylation [11].

In Y73-transformed cells vinculin and integrin are phosphorylated on tyrosine residues and the concentrations of PtdIns $3P$, PtdIns$(3,4)P_2$ and PtdIns$(3,4,5)P_3$ are increased [12].

Cancer

Moderate to strong expression of *YES1* has been detected at relatively low frequency in a variety of cancers including fibrosarcoma, malignant lymphoma, malignant melanoma, glioblastoma, breast cancer, colorectal cancer, head and neck cancer, renal cancers, lung cancers, gastric carcinoma and stomach cancer [13–16].

In animals

Y73 and ESV induce sarcomas in chickens [17].

In vitro

Y73 and ESV transform fibroblasts [18].

TRANSCRIPTIONAL REGULATION

The *YES* promoter contains six GC box-like sequences but no TATA box [19]. Four of the GC boxes immediately 5' of the gene bind SP1 and affect *YES* transcription.

PROTEIN STRUCTURE

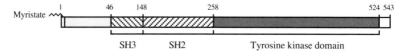

Human YES is 92% identical to chicken YES. v-YES differs from chicken YES by six substitutions and the replacement of eight amino acids at the extreme of the C-terminus of YES by three *env*-encoded residues. The latter modification may be the major feature responsible for the transforming properties of v-*yes* (see **SRC**).

SEQUENCE OF YES

```
  1  MGCIKSKENK  SPAIKYRPEN  TPEPVSTSVS  HYGAEPTTVS  PCPSSSAKGT
 51  AVNFSSLSMT  PFGGSSGVTP  FGGASSSFSV  VPSSYPAGLT  GGVTIFVALY
101  DYEARTTEDL  SFKKGERFQI  INNTEGDWWE  ARSIATGKNG  YIPSNYVAPA
151  DSIQAEEWYF  GKMGRKDAER  LLLNPGNQRG  IFLVRESETT  KGAYSLSIRD
201  WDEIRGDNVK  HYKIRKLDNG  GYYITTRAQF  DTLQKLVKHY  TEHADGLCHK
251  LTTVCPTVKP  QTQGLAKDAW  EIPRESLRLE  VKLGQGCFGE  VWMGTWNGTT
301  KVAIKTLKPG  TMMPEAFLQE  AQIMKKLRHD  KLVPLYAVVS  EEPIYIVTEF
351  MSKGSLLDFL  KEGDGKYLKL  PQLVDMAAQI  ADGMAYIERM  NYIHRDLRAA
401  NILVGENLVC  KIADFGLARL  IEDNEYTARQ  GAKFPIKWTA  PEAALYGRFT
451  IKSDVWSFGI  LQTELVTKGR  VPYPGMVNRE  VLEQVERGYR  MPCPQGCPES
501  LHELMNLCWK  KDPDERPTFE  YIQSFLEDYF  TATEPQYQPG  ENL (543)
```

Domain structure

1–7	Necessary and sufficient for myristylation (Gly2)
8–96	Unique domain variable between non-membrane receptor tyrosine kinases
96–148	SH3 domain (underlined)
148–256	SH2 domain
256–524	Catalytic domain, which shares sequence homology with other tyrosine kinases
283–291 and 305	ATP binding site surrounding Lys302
396	Active site
426	Autophosphorylation site
525–543	Regulatory domain

DATABASE ACCESSION NUMBERS

	PIR	SWISSPROT	EMBL/GENBANK	REFERENCE
Human *YES1*	A26714	P07947	M15990	[20]

References
1 Sudol, M. et al. (1993) Oncogene 8, 823–831.
2 Semba, K. et al. (1985) Science 227, 1038–1040.
3 Reed, J.C. et al. (1986) Proc. Natl. Acad. Sci. USA 83, 3982–3986.
4 Sukegawa, J. et al. (1990) Oncogene 5, 611–614.
5 **Eiseman, E. and Bolen, J.B. (1990) Cancer Cells 2, 303–310.**
6 Zhao, Y.-H. et al. (1990) Oncogene 5, 1629–1635.
7 Kypta, R.M. et al. (1990) Cell 62, 481–492.
8 Kornbluth, S. et al. (1990) J. Virol. 64, 1584–1589.
9 Huang, M.-M. et al. (1991) Proc. Natl Acad. Sci. USA 88, 7844–7848.
10 Eiseman, E. and Bolen, J.B. (1992) Nature 355, 78–80.
11 Zhao, Y. et al. (1993) Mol. Cell. Biol. 13, 7507–7514.
12 Fukui, Y. et al. (1991) Oncogene 6, 407–411.
13 Sugawara, K. et al. (1991) Br. J. Cancer 63, 508–513.
14 Loganzo, F. et al. (1993) Oncogene 8, 2637–2644.

15 Park, J. et al. (1993) Oncogene 8, 2627–2635.
16 Seki, T. et al. (1985) Jpn J. Cancer Res. (Gann) 76, 907–910.
17 Kawai, S. et al. (1980) Proc. Natl Acad. Sci. USA 77, 6199–6203.
18 Ghysdael, J. et al. (1981) Virology 111, 386–400.
19 Matsuzawa, Y. et al. (1991) Oncogene 6, 1561–1567.
20 Sukegawa, J. et al. (1987) Mol. Cell. Biol. 7, 41–47.

TUMOUR SUPPRESSOR GENES

TUMOUR SUPPRESSOR GENES

The existence of what are now variously known as tumour suppressor genes, recessive oncogenes, anti-oncogenes or growth suppressor genes was originally inferred from the finding that when tumorigenic and non-tumorigenic cells were fused in culture the resulting hybrids were generally non-tumorigenic [1]. When such hybrid cells do give rise to tumours in animals this usually involves the loss of a specific chromosome derived from the non-tumorigenic cell. In many spontaneously arising tumours, individual chromosomes or specific regions of a chromosome are lost or deleted.

These observations suggest the existence of a substantial class of tumour suppressor genes, the normal function of which is to govern cell proliferation, and indicate that when non-tumorigenic hybrids are formed from two different tumorigenic cells genetic complementation may be occurring. The two best understood tumour suppressor genes are the retinoblastoma (*RB1*) gene and *TP53/P53*: the properties of these and of other emerging potential tumour suppressor genes are summarized below. *RB1* provides the classical model for a recessive tumour suppressor gene in that both paternal and maternal copies of the gene must be inactivated for the tumour to develop. For *P53* and some other tumour suppressor genes, mutation at one allele may be sufficient to give rise to the altered cell phenotype.

Reference
1   Knudson, A.G. (1993) Proc. Natl Acad. Sci. USA 90, 10914–10921.

APC, MCC

IDENTIFICATION

Familial adenomatosis polyposis (FAP) arises from the inheritance of one abnormal *APC* (*a*denomatous *p*olyposis *c*oli) allele. The incidence is 1 in 8000 and it causes the development of hundreds of colonic polyps in early life and leads, in untreated individuals, to colorectal cancer. *APC* is mutated in the germline of FAP patients; virtually all mutations inactivate the gene [1]. Variant alleles of *APC* are also involved in the attenuated form of familial adenomatosis polyposis (AAPC). The locus is involved in other forms of colorectal cancers, although in these cases the incidence of allelic losses from chromosome 5q is very variable [2], and in gastric carcinomas [3]. The *MCC* (*m*utated in *c*olorectal *c*ancer) gene, ~180 kb from *APC*, is not mutated in the germline but undergoes somatic mutations in FAP and colon cancer [4]. However, *MCC* may not function as an independent tumour suppressor gene in colorectal cancer [5]. Deletions in the 5q21 region also occur in ~25% of lung cancers [6]. FAP is inconsistently associated with characteristic patches of congenital hypertrophy of the retinal pigment epithelium (CHRPE), the extent of which correlates with the location of mutation in the APC gene [7].

RELATED GENES

No closely related genes but both *APC* and *MCC* contain heptad repeats that give predicted coiled-coil domains, similar to those in myosins and keratins and the *SKI* family.

	APC	*MCC*
Nucleotides (kb)	120	170
Chromosome	5q21	5q21
Mass (kDa): predicted	312	93
expressed	~300	

Cellular location

Associated with detergent-insoluble cytoskeleton.

Tissue distribution

Probably ubiquitous.

PROTEIN FUNCTION

Unknown. APC forms dimers via the leucine zipper region and associates with the E-cadherin binding proteins α- and β-catenin [8]. Catenin–cadherin complexes comprise the adherens junction multiprotein complex that mediates adhesion, cytoskeletal anchoring and signalling, and catenin-APC complexes may play a role in regulating cell growth.

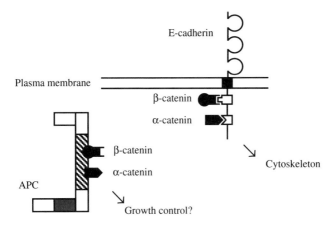

Transgenic mice homozygous for the null *APC* allele develop normally, indicating that in mice this gene is not essential for proliferation and differentiation. Animals with germline mutations of *APC* have a phenotype similar to that of FAP [9].

GENE STRUCTURE OF *APC*

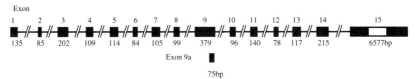

The alternatively spliced form (exon 9a) has a deletion that removes 101 amino acids. Isoforms lacking exon 7 have been detected in human and mouse cell lines. At least five isoforms arise from alternative splicing of 5′ non-coding sequences [10].

PROTEIN STRUCTURE

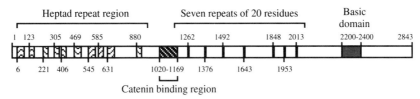

The initial amino acids of the 10 heptad repeats and the seven 20 residue repeats (consensus F–VE–TP–CFSR–SSLSSLS) are numbered. The last 14 amino acids of the fourth and the first seven amino acids of the fifth heptad repeats are present only in the longer gene product (containing exon 9). Full-length wild-type APC associates with truncated APC: the N-terminal 171 residues of APC are sufficient for this interaction, a domain that includes the first two heptad repeats [11,12].

APC germline mutations are usually point mutations or small deletions, insertions or splicing mutations leading to downstream termination, the most N-terminal being at codon 168. Mutations detected in AAPC are similar but are grouped nearer the 5' end of *APC*, the most C-terminal being at codon 157 [13]. Mutations between 1285 and 1465 correlate with profuse polyposis.

In CHRPE ocular lesions are present if *APC* is truncated after exon 9 but almost always absent if the mutation occurs before this exon [7].

SEQUENCE OF APC

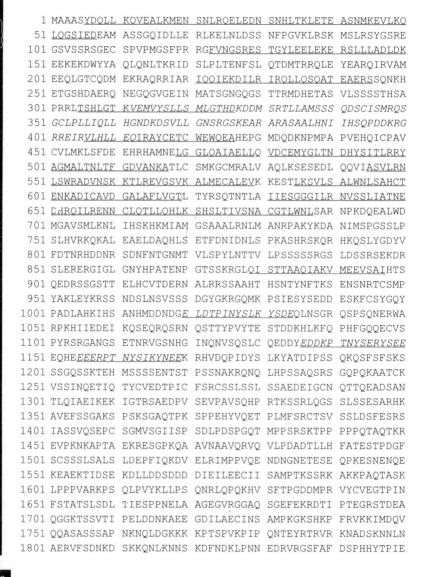

```
   1 MAAASYDQLL KQVEALKMEN SNLRQELEDN SNHLTKLETE ASNMKEVLKQ
  51 LQGSIEDEAM ASSGQIDLLE RLKELNLDSS NFPGVKLRSK MSLRSYGSRE
 101 GSVSSRSGEC SPVPMGSFPR RGFVNGSRES TGYLEELEKE RSLLLADLDK
 151 EEKEKDWYYA QLQNLTKRID SLPLTENFSL QTDMTRRQLE YEARQIRVAM
 201 EEQLGTCQDM EKRAQRRIAR IQQIEKDILR IRQLLQSQAT EAERSSQNKH
 251 ETGSHDAERQ NEGQGVGEIN MATSGNGQGS TTRMDHETAS VLSSSSTHSA
 301 PRRLTSHLGT KVEMVYSLLS MLGTHDKDDM SRTLLAMSSS QDSCISMRQS
 351 GCLPLLIQLL HGNDKDSVLL GNSRGSKEAR ARASAALHNI IHSQPDDKRG
 401 RREIRVLHLL EQIRAYCETC WEWQEAHEPG MDQDKNPMPA PVEHQICPAV
 451 CVLMKLSFDE EHRHAMNELG GLQAIAELLQ VDCEMYGLTN DHYSITLRRY
 501 AGMALTNLTF GDVANKATLC SMKGCMRALV AQLKSESEDL QQVIASVLRN
 551 LSWRADVNSK KTLREVGSVK ALMECALEVK KESTLKSVLS ALWNLSAHCT
 601 ENKADICAVD GALAFLVGTL TYRSQTNTLA IIESGGGILR NVSSLIATNE
 651 DHRQILRENN CLQTLLQHLK SHSLTIVSNA CGTLWNLSAR NPKDQEALWD
 701 MGAVSMLKNL IHSKHKMIAM GSAAALRNLM ANRPAKYKDA NIMSPGSSLP
 751 SLHVRKQKAL EAELDAQHLS ETFDNIDNLS PKASHRSKQR HKQSLYGDYV
 801 FDTNRHDDNR SDNFNTGNMT VLSPYLNTTV LPSSSSSRGS LDSSRSEKDR
 851 SLERERGIGL GNYHPATENP GTSSKRGLQI STTAAQIAKV MEEVSAIHTS
 901 QEDRSSGSTT ELHCVTDERN ALRRSSAAHT HSNTYNFTKS ENSNRTCSMP
 951 YAKLEYKRSS NDSLNSVSSS DGYGKRGQMK PSIESYSEDD ESKFCSYGQY
1001 PADLAHKIHS ANHMDDNDGE LDTPINYSLK YSDEQLNSGR QSPSQNERWA
1051 RPKHIIEDEI KQSEQRQSRN QSTTYPVYTE STDDKHLKFQ PHFGQQECVS
1101 PYRSRGANGS ETNRVGSNHG INQNVSQSLC QEDDYEDDKP TNYSERYSEE
1151 EQHEEEERPT NYSIKYNEEK RHVDQPIDYS LKYATDIPSS QKQSFSFSKS
1201 SSGQSSKTEH MSSSSENTST PSSNAKRQNQ LHPSSAQSRS GQPQKAATCK
1251 VSSINQETIQ TYCVEDTPIC FSRCSSLSSL SSAEDEIGCN QTTQEADSAN
1301 TLQIAEIKEK IGTRSAEDPV SEVPAVSQHP RTKSSRLQGS SLSSESARHK
1351 AVEFSSGAKS PSKSGAQTPK SPPEHYVQET PLMFSRCTSV SSLDSFESRS
1401 IASSVQSEPC SGMVSGIISP SDLPDSPGQT MPPSRSKTPP PPPQTAQTKR
1451 EVPKNKAPTA EKRESGPKQA AVNAAVQRVQ VLPDADTLLH FATESTPDGF
1501 SCSSSLSALS LDEPFIQKDV ELRIMPPVQE NDNGNETESE QPKESNENQE
1551 KEAEKTIDSE KDLLDDSDDD DIEILEECII SAMPTKSSRK AKKPAQTASK
1601 LPPPVARKPS QLPVYKLLPS QNRLQPQKHV SFTPGDDMPR VYCVEGTPIN
1651 FSTATSLSDL TIESPPNELA AGEGVRGGAQ SGEFEKRDTI PTEGRSTDEA
1701 QGGKTSSVTI PELDDNKAEE GDILAECINS AMPKGKSHKP FRVKKIMDQV
1751 QQASASSSAP NKNQLDGKKK KPTSPVKPIP QNTEYRTRVR KNADSKNNLN
1801 AERVFSDNKD SKKQNLKNNS KDFNDKLPNN EDRVRGSFAF DSPHHYTPIE
```

```
1851 GTPYCFSRND SLSSLDFDDD DVDLSREKAE LRKAKENKES EAKVTSHTEL
1901 TSNQQSANKT QAIAKQPINR GQPKPILQKQ STFPQSSKDI PDRGAATDEK
1951 LQNFAIENTP VCFSHNSSLS SLSDIDQENN NKENEPIKET EPPDSQGEPS
2001 KPQASGYAPK SFHVEDTPVC FSRNSSLSSL SIDSEDDLLQ ECISSAMPKK
2051 KKPSRLKGDN EKHSPRNMGG ILGEDLTLDL KDIQRPDSEH GLSPDSENFD
2101 WKAIQEGANS IVSSLHQAAA AACLSRQASS DSDSILSLKS GISLGSPFHL
2151 TPDQEEKPFT SNKGPRILKP GEKSTLETKK IESESKGIKG GKKVYKSLIT
2201 GKVRSNSEIS GQMKQPLQAN MPSISRGRTM IHIPGVRNSS SSTSPVSKKG
2251 PPLKTPASKS PSEGQTATTS PRGAKPSVKS ELSPVARQTS QIGGSSKAPS
2301 RSGSRDSTPS RPAQQPLSRP IQSPGRNSIS PGRNGISPPN KLSQLPRTSS
2351 PSTASTKSSG SGKMSYTSPG RQMSQQNLTK QTGLSKNASS IPRSESASKG
2401 LNQMNNGNGA NKKVELSRMS STKSSGSESD RSERPVLVRQ STFIKEAPSP
2451 TLRRKLEESA SFESLSPSSR PASPTRSQAQ TPVLSPSLPD MSLSTHSSVQ
2501 AGGWRKLPPN LSPTIEYNDG RPAKRHDIAR SHSESPSRLP INRSGTWKRE
2551 HSKHSSSLPR VSTWRRTGSS SSILSASSES SEKAKSEDEK HVNSISGTKQ
2601 SKENQVSAKG TWRKIKENEF SPTNSTSQTV SSGATNGAES KTLIYQMAPA
2651 VSKTEDVWVR IEDCPINNPR SGRSPTGNTP PVIDSVSEKA NPNIKDSKDN
2701 QAKQNVGNGS VPMRTVGLEN RLNSFIQVDA PDQKGTEIKP GQNNPVPVSE
2751 TNESSIVERT PFSSSSSSKH SSPSGTVAAR VTPFNYNPSP RKSSADSTSA
2801 RPSQIPTPVN NNTKKRDSKT DSTESSGTQS PKRHSGSYLV TSV (2843)
```

Domain structure

1–55	Region sufficient for APC homodimerization
1–730	Leucine-rich region
7–72 and 185–227	Potential coil
312–412	101 amino acids deleted in the alternatively spliced form (italics)
6–57, 123–150, 221–245, 305–326, 406–426, 469–517, 545–579, 585–619, 631–687, 880–897	10 heptad repeat regions (underlined)
731–2832	Serine-rich region
1020–1034, 1136–1150 and 1155–1169	Three imperfect 15 amino acid repeats, any one of which is sufficient to bind catenins (underlined italics)
1131–1156 and 1558–1577	Aspartate/glutamate-rich (acidic) region
1866–1893	Highly charged region

Variants in FAP patients: Arg414→Cys, Glu911→Gly, Thr1313→Ala. The most common mutation is a deletion at codon 1309 and other mutations have been detected at codons 764, 1061, 1323, 1368, 1464 and 1537 [14].

Variants in gastric adenoma: Deletions at codons 1156–1157, 1191; insertion at codon 1196; Gly817→Cys, Ile880→Thr, Asn942→Asp, Gly1120→Glu, Arg1171→His, Phe1197→Ser, Ile1259→Thr, Thr1301→Ser, Gly1312→Glu, Val1326→Ala.

SEQUENCE OF MCC

```
  1  MNSGVAMKYG NDSSAELSEL HSAALASLKG DIVELNKRLQ QTERERDLLE
 51  KKLAKAQCEQ SHLMREHEDV QERTTLRYEE RITELHSVIA ELNKKIDRLQ
101  GTTIREEDEY SELRSELSQS QHEVNEDSRS MDQDQTSVSI PENQSTMVTA
151  DMDNCSDLNS ELQRVLTGLE NVVCGRKKSS CSLSVAEVDR HIEQLTTASE
201  HCDLAIKTVE EIEGVLGRDL YPNLAEERSR WEKELAGLRE ENESLTAMLC
251  SKEEELNRTK ATMNAIREER DRLRRRVREL QTRLQSVQAT GPSSPGRLTS
301  TNRPINPSTG ELSTSSSSND IPIAKIAERV KLSKTRSESS SSDRPVLGSE
351  ISSIGVSSSV AEHLAHSLQD CSNIQEIFQT LYSHGSAISE SKIREFEVET
401  ERLNSRIEHL KSQNDLLTIT LEECKSNAER MSMLVGKYES NATALRLALQ
451  YSEQCIEAYE LLLALAESEQ SLILGQFRAA GVGSSPGDQS GDENITQMLK
501  RAHDCRKTAE NAAKALLMKL DGSCGGAFAV AGCSVQPWES LSSNSHTSTT
551  SSTASSCDTE FTKEDEQRLK DYIQQLKNDR AAVKLTMLEL ESIHIDPLSY
601  DVKPRGDSQR LDLENAVLMQ ELMAMKEEMA ELKAQLYLLE KEKKALELKL
651  STREAQEQAY LVHIEHLKSE VEEQKEQRMR SLSSTSSGSK DKPGKECADA
701  ASPALSLAEL RTTCSENELA AEFTNAIRRE KKLKARVQEL VSALERLTKS
751  SEIRHQQSAE FVNDLKRANS NLVAAYEKAK KKHQNKLKKL ESQMMAMVER
801  HETQVRMLKQ RIALLEEENS RPHTNETSL (829)
```

Domain structure

220–243 Similarity to amino acids 249 to 272 of the G protein coupled M3 muscarinic acetylcholine receptor (italics)

Variants in colorectal cancer: Arg267→Leu, Pro486→Leu, Ser490→Leu, Arg506→Gln, Ala698→Val.

DATABASE ACCESSION NUMBERS

	PIR	SWISSPROT	EMBL/GENBANK	REFERENCES
Human *APC*	A37261	P25054	M74088	15
Human *MCC*	A33166, A38434	P23508	M62397	16

References

1 Miyoshi, Y. et al. (1992) Proc. Natl Acad. Sci. USA 89, 4452–4456.
2 **Fearon, E.R. and Vogelstein, B. (1990) Cell 61, 759–767.**
3 Tamura, G. (1994) Cancer Res. 54, 1149–1151.
4 **Bourne, H.R. (1991) Nature 353, 696–698.**
5 Curtis, L.J. et al. 1994) Hum. Mol. Genetics 3, 443–446.
6 Ashton-Rickardt, P.G. et al. (1991). Oncogene 6, 1881–1886.
7 Olschwang, S. et al. (1993) Cell 75, 959–968.
8 Su, L.-K. et al. (1993) Science 262, 1734–1737.
9 Su, L.-K. et al. (1992) Science 256, 668–670.
10 Horii, A. et al. (1993) Hum. Mol. Genetics 2, 283–287.
11 Smith, K.J. et al. (1993) Proc. Natl Acad. Sci. USA 90, 2846–2850.
12 Su, L.-K. et al. (1993) Cancer Res. 53, 2728–2731.
13 Spiro, L. et al. (1993) Cell 75, 951–957.
14 Gayther, S.A. et al. (1994) Hum. Mol. Genet. 3, 53–56.
15 Joslyn, G. et al. (1991) Cell 66, 601–613.
16 Kinzler, K.W. et al. (1991) Science 251, 1366–1370.

CMAR/CAR

The *CMAR/CAR* gene (cell adhesion regulator; chromosome 16q) encodes a protein containing an N-terminal myristylation signal and a C-terminal tyrosine kinase phosphorylation consensus sequence that enhances cell attachment to collagen types I and IV and laminin [1]. CAR is unrelated to any known integrins nor does it modulate the expression of integrin heterodimers. The high levels of allelic loss on 16q that occur in breast and prostate cancers indicate that *CAR* may be a tumour suppressor gene, its normal function being to repress tissue invasiveness.

SEQUENCE OF CMAR/CAR

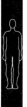

```
 1   MLRGSDMKGP CEPIVLSPAA LSSSSLINGA SQAQALGSGG LTTAPCCHVD
51   WCKLRTSCWS SHACSVGDAL VFTALRIVEI LY (82)
```

Domain structure

1–5   Myristylation site (italics)
76–82 Tyrosine phosphorylation site (underlined)

Reference
1 Pullman, W.E. and Bodmer, W.F. (1992) Nature 356, 529–532; correction ibid 361, 564.

DCC

Allelic loss of chromosomes 17p or 18q occurs in 70% of colorectal carcinomas and with high frequency in ovarian adenocarcinomas [1]. The 17p region contains *P53*; the 18q region contains a putative tumour suppressor gene, *DCC* (*d*eleted in *c*olorectal *c*arcinomas, 18q21–qter) [2] and also includes *BCL2* and *YES1*. The predicted sequence of the DCC protein is homologous to neural cell adhesion molecules (N-CAMs). Its reduced expression or allelic loss in colorectal, gastric, pancreatic, oesophageal, breast, haematological and glial malignancies [3] may reflect alterations in cellular attachment; antisense RNA to *DCC* inhibits cell adhesion *in vitro* [4]. In addition to mutations in *P53*, *DCC*, *APC* and *MCC*, colorectal carcinomas also accumulate mutations in *RAS*. Mutations in *DCC* also occur in breast carcinomas [5]. At least four scrambled transcripts are present at low concentrations in normal and neoplastic cells in which *DCC* exons are joined accurately at consensus splice sites but in a different order to that in the primary transcript [6]. *DCC* expression is reduced in HPV-18 immortalized human keratinocytes transformed to tumorigenicity by nitrosomethylurea [7].

SEQUENCE OF DCC

```
   1 MENSLRCVWV PKLAFVLFGA SLLSAHLQVT GFQIKAFTAL RFLSEPSDAV
  51 TMRGGNVLLD CSAESDRGVP VIKWKKDGIH LALGMDERKQ QLSNGSLLIQ
 101 NILHSRHHKP DEGLYQCEAS LGDSGSIISR TAKVAVAGPL RFLSQTESVT
 151 AFMGDTVLLK CEVIGEPMPT IHWQKNQQDL TPIPGDSRVV VLPSGALQIS
 201 RLQPGDIGIY RCSARNPASS RTGNEAEVRI LSDPGLHRQL YFLQRPSNVV
 251 AIEGKDAVLE CCVSGYPPPS FTWLRGEEVI QLRSKKYSLL GGSNLLISNV
 301 TDDDSGMYTC VVTYKNENIS ASAELTVLVP PWFLNHPSNL YAYESMDIEF
 351 ECTVSGKPVP TVNWMKNGDV VIPSDYFQIV GGSNLRILGV VKSDEGFYQC
 401 VAENEAGNAQ TSAQLIVPKP AIPSSSVLPS APRDVVPVLV SSRFVRLSWR
 451 PPAEAKGNIQ TFTVFFSREG DNRERALNTT QPGSLQLTVG NLKPEAMYTF
 501 RVVAYNEWGP GESSQPIKVA TQPELQVPGP VENLQAVSTS PTSILITWEP
 551 PAYANGPVQG YRLFCTEVST GKEQNIEVDG LSYKLEGLKK FTEYSLRFLA
 601 YNRYGPGVST DDITVVTLSD VPSAPPQNVS LEVVNSRSIK VSWLPPPSGT
 651 QNGFITGYKI RHRKTTRRGE METLEPNNLW YLFTGLEKGS QYSFQVSAMT
 701 VNGTGPPSNW YTAETPENDL DESQVPDQPS SLHVRPQTNC IIMSWTPPLN
 751 PNIVVRGYII GYGVGSPYAE TVRVDSKQRY YSIERLESSS HYVISLKAFN
 801 NAGEGVPLYE SATTRSITDP TDPVDYYPLL DDFPTSVPDL STPMLPPVGV
 851 QAVALTHDAV RVSWADNSVP KNQKTSEVRL YTVRWRTSFS ASAKYKSEDT
 901 TSLSYTATGL KPNTMYEFSV MVTKNRRSST WSMTAHATTY EAAPTSAPKD
 951 FTVITREGKP RAVIVSWQPP LEANGKITAY ILFYTLDKNI PIDDWIMETI
1001 SGDRLTHQIM DLNLDTMYYF RIQARNSKGV GPLSDPILFR TLKVEHPDKM
1051 ANDQGRHGDG GYWPVDTNLI DRSTLNEPPI GQMHPPHGSV TPQKNSNLLV
1101 IIVVTVGVIT VLVVVIVAVI CTRRSSAQQR KKRATHSAGK RKGSQKDLRP
1151 PDLWIHHEEM EMKNIEKPSG TDPAGRDSPI QSCQDLTPVS HSQSETQLGS
1201 KSTSHSGQDT EEAGSSMSTL ERSLAARRAP RAKLMIPMDA QSNNPAVVSA
1251 IPVPTLESAQ YPGILPSPTC GYPHPQFTLR PVPFPTLSVD RGFGAGRSQS
1301 VSEGPTTQQP PMLPPSQPEH SSSEEAPSRT IPTACVRPTH PLRSFANPLL
1351 PPPMSAIEPK VPYTPLLSQP GPTLPKTHVK TASLGLAGKA RSPLLPVSVP
1401 TAPEVSEESH KPTEDSANVY EQDDLSEQMA SLEGLMKQLN AITGSAF (1447)
```

Mutations in DCC detected in oesophageal carcinomas [8]: Met[168]$\to$ Thr; Arg[201] $\to$ Gly. Increased frequency of mutation appears to correlate with distance of lymph node metastasis from the primary tumour.

DATABASE ACCESSION NUMBERS

	PIR	SWISSPROT	EMBL/GENBANK	REFERENCE
Human	DCC		Hsdccg X76132	9

References

1 Chenevix-Trench, G. et al. (1992) Oncogene 7, 1059–1065.
2 Fearon, E.R. et al. (1990) Science 247, 49–56.
3 Scheck, A.C. and Coons, S.W. (1993) Cancer Res. 53, 5605–5609.
4 Narayanan, R. et al. (1992) Oncogene 7, 553–561.
5 Devilee, P. et al. (1991) Oncogene 6, 311–315.
6 **Nigro, J.M.** et al. **(1991) Cell 64, 607–613.**
7 Klingelhutz, A.J. et al. (1993) Oncogene 8, 95–99.
8 Miyake, S. et al. (1994) Cancer Res., 54, 3007-3010.
9 Hedrick L. et al. (1993) Unpublished.

Inhibin A and inhibin B are growth factors that suppress the secretion of follicle stimulating hormone (FSH). Both forms of inhibin contain an α subunit linked via one or more disulphide bridges to one of two types of β subunit (βA or βB).

Transgenic mice homozygous for the null allele of α-inhibin develop normally but all animals, both male and female, eventually develop mixed or incompletely differentiated gonadal stromal tumours [1]. Thus inhibin is not essential for normal sexual differentiation and development in the mouse but is a negative regulator of gonadal stromal cell proliferation.

Reference
1   Matzuk, M.M. et al. (1992) Nature 360, 313–319.

MLH1, MSH2 (Hereditary Nonpolyposis Colon Cancer (HNPCC))

This disease is the most common hereditary colon cancer susceptibility for which a candidate gene has been detected, the defective gene being carried by ~1/200 individuals and being responsible for ~15% of all colon cancers. Two HNPCC loci have been detected, *MSH2* and *MLH1*.

MSH2 (chromosome 2p22–21) was cloned by PCR amplification of degenerate oligonucleotide primers that hybridize to highly conserved regions of bacterial *MutS/HexA* and *Saccharomyces. cerevisiae MSH2*. It encodes a member of the MutS mismatch repair protein superfamily that bind to mismatched nucleotides in DNA and is closely related to *S. cerevisiae* MSH2. Mismatch repair systems play a major role in preventing mutations during DNA replication and HNPCC patients have germline mutations in *MSH2* at an intronic splice acceptor site presumed to cause aberrant mRNA processing [1].

MLH1 (chromosome 3p21.3–p23) is homologous to the bacterial mismatch repair protein MutL and its product is similar to the yeast mismatch repair protein MLH1 [2]. Mis-sense mutations in MLH1 occur in individuals with chromosome 3-linked HNPCC.

SEQUENCE OF MSH2

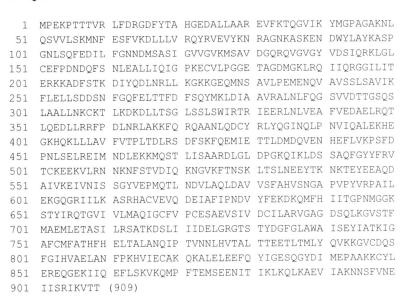

```
  1  MPEKPTTTVR  LFDRGDFYTA  HGEDALLAAR  EVFKTQGVIK  YMGPAGAKNL
 51  QSVVLSKMNF  ESFVKDLLLV  RQYRVEVYKN  RAGNKASKEN  DWYLAYKASP
101  GNLSQFEDIL  FGNNDMSASI  GVVGVKMSAV  DGQRQVGVGY  VDSIQRKLGL
151  CEFPDNDQFS  NLEALLIQIG  PKECVLPGGE  TAGDMGKLRQ  IIQRGGILIT
201  ERKKADFSTK  DIYQDLNRLL  KGKKGEQMNS  AVLPEMENQV  AVSSLSAVIK
251  FLELLSDDSN  FGQFELTTFD  FSQYMKLDIA  AVRALNLFQG  SVVDTTGSQS
301  LAALLNKCKT  LKDKDLLTSG  LSSLSWIRTR  IEERLNLVEA  FVEDAELRQT
351  LQEDLLRRFP  DLNRLAKKFQ  RQAANLQDCY  RLYQGINQLP  NVIQALEKHE
401  GKHQKLLLAV  FVTPLTDLRS  DFSKFQEMIE  TTLDMDQVEN  HEFLVKPSFD
451  PNLSELREIM  NDLEKKMQST  LISAARDLGL  DPGKQIKLDS  SAQFGYYFRV
501  TCKEEKVLRN  NKNFSTVDIQ  KNGVKFTNSK  LTSLNEEYTK  NKTEYEEAQD
551  AIVKEIVNIS  SGYVEPMQTL  NDVLAQLDAV  VSFAHVSNGA  PVPYVRPAIL
601  EKGQGRIILK  ASRHACVEVQ  DEIAFIPNDV  YFEKDKQMFH  IITGPNMGGK
651  STYIRQTGVI  VLMAQIGCFV  PCESAEVSIV  DCILARVGAG  DSQLKGVSTF
701  MAEMLETASI  LRSATKDSLI  IIDELGRGTS  TYDGFGLAWA  ISEYIATKIG
751  AFCMFATHFH  ELTALANQIP  TVNNLHVTAL  TTEETLTMLY  QVKKGVCDQS
801  FGIHVAELAN  FPKHVIECAK  QKALELEEFQ  YIGESQGYDI  MEPAAKKCYL
851  EREQGEKIIQ  EFLSKVKQMP  FTEMSEENIT  IKLKQLKAEV  IAKNNSFVNE
901  IISRIKVTT  (909)
```

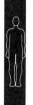

SEQUENCE OF MLH1

```
  1  MSFVAGVIRR  LDETVVNRIA  AGEVIQRPAN  AIKEMIENCL  DAKSTSIQVI
 51  VKEGGLKLIQ  IQDNGTGIRK  EDLDIVCERF  TTSKLQSFED  LASISTYGFR
101  GEALASISHV  AHVTITTKTA  DGKCAYRASY  SDGKLKAPPK  PCAGNQGTQI
151  TVEDLFYNIA  TRRKALKNPS  EEYGKILEVV  GRYSVHNAGI  SFSVKKQGET
201  VADVRTLPNA  STVDNIRSIF  GNAVSRELIE  IGCEDKTLAF  KMNGYISNAN
251  YSVKKCIFLL  FINHRLVEST  SLRKAIETVY  AAYLPKNTHP  FLYLSLEISP
301  QNVDVNVHPT  KHEVHFLHEE  SILERVQQHI  ESKLLGSNSS  RMYFTQTLLP
351  GLAGPSGEMV  KSTTSLTSSS  TSGSSDKVYA  HQMVRTDSRE  QKLDAFLQPL
401  SKPLSSQPQA  IVTEDKTDIS  SGRARQQDEE  MLELPAPAEV  AAKNQSLEGD
451  TTKGTSEMSE  KRGPTSSNPR  KRHREDSDVE  MVEDDSRKEM  TAACTPRRRI
501  INLTSVLSLQ  EEINEQGHEV  LREMLHNHSF  VGCVNPQWAL  AQHQTKLYLL
551  NTTKLSEELF  YQILIYDFAN  FGVLRLSEPA  PLFDLAMLAL  DSPESGWTEE
601  DGPKEGLAEY  IVEFLKKKAE  MLADYFSLEI  DEEGNLIGLP  LLIDNYVPPL
651  EGLPIFILRL  ATEVNWDEEK  ECFESLSKEC  AMFYSIRKQY  ISEESTLSGQ
701  QSEVPGSIPN  SWKWTVEHIV  YKALRSHILP  PKHFTEDGNI  LQLANLPDLY
751  KVFERC  (756)
```

DATABASE ACCESSION NUMBERS

	PIR	*SWISSPROT*	*EMBL/GENBANK*	*REFERENCES*
Human *MLH1*			U07343	*2*
Human *MSH2*				*1*

References
1 Fishel, R. et al. (1993) Cell 75, 1027–1038.
2 Bronner, C.E. et al. (1994) Nature 368, 258–261.

MTS1, MTS2

Multiple tumour suppressor 1 (MTS1, chromosome 9p21) encodes p16 (148 amino acids), an inhibitor of cyclin-dependent kinase 4 [1, 2]. Thus MTS1 competes with D cyclins, one of which (cyclin D1) has oncogenic capacity, in binding to CDK4. Mutations in MTS1 have been detected in ~75% of a wide variety of human tumour cell lines. However, mutations in p16 may be upt to three times less frequent in primary tumours, the discrepancy possibly reflecting tumour type and/or the ease with which specific cell lines can be established [4].

MTS1 has three exons (126, 307 and 11 bp). MTS2 is an adjacent gene containing a region of 93% identity to MTS1.

SEQUENCE OF MTS1

```
  1  MEPSADWLAT AAARGRVEEV RALLEAVALP NAPNSYGRRP IQVMMMGSAR
 51  VAELLLLHGA EPNCADPATL TRPVHDAARE GFLDTLVVLH RAGARLDVRD
101  AWGRLPVDLA EELGHRDVAR YLRAAAGGTR GSNHARIDAA EGPSDIPD(148)
```

Mutations in MTS1 in melanoma cell lines: Gln42→stop, Arg50→stop, Arg72→stop, Gly81→Ser, Trp102→stop, Pro106→Leu, Ala140→Thr, and frameshift deletions at Ser35, Arg50 and Leu89.

DATABASE ACCESSION NUMBERS

	PIR	SWISSPROT	EMBL/GENBANK	REFERENCE
Human MTS1		L27211	HSCDK4X	3

References
1 Kamb, A. et al. (1994) Science 264, 436–440.
2 Nobori, T. et al. (1994) Nature 368, 753–756.
3 Serrano, M. et al. (1994) Nature 366, 704–707.
4 Spruck, C.H. et al. (1994) Nature 370, 183–184.

IDENTIFICATION

The most frequent forms of neurofibromatosis are peripheral neuro-fibromatosis (NF1) and central neurofibromatosis (NF2). NF1 (von Recklinghausen neurofibromatosis) affects ~1 in 3 500 individuals and arises in cells derived from the embryonic neural crest, causing benign growths including neurofibromas and cafe-au-lait spots on the skin, phaeochromocytomas and malignant Schwannomas and neurofibro-sarcomas. The NF1 gene is always inherited as a mutant allele, unlike RB1. Mutations NF2 (incidence 1 in 40 000) give rise to acoustic neuromas, Schwann cell-derived tumours and meningiomas [1] and also occur in some breast carcinomas [2].

RELATED GENES

NF1 is highly conserved and has regions of homology with *Saccharomyces cerevisiae* IRA1 and IRA2, mammalian GTPase-activating protein (GAP) and with the microtubule-associated proteins MAP2 and TAU.

The *NF2* gene product merlin (moesin–ezrin–radixin-like protein) shares 45–47% amino acid identity with the cytoskeleton-associated proteins from which its name is derived [3].

	NF1 (neurofibromin)	NF2 (merlin)
Nucleotides (kb)	300	
Chromosome	17q11.2	22q12
Mass (kDa): predicted	327	69
expressed	250	

Cellular location

NF1: Particulate cellular fraction. NF2: Cytoskeleton/plasma membrane.

Tissue distribution

Neurofibromin is found in most tissues. Merlin is detected in *NF2* lymphoblast cell lines. Neurofibromin is highly expressed in brain [4]. An alternatively spliced *NF1* gene product (type II) is widely expressed in vertebrates [5] and has been reported to be differentially expressed in neuronal cells stimulated to differentiate by retinoic acid [6] and in brain tumours [7].

PROTEIN FUNCTION

Neurofibromin contains a GAP-related domain (NF1 GRD) that stimulates the GTPase activity of normal but not oncogenic RAS [8,9]. In tumour cells from NF1 patients RAS is activated even though p120^{GAP} is present [10]. *RAS* appears to promote *NF1*-linked malignancy and *NF1* itself may function as a recessive oncogene, its normal gene product converting RAS to the inactive form. Neurofibromin interacts with the effector domain of RAS, however, and may thus be the target of RAS rather than its regulator (see **RAS**). Neurofibromin GAP activity is inhibited by arachidonate, phosphatidate or PtdIns(4,5)P_2, to which p120^{GAP} is insensitive, and by tubulin [11,12]. Neurofibromin undergoes serine/threonine phosphorylation in cells stimulated by growth factors.

Non-overlapping germline deletions in the merlin gene in two independent families that remove the N-terminus or the C-terminus suggests that merlin is the *NF2* tumour suppressor [3].

NF1 GENE STRUCTURE

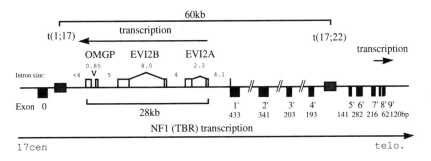

In *NF1* patients two translocations (t(1;17) and t(17;22), shaded boxes) and a number of deletions have been detected in the *NF1* (or translocation breakpoint (*TBR*)) gene. The breakpoints flank a 60 kb segment of DNA that contains the *EV12A*, *EVI2B* and oligodendrocyte-myelin glycoprotein (*OMGP*) loci [13,14]. *EV12A*, *EVI2B* and *OMGP* have the same transcriptional orientation, similar genomic organization and are contained within one intron of *NF1*, which is transcribed from the opposite strand. Some but not all of the deletions detected in *NF1* affect the *EV12A*, *EV12B* or *OMPG* genes. Nine of the 49 *NF1* exons (black boxes) are represented (designated here as 0 and 1'–9').

SEQUENCE OF NEUROFIBROMIN

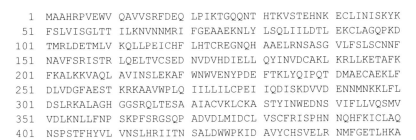

```
  1  MAAHRPVEWV QAVVSRFDEQ LPIKTGQQNT HTKVSTEHNK ECLINISKYK
 51  FSLVISGLTT ILKNVNNMRI FGEAAEKNLY LSQLIILDTL EKCLAGQPKD
101  TMRLDETMLV KQLLPEICHF LHTCREGNQH AAELRNSASG VLFSLSCNNF
151  NAVFSRISTR LQELTVCSED NVDVHDIELL QYINVDCAKL KRLLKETAFK
201  FKALKKVAQL AVINSLEKAF WNWVENYPDE FTKLYQIPQT DMAECAEKLF
251  DLVDGFAEST KRKAAVWPLQ IILLILCPEI IQDISKDVVD ENNMNKKLFL
301  DSLRKALAGH GGSRQLTESA AIACVKLCKA STYINWEDNS VIFLLVQSMV
351  VDLKNLLFNP SKPFSRGSQP ADVDLMIDCL VSCFRISPHN NQHFKICLAQ
401  NSPSTFHYVL VNSLHRIITN SALDWWPKID AVYCHSVELR NMFGETLHKA
```

```
 451 VQGCGAHPAI RMAPSLTFKE KVTSLKFKEK PTDLETRSYK YLLLSMVKLI
 501 HADPKLLLCN PRKQGPETQG STAELITGLV QLVPQSHMPE IAQEAMEALL
 551 VLHQLDSIDL WNPDAPVETF WEISSQMLFY ICKKLTSHQM LSSTEILKWL
 601 REILICRNKF LLKNKQADRS SCHFLLFYGV GCDIPSSGNT SQMSMDHEEL
 651 LRTPGASLRK GKGNSSMDSA AGCSGTPPIC RQAQTKLEVA LYMFLWNPDT
 701 EAVLVAMSCF RHLCEEADIR CGVDEVSVHN LLPNYNTFME FASVSNMMST
 751 GRAALQKRVM ALLRRIEHPT AGNTEAWEDT HAKWEQATKL ILNYPKAKME
 801 DGQAAESLHK TIVKRRMSHV SGGGSIDLSD TDSLQEWINM TGFLCALGGV
 851 CLQQRSNSGL ATYSPPMGPV SERKGSMISV MSSEGNADTP VSKFMDRLLS
 901 LMVCNHEKVG LQIRTNVKDL VGLELSPALY PMLFNKLKNT ISKFFDSQGQ
 951 VLLTDTNTQF VEQTIAIMKN LLDNHTEGSS EHLGQASIET MMLNLVRYVR
1001 VLGNMVHAIQ IKTKLCQLVE VMMARRDDLS FCQEMKFRNK MVEYLTDWVM
1051 GTSNQAADDD VKCLTRDLDQ ASMEAVVSLL AGLPLQPEEG DGVELMEAKS
1101 QLFLKYFTLF MNLLNDCSEV EDESAQTGGR KRGMSRRLAS LRHCTVLAMS
1151 NLLNANVDSG LMHSIGLGYH KDLQTRATFM EVLTKILQQG TEFDTLAETV
1201 LADRFERLVE LVTMMGDQGE LPIAMALANV VPCSQWDELA RVLVTLFDSR
1251 HLLYQLLWNM FSKEVELADS MQTLFRGNSL ASKIMTFCFK VYGATYLQKL
1301 LDPLLRIVIT SSDWQHVSFE VDPTRLEPSE SLEENQRNLL QMTEKFFHAI
1351 ISSSSEFPPQ LRSVCHCLYQ VVSQRFPQNS IGAVGSAMFL RFINPAIVSP
                                   ΔΔ
1401 YEAGILDKKP PPRIERGLKL MSKILQSIAN HVLFTKEEHM RPFNDFVKSN
1451 FDAARRFFLD IASDCPTSDA VNHSLSFISD GNVLALHRLL WNNQEKIGQY
1501 LSSNRDHKAV GRRPFDKMAT LLAYLGPPEH KPVADTHWSS LNLTSSKFEE
1551 FMTRHQVHEK EEFKALKTLS IFYQAGTSKA GNPIFYYVAR RFKTGQINGD
1601 LLIYHVLLTL KPYYAKPYEI VVDLTHTGPS NRFKTDFLSK WFVVFPGFAY
1651 DNVSAVYIYN CNSWVREYTK YHERLLTGLK GSKRLVFIDC PGKLAEHIEH
1701 EQQKLPAATL ALEEDLKVFH NALKLAHKDT KVSIKVGSTA VQVTSAERTK
1751 VLGQSVFLND IYYASEIEEI CLVDENQFTL TIANQGTPLT FMHQECEAIV
1801 QSIIHIRTRW ELSQPDSIPQ HTKIRPKDVP GTLLNIALLN LGSSDPSLRS
1851 AAYNLLCALT CTFNLKIEGQ LLETSGLCIP ANNTLFIVSI SKTLAANEPH
1901 LTLEFLEECI SGFSKSSIEL KHLCLEYMTP WLSNLVRFCK HNDDAKRQRV
1951 TAILDKLITM TINEKQMYPS IQAKIWGSLG QITDLLDVVL DSFIKTSATG
2001 GLGSIKAEVM ADTAVALASG NVKLVSSKVI GRMCKIIDKT CLSPTPTLEQ
2051 HLMWDDIAIL ARYMLMLSFN NSLDVAAHLP YLFHVVTFLV ATGPLSLRAS
2101 THGLVINIIH SLCTCSQLHF SEETKQVLRL SLTEFSLPKF YLLFGISKVK
2151 SAAVIAFRSS YRDRSFSPGS YERETFALTS LETVTEALLE IMEACMRDIP
2201 TCKWLDQWTE LAQRFAFQYN PSLQPRALVV FGCISKRVSH GQIKQIIRIL
2251 SKALESCLKG PDTYNSQVLI EATVIALTKL QPLLNKDSPL HKALFWVAVA
2301 VLQLDEVNLY SAGTALLEQN LHTLDSLRIF NDKSPEEVFM AIRNPLEWHC
2351 KQMDHFVGLN FNSNFNFALV GHLLKGYRHP SPAIVARTVR ILHTLLTLVN
2401 KHRNCDKFEV NTQSVAYLAA LLTVSEEVRS RCSLKHRKSL LLTDISMENV
2451 PMDTYPIHHG DPSYRTLKET QPWSSPKGSE GYLAATYPTV GQTSPRARKS
2501 MSLDMGQPSQ ANTKKLLGTR KSFDHLISDT KAPKRQEMES GITTPPKMRR
2551 VAETDYEMET QRISSSQQHP HLRKVSVSES NVLLDEEVLT DPKIQALLLT
2601 VLATLVKYTT DEFDQRILYE YLAEASVVFP KVFPVVHNLL DSKINTLLSL
2651 CQDPNLLNPI HGIVQSVVYH EESPPQYQTS YLQSFGFNGL WRFAGPFSKQ
2701 TQIPDYAELI VKFLDALIDT YLPGIDEETS EESLLTPTSP YPPALQSQLS
2751 ITANLNLSNS MTSLATSQHS PGIDKENVEL SPTTGHCNSG RTRHGSASQV
                            Δ
2801 QKQRSAGSFK RNSIKKIV (2818)
```

310

Domain structure

1264–1290, 1345–1407 and 1415–1430 — Regions of similarity to the GAP family (italics)

583–586, 815–818, 873–876, 2236–2239, 2573–2576 and 2810–281 — Six potential cAMP-dependent protein kinase recognition sites (underlined)

2549–2556 — Potential tyrosine kinase recognition site (underlined italics)

Alternative processing causes insertion of an additional 18 (ASLPCSNSAVFMQLFPHQ (Δ)) or 21 (ATCHSLLNKATVKEKKENKKS ($\Delta\Delta$)) amino acids, respectively. The 21 amino acid insertion decreases GTPase activity [5].

Substitution of Lys1423, detected in colon adenocarcinoma, myelodysplastic syndrome, anaplastic astrocytoma and NF1, decreases GAPase activity without affecting the binding affinity for RAS.GTP [15,16].

Mutation of Phe1434 or Lys1436 in NF1 confers the capacity to suppress the action of oncogenic RAS in v-*ras*-transformed NIH 3T3 cells [17].

SEQUENCE OF MERLIN

```
  1  MAGAIASRMS FSSLKRKQPK TFTVRIVTMD AEMEFNCEMK WKGKDLFDLV
 51  CRTLGLRETW FFGLQYTIKD TVAWLKMDKK VLDHDVSKEE PVTFHFLAKF
101  YPENAEEELV QEITQHLFFL QVKKQILDEK IYCPPEASVL LASYAVQAKY
151  GDYDPSVHKR GFLAQEELLP KRVINLYQMT PEMWEERITA WYAEHRGRAR
201  DEAEMEYLKI AQDLEMYGVN YFAIRNKKGT ELLLGVDALG LHIYDPENRL
251  TPKISFPWNE IRNISYSDKE FTIKPLDKKI DVFKFNSSKL RVNKLILQLC
301  IGNHDLFMRR RKADSLEVQQ MKAQAREEKA RKQMERQRLA REKQMREEAE
351  RTRDELERRL LQMKEEATMA NEALMRSEET ADLLAEKAQI TEEEAKLLAQ
401  KAAEAEQEMQ RIKATAIRTE EEKRLMEQKV LEAEVLALKM AEESERRAKE
451  ADQLKQDLQE AREAERRAKQ KLLEIATKPT YPPMNPIPAP LPPDIPSFNL
501  IGDSLSFDFK DTDMKRLSME IEKEKVEYME KSKHLQEQLN ELKTEIEALK
551  LKERETALDI LHNENSDRGG SSKHNTIKKL TLQSAKSRVA FFEEL (595)
                                 P QAQGRRPICI (590)
```

Domain structure

1–350 — Moesin–ezrin–radixin homology domain
580–590 — Alternative C-terminal 11 amino acids (italics) [2]

Mutations detected in vestibular schwannoma: in-frame deletions of nucleotides 676–810, 364–447, 115–240 (113–238), 364–447, 886–999 (888–1001), 358–375, 433–489 and 1575–1737 causing stop (1793).

Mutations detected in breast carcinoma: Ile273→Phe; deletion 600–810 causing stop (884).

Mutations detected in melanoma: Lys364→Ile; in-frame deletions of nucleotides 1000–1086 (1003–1089), 1504–1731 (1501–1728), and 361–445 causing stop (518), 1447–1571 causing stop (1646), 1123–1265 causing stop (1323) and 616 causing stop (623).

DATABASE ACCESSION NUMBERS

	PIR	SWISSPROT	EMBL/GENBANK	REFERENCES
Human *NF1*	A35222, A35605	P21359	M82814, M89914	18
Human *NF2*			L11353	3
			Schwannom	
			Z22664	19

References

1 Ruttledge, M.H. et al. (1994) Nature Genetics 6, 180–184.
2 Bianchi, A.B. et al. (1994) Nature Genetics 6, 185–192.
3 Trofatter, J.A. et al. (1993) Cell 72, 791–800.
4 Hattori, S. et al. (1992) Oncogene 7, 481–485.
5 Andersen, L.B. et al. (1993) Mol. Cell. Biol. 13, 487–495.
6 Nishi, T. et al. (1991) Oncogene 6, 1555–1559.
7 Suzuki, Y. et al. (1991) Biochem. Biophys. Res. Commun. 181, 95–961.
8 Bollag, G. and McCormick, F. (1991) Nature 351, 576–579.
9 Dibattiste, D. et al. (1993) Oncogene 8, 637–643.
10 Basu, T.N. et al. (1992) Nature 356, 713–715.
11 Golubic, M. et al. (1991) EMBO J. 10, 2897–2903.
12 Bollag, G. et al. (1993) EMBO J.,12, 1923–1927.
13 Cawthon, R.M. et al. (1991) Genomics 9, 446–460.
14 Viskochil, D. et al. (1991) Mol. Cell. Biol. 11, 906–912.
15 Li, Y. et al. (1992) Cell 69, 275–281.
16 Gutmann, D.H. et al. (1993) Oncogene 8, 761–769.
17 Nakafuku, M. et al. (1993) Proc. Natl Acad. Sci. USA 90, 6706–6710.
18 Marchuk, D.A. et al. (1991) Genomics 11, 931–940.
19 Rouleau, G.A. et al. (1993) Nature 363, 515–521.

P53

IDENTIFICATION

Chromosome 17p is frequently lost in human cancers and in most tumours that have been examined point mutations have occurred in one allelle of the *TP53* (*t*umour *p*rotein 53)/*P53* gene [1,2]. In Li–Fraumeni syndrome the mutated gene is transmitted in the germ line and this autosomal dominant syndrome is characterized by the occurrence of a variety of mesenchymal and epithelial neoplasms at multiple sites.

Nucleotides (kb)	12.5
Chromosome	17p13.1
Mass (kDa): predicted	43.5
expressed	p53

Cellular location

Nucleus. Detectable at the plasma membrane during mitosis in normal and transformed cells [3,4]. The conformational phenotype (see below) may determine its location [5] and in glioblastomas different mutations at the same codon modulate cytoplasmic/nuclear distribution [6].

Tissue distribution

Ubiquitous. In most transformed and tumour cells the concentration of p53 is increased five- to 100-fold [7] over the minute concentration in normal cells (~1000 molecules/cell), principally due to the half-life of the mutant forms (4 h) compared with that of the wild-type (20 min). High concentrations of p53 protein are transiently expressed in human epidermis and superficial dermal fibroblasts following mild ultraviolet irradiation[8].

PROTEIN FUNCTION

Transcriptional regulation

p53 binds to a DNA consensus sequence, the p53 response element, comprising two copies of 5'-PuPuPuC(^{A}/$_T$)(^{T}/$_A$)GPyPy-3' separated by 0–13bp [9]. Wild-type p53 has weak sequence-specific DNA binding activity that is strongly enhanced by factors acting on its C-terminal regulatory domain. Oligomerization of p53 is necessary for sequence specific DNA binding [10]. However, monomeric wild-type p53 expresses *trans*-activation activity even though it shows undetectable binding to DNA.

Factors enhancing p53 binding to DNA	Sequences to which p53 binds
Phosphorylation by casein kinase II	WAF1
mAb binding	MDM2
Escherichia coli dnaK	GADD45
Deletion of the C-terminus [11]	Human ribosomal gene cluster (RGC)
	ErbA-1 [12]
	Mouse muscle creatine kinase gene (MCK)
	Mouse endogenous retrovirus-like element (GLN LTR) [13]
	SV40 [14]

The first 42 amino acids of p53 comprise the minimum region sufficient for the powerful *trans*-activating function in p53/GAL4 fusion proteins [15–17]. Transcriptional activation by these proteins is prevented by mutant p53 proteins or by adenovirus E1B and inhibition of *trans*-activation by p53 correlates with transformation of primary cells by E1B in cooperation with E1A [18]. SV40 T antigen and HPV-16 E6 protein also inhibit *trans*-activation by wild-type p53 [19,20]. *Trans*-activation by p53 is enhanced by the presence of a GC_3 element (GCCCGGGC) adjacent to the consensus sequence to which a distinct factor may bind [12].

Genes repressed by p53

p53 suppresses transcription of a variety of genes that lack a p53 response element:

β-actin
BCL2
DNA polymerase α
Fos
Human IL6
Jun
Mybb [21, 22]
Porcine MHC class I gene [23, 24]
Proliferating cell nuclear antigen (PCNA)
Retinoblastoma (RB1) [25,2 6]
P-glycoprotein promoter (regulates the expression of the gene responsible for acquisition of the multidrug resistance (MDR) phenotype) [27]

Some of these effects may be mediated by the binding of wild-type (but not mutant p53) to human TATA-binding protein (TBP) and *in vitro* this inhibits transcription from minimal promoters [28–30]. p53 also interacts with CCAAT binding factor (CBF) to repress transcription from the HSP70 promoter [31].

Proteins associating with p53

Cellular proteins

CCAAT binding factor (CBF) [31]

HPV E6/p53 interaction mediator (E6-AP)

Heat shock protein 70 (HSP70)

Cellular oncoprotein MDM2

Replication protein A (RPA)

Transcription factor ERCC3
Transcription factor SP1 [34]
TATA binding protein (TBP)
Wilms' tumour protein (WT1)
p45, p56, p70 and other proteins in
non-small cell lung carcinoma cells [35]

Viral proteins

Adenovirus type 5 E1B

Epstein–Barr nuclear antigen 5
(EBNA-5) [32]

Epstein–Barr BZLF1 (Z)
protein [33]

Human papillomavirus type
16/18 E6 (HPV16/18 E6)

Simian virus 40 large T antigen
(SV40 T Ag)

Hepatitis B virus X protein

p53 binds via its acidic activation domain to the N-terminal region of the 90 kDa product of the murine double minute 2 (*Mdm2*) gene in intact cells and *in vitro* the formation of this complex inhibits p53-mediated *trans*-activation [36–39]. The expression of *Mdm2* is itself induced by p53, e.g. following ultraviolet irradiation [40], which may serve to autoregulate p53 activity in normal cells [41]. MDM2 is amplified in 36% of human sarcomas analysed and the overexpression of this gene may enable p53-regulated growth control to be over-ridden in these tumours.

P53 and the cell growth cycle

When 3T3 cells are stimulated by TPA or serum there is a 10- to 20-fold rise in *P53* mRNA within 6 h. Transcription of $p34^{CDC2}$, a critical regulator of mammalian cell cycle progression, also increases in serum-stimulated fibroblasts, reaching a maximum after 18 h, shortly before S phase. p53 is phosphorylated by $p34^{CDC2}$ when the latter is complexed with either p60 (cyclin A) or cyclin B [42,43]. These two active forms of p34 occur in late G_1 and M phases of the cell cycle, respectively, and the fact that, in addition to p53, $p105^{RB1}$ and SV40 T antigen are substrates, suggests that either suppressing the action of these proteins or redirecting their activity is a crucial requirement for both DNA synthesis and mitosis to occur.

p53 regulates the normal cell growth cycle by activating transcription of genes that control progression through the cycle and of other genes that cause arrest in G_1 when the genome is damaged [44]. A key regulator of

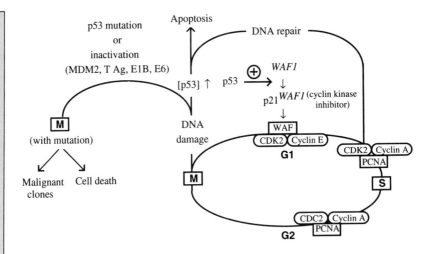

normal proliferation is *WAF1* (*w*ild-type p53-*a*ctivated *f*ragment *1*), the expression of which is induced by wild-type but not mutant p53 acting via a p53 response element. p21^WAF1 is present in cyclin-dependent kinase (CDC2/CDK)/cyclin complexes in normal cells, but not in some cancer cell lines, and functions as a CDK inhibitor to block progression through the cell cycle. It is expressed in cells undergoing either G_1 arrest or apoptosis by p53-dependent mechanisms [45].

The *GADD* (*G*rowth *A*rrest on *D*NA *D*amage) genes are induced in a wide variety of mammalian cells by DNA-damaging agents or other causes of growth arrest [46] and wild-type but not mutant p53 also induces *GADD45* transcription via a p53 response element. Thus p53 may function through *GADD45* to inhibit progression to S phase. The accumulation of p53 may merely inhibit the cell cycle until damaged DNA has been repaired or, if sustained, cause the activation of programmed cell death. The latter mechanism is consistent with the finding that expression of wild-type p53 (or p105^RB1) can mediate apoptosis in the absence of appropriate differentiation or proliferation signals and that extended survival without growth factors is conferred by the expression of mutant forms of p53 that act as dominant negative inhibitors of the wild-type protein [47]. The inactivation of p53 may thus permit replication of damaged DNA and promote the development of malignant cell clones, as occurs with high frequency in *P53* null mice and in patients with Li–Fraumeni syndrome.

These observations are consistent with transgenic mouse studies, indicating that p53 is not essential for cell growth control during early development but inhibition of DNA synthesis induces nuclear accumulation of p53 that correlates with arrest in G_1.

Cancer

P53 is the most commonly mutated gene in spontaneously occurring human cancers. Mutations arise with an average frequency of 70% but the incidence varies from zero in carcinoid lung tumours [48] to 97% in primary melanomas [49]. Cervical carcinomas expressing HPV DNA sequences normally co-express wild-type *P53* mRNA, mutant *P53* being present in the absence of HPV DNA [50], although *P53* mutations do occur in some HPV-associated cancers [51] and mutant *P53* can convert HPV-immortalized cells to a more transformed state [52]. p53 binds to the HPV E6 protein [53] and this interaction with the oncogenic E6 protein targets the suppressor form of p53 for ubiquitin-mediated degradation [54,55].

In animals

Disruption of *P53* by proviral insertion of murine leukaemia viruses has been detected in erythroid and lymphoid tumours [56].

In vitro

Mutant (but not wild-type) *P53* plus *Ras* transforms primary rat embryo fibroblasts [57] and mutant *P53*, like E1A, can immortalize cells. In transfected primary fibroblasts expression of wild-type *P53* inhibits the ability of mutant *P53* plus *Ras* (or E1A plus *Ras*) to cause transformation. The transfection of some breast carcinoma, osteosarcoma, colorectal carcinoma and glioblastoma cell lines that carry mutations in *P53* with a wild-type *P53* gene suppresses growth [58–60]. The tumorigenicity of breast carcinoma cell lines that harbour mutations in both *P53* and *RB1* genes is reduced by the expression of wild-type forms of either *P53* or *RB1* [61]. These *in vitro* findings are consistent with the occurrence of *trans*-dominant mutations in *P53*, as are those from analysis of a number of animal and human tumours.

In cells transformed by SV40 or adenovirus and in tumours induced by these viruses, p53 is found in an oligomeric complex with SV40 large T antigen or with adenovirus type 5 E1B-55 kDa protein.

Transgenic animals

Mice homozygous for the null allele develop normally but are predisposed to spontaneous tumour formation at an early age [62]. However, tumour development in *P53*-deficient mice is sporadic, indicating that additional genetic or epigenetic events are required. Fibroblasts from *P53*-deficient mice have accelerated growth properties *in vitro* and are genetically unstable [63].

GENE STRUCTURE

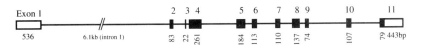

The *P53* promoter lacks a TATA or CAAT sequence but contains potential nuclear factor 1 (NF1) and p53 factor 1 (PF1) binding sites [24] and a helix–loop–helix consensus binding sequence [64]. In the murine promoter the latter element is required for full promoter activity and it contains the sequence CACGTG which is the recognition site for the transcription factors MYC/MAX, USF and TFE3 [65]. The region between +22 and +67 is involved in *trans*-activation of the *P53* promoter by p53 itself [66]. A strong promoter is present within intron 1 [67] and intron 4 binds a protein that is necessary for transformation by p53 [68]. Intron 4 is essential for *P53* expression in transgenic mice [69]. Differentiating mouse erythroleukaemia cells accumulate antisense RNA to the first intron that may be involved in the downregulation of *P53* mRNA [70].

A large number of *P53* mutations lead to single substitutions of a nucleic acid base pair [71] but ~10% of human cancers are characterized by deletions or insertions in this gene [72]. Normal and epidermal carcinoma cells express an alternatively spliced RNA at ~30% of the level of the normal transcript that contains an additional 96 bases derived from intron 10 [73]. Somatic mutations have been detected in most exons although the vast majority occur between exons 5 and 8. Exons 7 and 8 are the most frequent site of germline mutations. Germline mutations in intron 5 and exon 7 that create truncated proteins have been detected in a families with early onset breast–ovarian cancer [74,75].

PROTEIN STRUCTURE

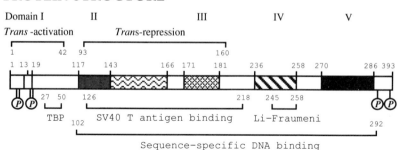

p53 forms stable homo-oligomers that principally result from the α helix (334–356) and basic regions (363–386) of the C-terminus [76-79].

The "hot-spot" in exon 7 for Li–Fraumeni germline mutations is indicated; some Li–Fraumeni families have also been identified with *P53* mutations outside exon 7 [80, 81]. Mutations at codons 141 or 175 abolish *trans*-activation potential whereas mutations at 248 or 273 result in substantial enhancement [82]. In hepatocellular carcinomas (HCCs) there is a mutational hot-spot at codon 249 [83, 84] that may be caused by exposure to hepatitis B virus (HBV) and aflatoxin B_1. Other mutations occur in HCCs from patients who have not been exposed to HBV or AFB_1 that frequently cause overexpression of the mutant protein [85]. HBV X protein complexes with wild-type p53 and inhibits its sequence-specific DNA binding *in vitro*. This interaction also prevents association of p53 with the general transcription factor ERCC3 that is involved in nucleotide excision repair [86].

Mutations are mainly clustered in four domains that are highly conserved among vertebrates, involving exons 5–10 (amino acids 120–290). The resultant mutant proteins fail to bind mAb PAb246 (which recognizes an epitope between amino acids 88 and 109 of wild-type p53), bind to DNA or to SV40 T antigen with much reduced affinity but bind with high affinity to the HSP70 protein via the C-terminal 28 amino acids of p53 [87]. In cells transformed by *Ras* with *P53*, mutant p53 protein occurs in a trimeric complex with the heat shock protein and wild-type p53. Mutations producing an abnormal protein that inhibits the function of its normal allelic gene product by formation of mutant/wild-type protein complexes are called *trans*-dominant mutations.

Mutations in p53 may (1) be of the dominant negative type when the protein overrides the action of the suppressor wild-type p53 or (2) result in the loss of suppressor function or (3) result in a protein that functions as a tumour promoter [76,88].

SEQUENCE OF P53

```
  1   MEEPQSDPSV EPPLSQETFS DLWKLLPENN VLSPLPSQAM DDLMLSPDDI
 51   EQWFTEDPGP DEAPRMPEAA PPVAPAPAAP TPAAPAPAPS WPLSSSVPSQ
101   KTYQGSYGFR LGFLHSGTAK SVTCTYSPAL NKMFCQLAKT CPVQLWVDST
151   PPPGTRVRAM AIYKQSQHMT EVVRRCPHHE RCSDSDGLAP PQHLIRVEGN
201   LRVEYLDDRN TFRHSVVVPY EPPEVGSDCT TIHYNYMCNS SCMGGMNRRP
251   ILTIITLEDS SGNLLGRNSF EVRVCACPGR DRRTEEENLR KKGEPHHELP
301   PGSTKRALPN NTSSSPQPKK KPLDGEYFTL QIRGRERFEM FRELNEALEL
351   KDAQAGKEPG GSRAHSSHLK SKKGQSTSRH KKLMFKTEGP DSD (393)
```

Domain structures

1–75	Acidic: predicted α helix
6, 9, 15, 37, 315, 392	Major phosphorylation sites [89]
75–150	Proline-rich, hydrophobic
102–292	Sequence-specific DNA binding [90,91]
135–179 & 238–277	Putative Zn^{2+} binding domains (underlined) [87]
126–218	T Antigen binding region mapped by mutagenesis [92]
313–322	Nuclear localization signal
323–393	C-terminus: highly basic containing helix–coil–helix motifs: forms stable tetramers and binds DNA non-specifically [90, 91]
389	5.8S rRNA attachment site [93, 94]
392	Casein kinase II phosphorylation [11]
15, 37	Phosphorylated *in vitro* by the protein kinase DNA-PK [95]

Common mutations occurring in human cancers: Lys132→Asn, Met133→Leu, Phe134→Leu, Cys135→Tyr, Cys141→Tyr, Pro151→Ser, Ala159→Pro, Arg175→His, His179→Tyr, Asn239→Ser, Asn247→Ile, Arg248→Thr/Trp, Arg249→Pro/Leu, Val272→Met, Arg273→His/Leu/Pro, Asp281→Gly.

Other mutations occurring in human cancers: Pro72→Arg, Ala79→Thr, Ser94→Thr, Pro151→Thr, Pro153→Thr, Arg156→Pro, Val157→Ser, 172–186 deletion, Val173→Glu, Arg175→Cys, Pro177/His178Pro/His/Pro/His/Pro, Arg181→Leu, Arg213→Gln, Ile232→Thr, Tyr234→His, Cys238→Phe,Ser240→Ile, Ser241→Phe, Gly245→Cys, Arg249→Ser, Leu252→Pro, Leu257→Gln, Glu258→Lys, Arg273→His, Val274→Phe, Arg280→Thr, Asp281→Val, Thr284→Ala.

Two germline mutations at codon 257 detected in breast cancers (Leu→Gln and frame-shift → 87 abnormal C-terminal amino acids) [75].

Polymorphisms have been detected at codons 21, 36, 72 and 213.

DATABASE ACCESSION NUMBERS

	PIR	SWISSPROT	EMBL/GENBANK	REFERENCES
Human *TP53*	A25224	P04637	K03199	*96*
	A25397		X01405	*97*
	B25397		X02469	*98–100*
	JT0436			*101–104*

References

1 Donehower, L.A. and Bradley, A. (1993) Biochim. Biophys. Acta 1155, 181–205.
2 Vogelstein, B. and Kinzler, K.W. (1992) Cell 70, 523–526.
3 Milner, J. and Cook, A. (1986) Virology 150, 265–269.
4 Shaulsky, G. et al. (1990) Oncogene 5, 1707–1711.
5 Zerrahn, J. et al. (1992) Oncogene 7, 1371–1381.
6 Ali, I.U. et al. (1994) Cancer Res. 54, 1–5.
7 Hassapoglidou, S. et al. (1993) Oncogene 8, 1501–1509.
8 Hall, P.A. et al. (1993) Oncogene 8, 203–207.
9 El-Deiry, W.S. et al. (1992) Nature Genetics 1, 45–49.
10 Hainaut, P. et al. (1994) Oncogene 9, 299–303.
11 Hupp, T.R., et al. (1992) Cell 71, 875–886.
12 Shiio, Y. et al. (1993) Oncogene 8, 2059–2065.
13 Zauberman, A. et al. (1993) EMBO J. 12, 2799–2808.
14 Bargonetti, J. et al. (1992) Genes Devel. 6, 1886–1898.
15 Fields, S. and Jang, S.K. (1990) Science 249, 1046–1049.
16 Raycroft, L. et al. (1990) Science 249, 1049–1051.
17 Unger, T. et al. (1992) EMBO J. 11, 1383–1390.
18 Yew, P.R. and Berk, A.J. (1992) Nature 357, 82–85.
19 Mietz, J.A. et al. (1992) EMBO J. 11, 5013–5020.
20 Band, V. et al. (1993) EMBO J. 12, 1847–1852.
21 Mercer, W.E. et al. (1991) Proc. Natl Acad. Sci. USA 88, 1958–1962.
22 Lin, D. et al. (1992) Proc. Natl Acad. Sci. USA 89, 9210–9214.
23 Santhanam, U. et al. (1991) Proc. Natl Acad. Sci. USA 88, 7605–7609.
24 Ginsberg, D. et al. (1991) Proc. Natl Acad. Sci. USA 88, 9979–9983.
25 Shiio, Y. et al. (1992) Proc. Natl Acad. Sci. USA 89, 5206–5210.
26 Jackson, P. et al. (1993) Oncogene 8, 589–597.

27 Zastawny, R.L. et al. (1993) Oncogene 8, 1529–1535.
28 Seto, E. et al. (1992) Proc. Natl Acad. Sci. USA 89, 12028–12032.
29 Mack, D.H. et al. (1993) Nature 363, 281–283.
30 Liu, X. et al. (1993) Mol. Cell. Biol. 13, 3291–3300.
31 Agoff, S.N. et al. (1993) Science 259, 84–87.
32 Szekely, L. et al. (1993) Proc. Natl Acad. Sci. USA 90, 5455–5459.
33 Zhang, Q. et al. (1994) Mol. Cell. Biol. 14, 1929–1938.
34 Borellini, F. and Glazer, R.I. (1993) J. Biol. Chem. 268, 7923–7928.
35 Maxwell, S.A. and Roth, J.A. (1993) Oncogene 8, 3421–3426.
36 Momand, J. et al. (1992) Cell 69, 1237–1245.
37 Oliner, J.D. et al. (1993) Nature 362, 857–860.
38 Chen, J. et al. (1993) Mol. Cell. Biol. 13, 4107–4114.
39 Haines, D.S. et al. (1994) Mol. Cell. Biol. 14, 1171–1178.
40 Perry, M.E. et al. (1994) Proc. Natl Acad. Sci. USA 90, 11623–11627.
41 Juven, T. et al. (1993) Oncogene 8, 3411–3416.
42 Sturzbecher, H.-W. et al. (1990) Oncogene 5, 795–801.
43 Bischoff, J.R. et al. (1990) Proc. Natl Acad. Sci. USA 87, 4766–4770.
44 **Lane, D.P. (1992) Nature 358, 15–16.**
45 El-Deiry, W.S. et al. (1994) Cancer Res. 54, 1169–1174.
46 Kastan, M.B. et al. (1992) Cell 71, 587–597.
47 Gottlieb, E. et al. (1994) EMBO J. 13, 1368–1374.
48 Iggo, R. et al. (1990) Lancet 335, 675–679.
49 Akslen, L.A. and Morkve, O. (1992) Int. J. Cancer 52, 13–16.
50 Crook, T. et al. (1991) Oncogene 6, 873–875.
51 Crook, T. and Vousden, K.H. (1992) EMBO J. 11, 3935–3940.
52 Chen, T.-M. et al. (1993) Oncogene 8, 1511–1518.
53 Huibregtse, J.M. et al. (1993) Mol. Cell. Biol. 13, 775–784.
54 Scheffner, M. et al. (1990) Cell 63, 1129–1136.
55 Crook, T. et al. (1994) Oncogene 9, 1225–1230.
56 Munroe, D.G. et al. (1990) Mol. Cell. Biol. 10, 3307–3313.
57 Finlay, C. et al. (1989) Cell 57, 1083–1093.
58 Baker, S.J. et al. (1990) Science 249, 912–915.
59 Diller, L. et al. (1990) Mol. Cell. Biol. 10, 5772–5781.
60 Mercer, W.E. et al. (1990) Proc. Natl Acad. Sci. USA 87, 6166–6170.
61 Wang, N.P. et al. (1993) Oncogene 8, 279–288.
62 Donehower, L.A. et al. (1992) Nature 356, 215–221.
63 Harvey, M. et al. (1993) Oncogene 8, 2457–2467.
64 Ronen, D. et al. (1991) Proc. Natl Acad. Sci. USA 88, 4128–4132.
65 Reisman, D. and Rotter, V. (1993) Nucl. Acids Res. 21, 345–350.
66 Deffie, A. et al. (1993) Mol. Cell. Biol. 13, 3415–3423.
67 Reisman, D. (1988). Proc. Natl Acad. Sci. USA 85, 5146–5150.
68 Beenken, S.W. et al. (1991) Nucl. Acids Res. 19, 4747–4752.
69 Lozano-G. and Levine, A.J. (1991) Mol. Carcinogen. 4, 3–9.
70 Khochbin, S. and Lawrence, J.-J. (1989) EMBO J. 8, 4107–4114.
71 **Hollstein, M. et al. (1991) Science 253, 49–53.**
72 Jego, N. et al. (1993) Oncogene 8, 209–213.
73 Han, K.-A. and Kulesz-Martin, M.F. (1992) Nucl. Acids Res. 20, 1979–1981.
74 Jolly, K.W. et al. (1994) Oncogene 9, 97–102.

75 Mazoyer et al. (1994) Oncogene 9, 1237–1239.
76 Milner, J. and Medcalf, E.A. (1991) Cell 65, 765–774.
77 Sturzbecher, H.-W. et al. (1992) Oncogene 7, 1513–1523.
78 Friedman, P.N. et al. (1993) Proc. Natl Acad. Sci. USA 90, 3319–3323.
79 Iwabuchi, K. et al. (1993) Oncogene 8, 1693–1696.
80 Prosser, J. et al. (1992) Br. J. Cancer 65, 527–528.
81 Srivastava, S. et al. (1990) Nature 348, 747–749.
82 Miller, C.W. et al. (1993) Oncogene 8, 1815–8124.
83 Hsu, I.C. et al. (1991) Nature 350, 427–428.
84 Bressac, B. et al. (1991) Nature 350, 429–431.
85 Volkmann, M. et al. (1994) Oncogene 9, 195–204.
86 Wang, X.W. et al. (1994) Proc. Natl Acad. Sci. USA 91, 2230–2234.
87 Hainaut, P. and Milner, J. (1992) EMBO J. 11, 3513–3520.
88 Halazonetis, T. et al. (1993) EMBO J. 12, 1021–1028.
89 Wang, Y. and Eckhart, W. (1992) Proc. Natl Acad. Sci. USA 89, 4231–4235.
90 Pavletich, N.P. et al. (1994) Genes Devel. 7, 2556–2564.
91 Wang, Y. et al. (1994) Genes Devel. 7, 2575–2586.
92 Ruppert, J.M. and Stillman, B. (1993) Mol. Cell. Biol. 13, 3811–3820.
93 Samad, A. and Carroll, R.B. (1991) Mol. Cell. Biol. 11, 1598–1606.
94 Fontoura, B.M.A. et al. (1992) Mol. Cell. Biol. 12, 5145–5151.
95 Lees-Miller, S.P. et al. (1992) Mol. Cell. Biol. 12, 5041–5049.
96 Harlow, E. et al. (1985) Mol. Cell. Biol. 5, 1601–1610.
97 Zakut-Houri, R. et al. (1985) Nature 306, 594–597.
98 Harris, N. et al. (1986) Mol. Cell. Biol. 6, 4650–4656.
99 Buchman, V.L. et al. (1988) Gene 70, 245–252.
100 Matlashewski, G. et al. (1984) EMBO J. 3, 3257–3262.
101 Addison, C. et al. (1990) Oncogene 5, 423–426.
102 Rodrigues, N.R. et al. (1990) Proc. Natl Acad. Sci. USA 87, 7555–7559.
103 Malkin, D. et al. (1990) Science 250, 1233–1238.
104 Hsu, I.C. et al. (1991) Nature 350, 427–428.

PKR (also called PK_{ds}, p68, dsI, P1 kinase or dsRNA-activated inhibitor (DAI)) is a cytoplasmic, ribosome-associated enzyme that is activated by double-stranded RNA. PKR is activated by dsRNA produced during viral replication and it phosphorylates the initiation factor eIF-2, thereby inhibiting protein synthesis. A number of viral genomes encode RNAs or proteins that inhibit the activation of PKR [1-4]. The overexpression of mutant, inactive PKR renders NIH 3T3 fibroblasts highly tumorigenic in nude mice [5,6]. This indicates that inactive *PKR* may function as a dominant negative tumour suppressor gene.

References

1 Imani, F. and Jacobs, B.L. (1988) Proc. Natl Acad. Sci. USA 85, 7887–7891.
2 Gunnery, S. et al. (1990) Proc. Natl Acad. Sci. USA 87, 8687–8691.
3 **Mathews, M.B. and Shenk, T. (1991) J. Virol. 65, 5657–5662.**
4 Davies, M.V. et al. (1992) J. Virol. 66, 1943–1950.
5 Koromilas, A.E. et al. (1992) Science 257, 1685–1689.
6 Meurs, E.F. et al. (1992) Proc. Natl Acad. Sci. USA 90, 232–236.

RB1

IDENTIFICATION

Retinoblastoma is a rare hereditary disease, occurring in 1 child in 20 000, that affects retina cell precursors. In 60% of the cases the condition is termed sporadic, when there is no family history of the disease and a single tumour occurs in one eye; in the remaining 40% of cases (familial or germinal retinoblastoma) tumours are bilateral and more than one independently derived tumour is frequently present. The disease is caused by the loss of both copies of the gene (*RB1*) by inactivating mutations resulting in null alleles. Familial retinoblastoma occurs because one of the alleles was mutated at conception with the other undergoing somatic mutation. In sporadic retinoblastoma both mutations occur somatically within one cell to give rise to a tumour clone [1, 2].

RELATED GENES

RB1 and *RB2* are members of the retinoblastoma gene family. *RB1* has regions of homology with p107 and the transcription factor TFIIB [3,4]. *RB2* encodes p130, the E1A-associated protein that also binds cyclins A and E [5].

Nucleotides (kb)	180
Chromosome	13q14.2
Mass (kDa): predicted	106
expressed	105

Cellular location

Nuclear matrix: some mutant forms cytoplasmic.

Tissue distribution

Ubiquitous.

PROTEIN FUNCTION

p105^{RB1} (RB1) binds to double-stranded DNA in a non-sequence-specific manner. It acts through a motif (the retinoblastoma control element, RCE) to repress *MYC* transcription in human keratinocytes (see **MYC**), to repress *FOS* transcription, to enhance transcription of insulin-like growth factor II and to regulate either positively or negatively the expression of *TGFβ$_1$* depending on cell type (see **FOS**). The transcription factor SP1 also interacts with the RCE and p105^{RB1} enhances the *trans*-activating capacity of Sp1 [6]. p105^{RB1} also negatively regulates expression of p34^{CDC2} [7].

p105^{RB1} interacts with a large number of proteins, many of which are transcription factors.

Proteins associating with p105^{RB1}

Cellular proteins

Cyclins D2, D3, B1 and C [8-10]

ATF-2 (transcription factor) [11]

DRTF-1 and PU.1 (transcription factors) [13]

E2F family transcription factors
(E2F, E2F-1, E2F-2, E2F-3) [14]

RBAP1 and RBAP2 [15,16]

RBAP46 [17]

RBP1 and RBP2 [18,19]

Lamin C [20]

MYC and MYCN [21]

p34^{CDC2} [22]

p48 [23]

Protein phosphatase PP-1α2 (type 1 catalytic subunit) [24]

Viral proteins

Adenovirus type 5 E1A

Epstein–Barr nuclear antigen 5
(EBNA-5) [12]

Human papillomavirus type 16
E7 (HPV16 E7)

Simian virus 40 large T antigen
(SV40 T Ag)

The prevention of normal p105^{RB1} function by E1A, T antigen and E7 appears to be a crucial common step in cell transformation by the corresponding DNA tumour viruses[25].

p105^{RB1} and cell proliferation

The phosphorylation of p105^{RB1} appears to be essential for progression through the cell cycle and inhibition of p105^{RB1} phosphorylation causes cell cycle arrest [26-29]. Phosphorylation of p105^{RB1} probably results from the activity of p33^{CDK2}/p58^{cyclinA} or p34^{CDC2}/p58^{cyclinA} [30], with which p105^{RB1} associates [22,31] and may result in activated transcription of thymidine kinase[32]. In a variety of human tumour cell lines each of the D-cyclins (D1, D2 and D3) form complexes with CDK4 and its close relative CDK6 but these complexes are not detectable in cells having a mutated *RB1* gene or in which the function of p105^{RB1} is compromised by the presence of a DNA tumour virus oncoprotein. Thus, as well a being a potential substrate for D-cyclin kinases, p105^{RB1} contributes to the formation or stability of such complexes [33] and directly regulates transcription of cyclin D1 [34].

Underphosphorylated p105^{RB1} also associates with the ubiquitous transcription factor E2F and the complex is dissociated by E1A, SV40 T antigen or HPV E7 [35-37]. The p105^{RB1}/E2F complex occurs in G$_1$ in human primary cells and tumour cell lines and functions as a transcriptional repressor in the presence of an additional factor, RBP60 [38,39]. One target of the p105^{RB1}/E2F complex is the *CDC2* promoter [7]. As the cells enter S phase, a second E2F complex forms containing the p105^{RB1}-related protein p107 and cyclin A [40,41].

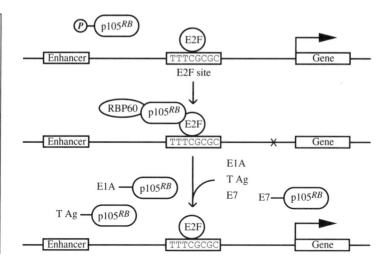

Cancer

The *RB1* gene is defective in all retinoblastomas and in a number of other cancers. Inactive *RB1* alleles are very common in small cell lung carcinoma, and they occur in 20–30% of non-small-cell lung cancers [42], bladder and pancreatic carcinomas and cell lines derived from human breast carcinomas [43–45]. Individuals with inherited retinoblastoma are also susceptible to malignant tumours in mesenchymal tissues, often osteosarcomas or soft tissue sarcomas.

The neoplastic phenotype of retinoblastoma, osteosarcoma, small cell lung carcinoma or human prostate carcinoma cells carrying inactivated *RB1* genes can be suppressed by transfection of a cloned *RB1* gene [47] and transfection of the *RB1* gene also arrests the growth of normal cells [48]. p105[RB1] suppresses transformation and metastasis induced in fibroblasts by *Neu*.

Transgenic animals

Mice carrying a homozygous mutation in the retinoblastoma gene die before the 16th day of gestation, indicating that *Rb-1* is essential for normal mouse development but not for cell proliferation and differentiation in the early stages of organogenesis [49, 50]. Heterozygous mice appear normal but almost invariably develop spontaneous pituitary tumours within the first 11 months[51]. The expression in transgenic mice of T antigen, which binds to p105[RB1], in the retina causes hereditable ocular tumours apparently identical to those of retinoblastoma[52].

GENE STRUCTURE

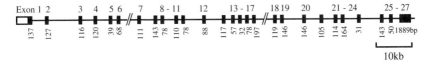

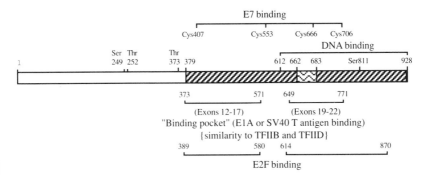

The region extending 600 bases upstream from the initiation codon includes potential AP-1, E2F/DRTF1 and ATF (CREB family) binding sites and three Sp1 sites to which RBF1 (distinct from SP1) binds. E2F1 *trans*-activates the *RB1* promoter via an E2F recognition sequence. *RB1* expression is negatively regulated by its own gene product acting via E2F [53].

Major deletions in the gene occur in 15–40% of retinoblastomas. More subtle effects are presumed to occur in all other cases, including (1) hypermethylation in the 5′ region of the gene which inhibits binding of ATF-like and RBF1 transcription factors [54], (2) point mutations in the ATF and Sp1 sites that are known to cause hereditary retinoblastoma [55], (3) a point mutation that results in the loss of exon 21 and inactivation of the protein, (4) Cys706 to Phe706 mutation in a small cell lung carcinoma line resulting in an underphosphorylated protein that does not bind to SV40 T Ag or E1A [56] but retains the capacity to bind MYC and MYCL proteins [57] and (5) loss of 103 nucleotides in the promoter preventing expression of *RB1* in human prostate tumours [58].

STRUCTURE OF (HUMAN) p105^*RB1*

The E1A and SV40 T antigen binding regions overlap sites of naturally occurring mutations, notably in exon 21 (bladder carcinoma and small cell lung carcinoma) and these regions also mediate E2F binding [59,60].

SEQUENCE OF P105^{RB1}

```
  1  MPPKTPRKTA ATAAAAAAEP PAPPPPPPPE EDPEQDSGPE DLPLVRLEFE
 51  ETEEPDFTAL CQKLKIPDHV RERAWLTWEK VSSVDGVLGG YIQKKKELWG
101  ICIFIAAVDL DEMSFTFTEL QKNIEISVHK FFNLLKEIDT STKVDNAMSR
151  LLKKYDVLFA LFSKLERTCE LIYLTQPSSS ISTEINSALV LKVSWITFLL
201  AKGEVLQMED DLVISFQLML CVLDYFIKLS PPMLLKEPYK TAVIPINGSP
251  RTPRRGQNRS ARIAKQLEND TRIIEVLCKE HECNIDEVKN VYFKNFIPFM
301  NSLGLVTSNG LPEVENLSKR YEEIYLKNKD LDARLFLDHD KTLQTDSIDS
351  FETQRTPRKS NLDEEVNVIP PHTPVRTVMN TIQQLMMILN SASDQPSENL
401  ISYFNNCTVN PKESILKRVK DIGYIFKEKF AKAVGQGCVE IGSQRYKLGV
451  RLYYRVMESM LKSEEERLSI QNFSKLLNDN IFHMSLLACA LEVVMATYSR
501  STSQNLDSGT DLSFPWILNV LNLKAFDFYK VIESFIKAEG NLTREMIKHL
551  ERCEHRIMES LAWLSDSPLF DLIKQSKDRE GPTDHLESAC PLNLPLQNNH
601  TAADMYLSPV RSPKKKGSTT RVNSTANAET QATSAFQTQK PLKSTSLSLF
651  YKKVYRLAYL RLNTLCERLL SEHPELEHII WTLFQHTLQN EYELMRDRHL
701  DQIMMCSMYG ICKVKNIDLK FKIIVTAYKD LPHAVQETFK RVLIKEEEYD
751  SIIVFYNSVF MQRLKTNILQ YASTRPPTLS PIPHIPRSPY KFPSSPLRIP
801  GGNIYISPLK SPYKISEGLP TPTKMTPRSR ILVSIGESFG TSEKFQKINQ
851  MVCNSDRVLK RSAEGSNPPK PLKKLRFDIE GSDEADGSKH LPGESKFQQK
901  LAEMTSTRTR MQKQKMNDSM DTSNKEEK (928)
```

Domain structures

10–18	Poly-alanine
20–29	Poly-proline
373–771	Binding pocket (binds T antigen and E1A)
373–579	Domain A
379–928	The minimal region necessary for growth suppression by p105^{RB1} [61]
407, 553, 666 and 706	Four of eight Cys residues in the "binding pocket": they are involved in E7 binding
580–639	Spacer
612–928	DNA binding activity[62]
640–771	Domain B
662–683	Leucine zipper motif (bold, underlined)
249–255, 354–359, 372–376, 567–568, 607–615, 787–791, 794–798, 806–814, 820–824, 826–827	Potential serine/threonine phosphorylation sites conserved between human and mouse (underlined)

DATABASE ACCESSION NUMBERS

	PIR	SWISSPROT	EMBL/GENBANK	REFERENCES
Human *RB1*	A39947	P06400	M15400	*63, 64*
	JS0276		M28419, M33647, X16439	*44, 65*

References

1 **Goodrich, D.W. and Lee, W.H. (1993) Biochim. Biophys. Acta 1155, 43–61.**
2 **Zacksenhaus, E. et al. (1993) Adv. Cancer Res. 61, 115–141.**
3 Ewen, M.E. et al. (1991) Cell 66, 1155–1164.
4 Zhu, L. et al. (1993) Genes Devel. 7, 1111–1125.
5 Li, Y. et al. (1993) Genes Devel. 7, 2366–2377.
6 Udvadia, A.J. et al. (1993) Proc. Natl Acad. Sci. USA 90, 3265–3269.
7 Dalton, S. et al. (1992) EMBO J. 11, 1797–1804.
8 Dowdy, S.F. et al. (1993) Cell 73, 499–511.
9 Ewen, M.E. et al. (1993) Cell 73, 487–497.
10 Kato, J. et al. (1993) Genes Devel. 7, 331–342.
11 Kim, S.-J. et al. (1992). Nature 358, 331–334.
12 Szekely, L. et al. (1993) Proc. Natl Acad. Sci. USA 90, 5455–5459.
13 Ouellette, M.M. et al. (1992) Oncogene 7, 1075–1081.
14 Lees, J.A. et al. (1993) Mol. Cell. Biol. 13, 7813–7825.
15 Helin, K. et al. (1992) Cell 70, 337–350.
16 Kaelin, W.G. et al. (1992) Cell 70, 351–364.
17 Huang, S. et al. (1991) Nature 350, 160–162.
18 Otterson, G.A. et al. (1993) Oncogene 8, 949–957.
19 Fattaey, A.R. et al. (1993) Oncogene 8, 3149–3156.
20 Seizinger et al., (1986) Nature 322, 644–647.
21 Hateboer, G. et al. (1993) Proc. Natl Acad. Sci. USA 90, 8489–8493.
22 Hu, Q. et al. (1992) Mol. Cell. Biol. 12, 971–980.
23 Qian, Y.-W. et al. (1993) Nature 364, 648–652.
24 Durfee, T. et al. (1993) Genes Devel. 7, 555–569.
25 Whyte, P. et al. (1988) Nature 334, 124–129.
26 Schonthal, A. and Feramisco, J.R. (1993) Oncogene 8, 433–441.
27 Alberts, A.S. et al. (1993) Proc. Natl Acad. Sci. USA 90, 388–392.
28 Ludlow, J.W. et al. (1993) Oncogene 8, 331–339.
29 Zhang, W. et al. (1992) Biochem. Biophys. Res. Commun. 184, 212–216.
30 Lin, B.T.-Y. et al. (1991) EMBO J. 10, 857–864.
31 Williams, R.T. et al. (1992) Oncogene 7, 423–432.
32 Dou, Q.-P. et al. (1992) Proc. Natl Acad. Sci. USA 89, 3256–3260
33 Bates, S. et al. (1994) Oncogene 9, 1633–1640.
34 Müller, H. et al. (1994) Proc. Natl Acad. Sci. USA 91, 2945–2949.
35 Chellappan, S.P. et al. (1992) Proc. Natl Acad. Sci. USA 89, 4549–4553.
36 Hamel, P.A. et al. (1992) Mol. Cell. Biol. 12, 3431–3438.
37 Pagano, M. et al. (1992) Oncogene 7, 1681–1686.
38 Weintraub, S.J. et al. (1992) Nature 358, 259–261.
39 Ray, S.K. et al. (1992) Mol. Cell. Biol. 12, 4327–4333.
40 Shirodkar, S. et al. (1992) Cell 68, 157–166.
41 Schwarz, J.K. et al. (1993) EMBO J. 12, 1013–1020.

42 Reissmann, P.T. et al. (1993) Oncogene 8, 1913–1919.

43 Horowitz, J.M. et al. (1990) Proc. Natl Acad. Sci. USA 87, 2775–2779.

44 Friend, S.H. et al. (1987) Proc. Natl Acad. Sci. USA 84, 9059–9063.

45 Weichselbaum, R.R. et al. (1988) Proc. Natl Acad. Sci. USA 85, 2106–2109.

46 Ruggeri, B. et al. (1992) Oncogene 7, 1503–1511.

47 Ookawa, K. et al. (1993) Oncogene 8, 2175–2181.

48 Fung, Y.-K.T. et al. (1993) Oncogene 8, 2659–2672.

49 Lee, E.Y.-H.P. et al. (1992) Nature 359, 288–294.

50 Jacks, T. et al. (1992) Nature 359, 295–300.

51 Hu, N. et al. (1994) Oncogene 9, 1021–1027.

52 Windle, J.J. et al. (1990) Nature 343, 665–669.

53 Shan, B. et al. (1994) Mol. Cell. Biol. 14, 299–309.

54 Ohtani-Fujita, N. et al. (1993) Oncogene 8, 1063–1067.

55 Sakai, T. et al. (1991) Nature 353, 83–86.

56 Kaye, F.J. et al. (1990) Proc. Natl Acad. Sci. USA 87, 6922–6926.

57 Kratzke, R.A. et al. (1992) J. Biol. Chem. 267, 25998–26003.

58 Bookstein, R. et al. (1990) Proc. Natl Acad. Sci. USA 87, 7762–7766.

59 Qian, Y. et al. (1992) Mol. Cell. Biol. 12, 5363–5372.

60 Hiebert, S.W. et al. (1993) Mol. Cell. Biol. 13, 3384–3391.

61 Qin, X.-Q. et al. (1992) Genes Devel. 6, 953–964.

62 Wang, N.P. et al. (1990) Cell Growth Differ. 1, 233–239.

63 Lee W.-H. et al. (1987) Science 235, 1394–1399.

64 Lee W.-H. et al. (1987) Nature 329, 642–645.

65 T'Ang, A. et al. (1989) Oncogene 4, 401–407.

VHL

Von Hippel–Lindau Disease (VHL)[1] is a dominantly inherited familial cancer syndrome that predisposes individuals most frequently to haemangioblastomas of the central nervous system and retina, renal cell carcinoma and phaeochromocytoma. The incidence at birth is at least 1/36 000.

RELATED GENES

VHL is highly conserved but has no significant homology to known proteins although it includes eight copies of a tandemly repeated pentamer similar to that present in the surface membrane protein of *Trypanosoma brucei*.

Nucleotides (kb)	<20
Chromosome	3p25–p26
Mass (kDa): predicted	28

Cellular location

Possibly plasma membrane.

Tissue distribution

Widely expressed. Only one of the two mRNA species is expressed in fetal brain and fetal kidney; both are expressed in adult tissues.

PROTEIN FUNCTION

Unknown. The repeated acidic domain may contribute to VHL involvement in signal transduction or cell–cell contacts.

SEQUENCE OF VHL

```
  1  PRLRYNSLRC WRILLRTRTA SGRLFPRARS ILYRARAKTT EVDSGARTQL
 51  RPASDPRIPR RPARVVWIAE GMPRRAENWD EAEVGAEEAG VEEYGPEEDG
101  GEESGAEESG PEESGPEELG AEEEMEAGRP RPVLRSVNSR EPSQVIFCNR
151  SPRVVLPVWL NFDGEPQPYP TLPPGTGRRI HSYRGHLWLF RDAGTHDGLL
201  VNQTELFVPS LNVDGQPIFA NITLPVYTLK ERCLQVVRSL VKPENYRRLD
251  IVRSLYEDLE DHPNVQKDLE RLTQERIAHQ RMGD (284)
```

Domain structure

85–124   Tandemly repeated acidic domain Gly–X–Glu–Glu–X (underlined)

Major deletions or insertions in the gene occur with high frequency (>12%) in VHL patients and mutations removing amino acids 153–154 or Ile146 (italics) have also been detected in VHL families. Mutations in sporadic renal cell carcinomas may replace residues 246–284 with 28 new amino acids, residues 238–284 with 32 new residues, residues 212–284 with 62 new residues or generate a truncated protein caused by mutation in codon 254.

DATABASE ACCESSION NUMBERS

	PIR	*SWISSPROT*	*EMBL/GENBANK*	*REFERENCE*
Human *VHL*			L15409	*1*

Reference
1 Latif, F. et al. (1993) Science 260, 1317–1320.

WT1

Wilms' tumour is an embryonal renal neoplasm that occurs in sporadic and familial forms and affects 1 in 10 000 children [1, 2]. Approximately 2% of Wilms' tumours occur in association with aniridia, genitourinary anomalies and mental retardation (WAGR syndrome) in which deletions of 11p13 were first detected.

RELATED GENES

WT1 is a member of the early growth response family (EGR1, EGR2, EGR3, EGR4).

Nucleotides (kb)	50
Chromosome	11p13
Mass (kDa): predicted	49
expressed	52/54

Cellular location

Nucleus.

Tissue distribution

WT1 is expressed in the developing kidney, gonads, spleen and mesothelium and brain [3,4].

PROTEIN FUNCTION

WT1 proteins are transcription factors that may play a crucial role in normal genitourinary development [5]. The minor forms repress transcription by binding to the sequence to which EGR1 binds as a transcriptional activator [6–8]. The major form (+KTS, see below) binds to a different DNA sequence [9].

Human PDGFA transcription is strongly repressed by WT1 interaction with two binding sites that lie 5' and 3' relative to the transcription start site [10,11]. When WT1 binds to only one of these sites it functions as a trans-activator. IGF2, which encodes an autocrine growth factor expressed at high levels in Wilms' tumour, may also be a target gene. IGF2 is expressed from the paternal allele in normal human fetal tissue but expression can occur biallelically in Wilms' tumour [12]. Many of the actions of IGF2 are mediated via the IGF1 receptor and WT1 can repress the activity of the IGF1R promoter [13]. The H19 gene is also monoallelically expressed in normal tissue but can show biallelic expression in Wilms' tumour [14] and transfection of H19 can suppress tumorigenicity [15]. Both IGF2 and H19 are located at 11p15 and the relaxation of genomic imprinting may therefore be involved in the development of Wilms' tumour.

Cancer

Wilms' tumour, like retinoblastoma, occurs in unilateral or bilateral early onset forms but may involve three loci rather than one. Deletions at 11p13 are associated with the bilateral form but in the sporadic forms allelic loss occurs at 11p15 (*WT2*), exclusively in the maternal allele, and a third locus may be involved in the familial forms. Insertion of a normal human chromosome 11 into Wilms' tumour cells causes reversion to normal, non-tumorigenic cells that correlates with the expression of the *QM* gene [16].

Transgenic animals

Homozygous mutation of the murine *Wt-1* gene causes embryonic lethality arising from the failure of kidney and gonad development [17].

In vitro

In transfected cells p53 interacts with WT1 and converts the *trans*-activating capacity of the latter to *trans*-repression [18]. WT1 also exerts a cooperative effect on p53 by enhancing its *trans*-activation of the muscle creatine kinase promoter (see *P53*).

GENE STRUCTURE

The alternatively spliced exons are cross-hatched. All four possible variants are expressed in normal developing kidney, with that including both alternative sequences being most common [19], and also in Wilms' tumours [20]. Variants having a three amino acid insertion at exon 9 cannot bind the *EGR* recognition element [8]. Mutations within intron 6 that lead to exon-skipping, resulting in transcripts either missing exon 6 or exons 5 and 6 [21], or within intron 9 that prevent alternative splicing, and in the zinc finger domains occur in Denys–Drash syndrome [22] and in Wilms' tumour DNA [23]. Mutations in exons 7 and 8 that generate truncated proteins lacking part of the zinc finger domain have also been detected in unilateral Wilms' tumours [24].

TRANSCRIPTIONAL REGULATION

The *WT1* promoter lacks TATA or CCAAT boxes, has a high GC content and contains four transcriptional start sites within a 32 bp region. There are 11 putative SP1 binding sites and several potential recognition sites for EGR, Pax-8 and GAGA-like factors [25]. WT1 binds to multiple sites in its own promoter to autoregulate transcription negatively [26]. Tissue-specific expression of *WT1* is modulated by an enhancer located >50 kb 3' of the promoter [27]. The *WT1* transcript can undergo RNA editing in which U^{839} is converted to C, causing Leu^{281} to be replaced by proline [28]. The WT1-Leu^{281} protein represses the EGR1 promoter ~30% more efficiently than WT1-Pro.

SEQUENCE OF WT1

```
  1  MGSDVRDLNA LLPAVPSLGG GGGCALPVSG AAQWAPVLDF APPGASAYGS
 51  LGGPAPPPAP PPPPPPPPHS FIKQEPSWGG AEPHEEQCLS AFTVHFSGQF
101  TGTAGACRYG PFGPPPPSQA SSGQARMFPN APYLPSCLES QPAIRNQGYS
151  TVTFDGTPSY GHTPSHHAAQ FPNHSFKHED PMGQQGSLGE QQYSVPPPVY
201  GCHTPTDSCT GSQALLLRTP YSSDNLYQMT SQLECMTWNQ MNLGATLKGV
251  AAGSSSSVKW TEGQSNHSTG YESDNHTTPI LCGAQYRIHT HGVFRGIQDV
301  RRVPGVAPTL VRSASETSEK RPFMCAYPGC NKRYFKLSHL QMHSRKHTGE
351  KPYQCDFKDC ERRFSRSDQL KRHQRRHTGV KPFQCKTCQR KFSRSDHLKT
401  HTRTHTGKTS EKPFSCRWPS CQKKFARSDE LVRHHNMHQR NMTKLQLAL (449)
```

Domain structure

27–83	Proline-rich domain
323–347, 353–377, 383–405, 414–438	Zinc finger (C_2H_2 type) regions (underlined)
250–266 and 408–410	Alternative splice regions (underlined italics). These introduce 17 amino acids after 249 or three amino acids between the third and fourth zinc fingers. The variant containing the KTS sequence is the predominant form in all cells that express WT1 [19].
84–179	Mediate *trans*-repression by the 429 amino acid form
180–294	Mediate *trans*-activation by the 429 amino acid form

Variant in a WT patient: Arg366→Cys.

Variants in Denys–Drash patients: Cys355→Tyr, Arg366→His, Arg394→Trp, Asp396→Asn/Gly, Cys360→Gly, Arg362→stop, His373→stop, His401→Tyr.

Mutation of Gly201 to Asp has been detected in a child with WAGR that converts WT1 from a transcriptional repressor to an activator [29].

DATABASE ACCESSION NUMBERS

	PIR	SWISSPROT	EMBL/GENBANK	REFERENCES
Human WT1	A34673, S08273	P19544	X51630	30
			M30393	5, 6
			M80217 to M80221	19
			M80228	31
			M80231/32; M74917	23, 24

References
1 van Heyningen, V. and Hastie, N.D. (1992) Trends Genet. 8, 16–21.
2 Haber, D.A. and Buckler, A.J. (1992) New Biol. 4, 97–106.
3 Huang, A. et al. (1990) Science 250, 991–994.
4 Pritchard-Jones, K. et al. (1990) Nature 346, 194–197.
5 Pelletier, J. et al. (1991) Cell 67, 437–447.
6 Call, K.M. et al. (1990) Cell 60, 509–520.
7 Morris, J.F. et al. (1991) Oncogene 6, 2339–2348.
8 Madden, S.L. et al. (1993) Oncogene 8, 1713–1720.
9 Bickmore, W.A. et al. (1992) Science 257, 235–237.
10 Gashler, A.L. et al. (1992) Proc. Natl Acad. Sci. USA 89, 10984–10988.
11 Wang, Z.-Y. et al. (1993) J. Biol. Chem. 268, 9172–9175.
12 Ogawa, O. et al. (1993) Nature 362, 749–751.
13 Werner, H. et al. (1993) Proc. Natl Acad. Sci. USA 90, 5828–5832.
14 Rainer, S. et al. (1993) Nature 362, 747–749.
15 Hao, Y. et al. (1993) Nature 365, 764–767.
16 Dowdy, S.F. et al. (1991) Nucl. Acids Res. 19, 5763–5769.
17 Kreidberg, J.A. et al. (1993) Cell 74, 679–691.
18 Maheswaran, S. et al. (1993) Proc. Natl Acad. Sci. USA 90, 5100–5104.
19 Haber, D.A. et al. (1991) Proc. Natl Acad. Sci. USA 88, 9618–9622.
20 Brenner, B. et al. (1992) Oncogene 7, 1431–1433.
21 Schneider, S. et al. (1993) Hum. Genet. 91, 599–604.
22 Bruening, W. et al. (1992) Nature Genomics 1, 144–148.
23 Little, M.H. et al. (1992) Proc. Natl Acad. Sci. USA 89, 4791–4795.
24 Baird, P.N. et al. (1992) Oncogene 7, 2141–2149.
25 Hofmann, W. et al. (1993) Oncogene 8, 3123–3132.
26 Rupprecht, H.D. et al. (1994) J. Biol. Chem. 269, 6198–6206.
27 Fraizer, G.C. et al. (1994) J. Biol. Chem. 269, 8892–8900.
28 Sharma, P.M. et al. (1994) Genes Devel. 8, 720–731.
29 Park, S. et al. (1993) Cancer Res. 53, 4757–4760.
30 Gessler, M. et al. (1990) Nature 343, 774–778.
31 Buckler, A.J. et al. (1991) Mol. Cell. Biol. 11, 1707–1712.

DNA
TUMOUR
VIRUSES

DNA TUMOUR VIRUSES

Within the genomes of some DNA tumour viruses genes have been identified the products of which will transform cells; that is, the oncogene product has evolved to stimulate cells after viral infection. These include simian vacuolating virus 40 (SV40), the human BK and JC papovaviruses, polyomavirus and adenovirus, each of which can transform a variety of types of cell *in vitro* and can be tumorigenic in appropriate host animals. These viruses are not oncogenic in humans although their oncoproteins function at least in part by binding to and thus inhibiting the normal activity of the products of tumour suppressor genes in target cells (*P53* and retinoblastoma). A similar strategy is followed by the oncogenic human papillomaviruses (see below). The Epstein–Barr herpesvirus carries one gene that is consistently expressed in Burkitt's lymphoma and another that is required for immortalization of primary B cells by EBV and is tumorigenic *in vitro*. For other DNA viruses (e.g. hepatitis B virus (HBV) and the herpesviruses HSV-1, HSV-2 and human cytomegalovirus) there is circumstantial evidence for their association with the development of a variety of human cancers and HBV is established as a causative agent in the vast majority of primary hepatocellular carcinomas that are responsible for up to 1 million deaths per annum worldwide [1,2]. However, the genomes of these viruses contain no known oncogenes, although the hepatitis B virus protein HBx *trans*-activates a variety of promoters commonly involved in transformation [3] and causes tumours in transgenic mice [4].

References

[1] Harris, C.C. (1990) Cancer Cells 2, 146–148.
[2] zur Hausen, H. (1991) Science 254, 1167–1173.
[3] Kekule, A.S. et al. (1993) Nature 361, 742–745.
[4] Kim, C.-M. et al. (1991) Nature 351, 317–320.

PAPILLOMAVIRUSES

There are over 60 human papillomavirus (HPV) genotypes [1] that colonize various stratified epithelia including the skin and oral and genital mucosa and induce the formation of self-limiting, benign tumours known as papillomas (warts) or condylomas. Viruses increase the division rate of infected stem cells in the epithelial basal layer and the viral genome replicates episomally in concert with the cell genome. As the keratinocytes terminally differentiate, synthesis of virally encoded late proteins causes cell death. Very infrequently this mechanism defaults and maligant tumours develop [2-4]. The genomes comprise "early" ORFs (E1–E8) and "late" ORFs (L1 and L2).

	E5	E6	E7
Mass (kDa): predicted (type16/18)	9.4/8.3	19.2/18.8	11.0/11.9
expressed	44	18	20

Cellular location

E5: Plasma membrane (homodimers). E6 and E7: Nucleus.

PROTEIN FUNCTION

E5 activates receptors for PDGFB, EGF and CSF1; E6 binds p53; and E7 binds p105^{RB1}.

Cancer

Eleven HPVs have been shown to be commonly associated with human tumours and DNA sequences of HPV-16 or HPV-18 are expressed in ~90% of all cervical carcinomas and HPV-16 DNA is present in 50% of anal cancers. HPV types 6 and 11 are frequently present together with types 16 and 18 in genital infections but are rarely detected in cervical malignancies. Thus infection with certain types of HPV constitutes an increased risk of the onset of some cancers. The HPV-16 long control region contains three binding sites for the cellular transcriptional repressor YY1. Point mutations in this region have been detected in episomal HPV-16 DNAs from cervical cancers that result in enhanced promoter activity [5].

E5

Expression of the HPV-16 E5 gene transforms 3T3-A31 cells and enhances their tumorigenicity. The transcription of Fos in 3T3-A31 cells in response to EGF, PDGF or serum is increased by expression of E5 [6]. This suggests that E5 may contribute to the early stages of tumorigenesis by enhancing proliferation in HPV-16 infected cells.

E6 and E7

E6 and E7 DNAs are detectable in all HPV-associated tumours. E2 is usually interrupted or deleted and the late genes are often missing. In some classes of tumours (e.g. cervical carcinomas) the E1, E6 and E7 ORFs of HPV DNA are usually integrated into the host chromosome (the ORFs of E2, E3, E4 and E5 are lost) whereas in others (e.g. squamous cell carcinomas) they are present in extrachromosomal form [7]. The expression of antisense E6/E7 renders HPV-containing cervical carcinoma cells non-tumorigenic [8].

The expression of HPV type 16 E6 and E7 oncogenes in the skin of transgenic mice promotes the development of epidermal cancers [9]. Expression of either HPV type 16 E6 or E7 genes in non-metastatic cell lines renders these cell metastatic in nude mice [10].

HPV-16 E6 and E7 proteins cooperate to immortalize human fibroblasts, keratinocytes or mammary epithelial cells [11,12]. Prolonged growth *in vitro* produces malignant clones from such immortalized cells [13]. Alternatively, the co-expression of v-*ras* with E7 transforms primary cells [14] and v-*ras* and E6 immortalize primary cells [15]. E7 functions as an immortalizing oncogene in that there is a continued requirement for its expression, together with *Ras*, to maintain the transformed phenotype [16]. However, this does not imply that E6 functions as a RAS protein. Binding of E7 to the retinoblastoma protein is necessary but not sufficient for co-transformation [17], although mutational analysis of the cottontail rabbit papillomavirus E7 protein indicates that its association with p105^{RB1} is not necessary for the viral induction of warts [18]. E7 also associates with p33^{CDK2} and cyclin A [19]. E7 is a weak mitogen for Swiss 3T3 fibroblasts in which its expression induces the appearance of the transcriptionally active form of E2F [20].

HPV-16 and HPV-18 E6 enhance the degradation rate of p53 via specific binding (see **Tumour Suppressor Genes, *P53***) and a fusion protein of the N-terminal half of HPV-16 E7 and full-length HPV-16 E6 promotes the degradation of p105^{RB1} [21].

Bovine papilloma virus 1 (BPV-1)

BPV-1 replicates episomally in fibroblasts *in vitro* and transforms the cells: replication with high efficiency requires the E1, E6 and E7 gene products. The E5 gene encodes a hydrophobic, 44 amino acid (7 kDa) protein that causes tumorigenic transformation of rodent fibroblasts [22]. In NIH 3T3 cells this involves activation of EGF and CSF1 receptors, independently of the presence of their ligands [23]. It is the smallest, known oncoprotein and microinjection into the nucleus of the 13 C-terminal amino acids of E5 activates DNA synthesis. The 30 amino acid N-terminus contains two cysteine residues essential for homodimerization and biological activity. In two cell lines, E5 has been shown to form an activating complex with PDGFRβ and to stimulate DNA synthesis [24]. Activation of its transforming capacity may require association with a 16 kDa cellular protein [25].

SEQUENCE OF HPV-16 E5

```
 1   MTNLDTASTT LLACFLLCFC VLLCVCLLIR PLLLSVSTYT SLIILVLLLW
51   ITAASAFRCF IVYIIFVYIP LFLIHTHARF LIT (83)
```

SEQUENCE OF HPV-18 E5

```
 1   MLSLIFLFCF CVCMYVCCHV PLLPSVCMCA YAWVLVFVYI VVITSPATAF
51   TVYVFCFLLP MLLLHIHAIL SLQ (73)
```

SEQUENCE OF HPV-16 E6

```
 1   MHQKRTAMFQ DPQERPRKLP QLCTELQTTI HDIILECVYC KQQLLRREVY
51   DFAFRDLCIV YRDGNPYAVC DKCLKFYSKI SEYRHYCYSL YGTTLEQQYN
101  KPLCDLLIRC INCQKPLCPE EKQRHLDKKQ RFHNIRGRWT GRCMSCCRSS
151  RTRRETQL (158)
```

Domain structure

37–73 and 110–146   Zinc finger domains (underlined)

SEQUENCE OF HPV-18 E6

```
 1   MARFEDPTRR PYKLPDLCTE LNTSLQDIEI TCVYCKTVLE LTEVFEFAFK
51   DLFVVYRDSI PHAACHKCID FYSRIRELRH YSDSVYGDTL EKLTNTGLYN
101  LLIRCLRCQK PLNPAEKLRH LNEKRRFHNI AGHYRGQCHS CCNRARQERL
151  QRRRETQV (158)
```

Domain structure

32–68 and 105–141   Zinc finger domains (underlined)

SEQUENCE OF HPV-16 E7

```
 1   MHGDTPTLHE YMLDLQPETT DLYCYEQLND SSEEEDEIDG PAGQAEPDRA
51   HYNIVTFCCK CDSTLRLCVQ STHVDIRTLE DLLMGTLGIV CPICSQKP (98)
```

Domain structure

21–30   p105^{RB1} binding region (underlined). An additional domain (amino acids 60–98) appears necessary to inhibit complex formation between p105^{RB1} and E2F [26].

58–61 and 91–94   C–XX–C motifs

31 and 32   Casein kinase II phosphorylation sites. Mutation in these regions inhibits transforming potential, although negative charge at these sites is not essential for p105^{RB1} binding [27]. HPV-16 E7 shows significant sequence homology with E1A, T Ag, MYC and the yeast mitotic regulator *cdc*25.

SEQUENCE OF HPV18 E7

```
  1  MHGPKATLQD IVLHLEPQNE IPVDLLCHEQ LSDSEEENDE IDGVNHQHLP
 51  ARRAEPQRHT MLCMCCKCEA RIKLVVESSA DDLRAFQQLF LNTLSFVCPW
101  CASQQ (105)
```

Domain structure

24–33   p105^{RB1} binding region (underlined)
63–66 and 98–101   C–XX–C motifs

SEQUENCE OF BPV-1 E5

```
  1  MPNLWFLLFL GLVAAMQLLL LLFLLLFFLV YWDHFECSCT GLPF (44)
```

Domain structure

6–30   Transmembrane region
32–44   Cellular DNA synthesis induction

DATABASE ACCESSION NUMBERS

	PIR	SWISSPROT	EMBL/GENBANK	REFERENCES
HPV-16 E5	A30016	P06927	K02718	28, 29
HPV-18 E5	F26251	P06792	X05015	30
HPV-16 E6	A30682	P03126	K02718	28
HPV-18 E6	G26251	P06463	X04354	30
			X05015, M20325	31, 32
			M26798, M26798	33, 34
HPV-16 E7		P03129	K02718	28, 35
HPV-18 E7	H26251	P06788	X05015	30
			M20324, M20325	32, 33
			M26798, M26798	
BPV-1 E5	B18151	P06928	X02346	36
	F18151, S12366		M20219	25, 37

References
[1] de Villiers, E.-M. (1989) J. Virol. 63, 4898–4903.
[2] **Campo, M.S. (1992) J. Gen. Virol. 73, 217–222.**

3   DiMaio, D. (1991) Adv. Cancer Res. 56, 133–159.
4   Galloway, D.A. and McDougall, J.K. (1989) Adv. Virus Res. 37, 125–171.
5   May, M. et al. (1994) EMBO J. 13, 1460–1466.
6   Leechanachai, P. et al. (1992) Oncogene 7, 19–25.
7   Cullen, A.P. et al. (1991) J. Virol. 65, 606–612.
8   von Knebel Doeberitz, M. et al. (1988) Cancer Res. 48, 3780–3786.
9   Lambert, P.F. et al. (1993) Proc. Natl Acad. Sci. USA 90, 5583–5587.
10 Chen, L. et al. (1993) Proc. Natl Acad. Sci. USA 90, 6523–6527.
11 Band, V. et al. (1990) Proc. Natl. Acad, Sci. USA 87, 463–467.
12 Hudson, J.B. et al. (1990) J. Virol. 64, 519–526.
13 Hurlin, P.J. et al. (1991) Proc. Natl. Acad, Sci. USA 88, 570–574.
14 Durst, M. et al. (1989) Virology 173, 767–771.
15 Storey, A. and Banks, L. (1993) Oncogene 8, 919–924.
16 Crook, T. et al. (1989) EMBO J. 8, 513–519.
17 Banks, L. et al. (1990) Oncogene 5, 1383–1389.
18 Defeo-Jones, D. et al. (1993) J. Virol. 67, 716–725.
19 Tommasino, M. et al. (1993) Oncogene 8, 195–202.
20 Morris, J.D.H. et al. (1993) Oncogene 8, 893–898.
21 Scheffner, M. et al. (1992) EMBO J. 2425–2431.
22 Settleman, J. et al. (1989) Mol. Cell. Biol. 9, 5563–5572.
23 Martin, P. et al. (1989) Cell 59, 21–32.
24 Petti, L., and DiMaio, D. (1992) Proc. Natl Acad. Sci. USA 6736–6740.
25 Goldstein, D.J. and Schlegel, R. (1990) EMBO J. 9, 137–145.
26 Huang, P.S. et al. (1993) Mol. Cell. Biol. 13, 953–960.
27 Firzlaff, J.M. et al. (1991) Proc. Natl Acad. Sci. USA 88, 5187–5191.
28 Seedorf, K. et al. (1985) Virology 145, 181–185.
29 Bubb, V. et al. (1988) Virology 163, 243–246.
30 Cole, S.T. and Danos, O. (1987) J. Mol. Biol. 193, 599–608.
31 Matlashewski, G. et al. (1986) J. Gen. Virol. 67, 1909–1916.
32 Inagaki, Y. et al. (1988) J. Virol. 62, 1640–1646.
33 Schneider-Gaedicke, A. and Schwarz, E. (1986) EMBO J. 5, 2285–2292.
34 Grossman, S.R. and Laimins, L.A. (1989) Oncogene 4, 1089–1093.
35 Phelps, W.C. et al. (1988) Cell 53, 539–547.
36 Schlegel, R. et al. (1986) Science 233, 464–467.
37 Petti, L. et al. (1991) EMBO J. 10, 845–856.

Epstein–Barr virus (EBV) is a herpesvirus of high incidence in humans that binds to the CR2 receptor for complement factor iC3b present only on B lymphocytes, follicular dendritic cells and B- and T-derived cell lines [1]. After infection the viral genome circularizes through its terminal repeats and in immortalized cells is latently maintained as an episomal molecule. Approximately 11 genes are expressed in latent infections [2]. Five regions of the genome encode latent poly(A) transcripts and these give rise to six different nuclear proteins (Epstein–Barr nuclear antigens (EBNAs) 1, 2, 3A, 3B and 3C and a leader protein (EBNA-LP)) and three viral membrane proteins (latent membrane proteins, LMPs 1, 2A and 2B). The switch to expressing most of the other genes is mediated by the virally encoded transcription factor Z (also called BZLF1, EB1, ZEBRA or Zta). Z Transcription can be enhanced by TPA, cross-linked cell-surface Ig or by its own protein product. The Z protein has a basic DNA binding domain homologous to that of FOS that binds to AP-1 sites and activates transcription of the EBV early genes BSLF2 and BMLF1 in some cell types (e.g. HeLa cells) but not others (e.g. Jurkat cells). Z also has a coiled coil-like dimerization domain, shares homology with C/EBP and binds to the same CCAAT sequence as C/EBP [3]. However, in Jurkat or Raji cells (an EBV⁺ B cell line), Z interacts synergistically with MYB to activate the BMRF1 promoter [4]. Z/MYB binds through the interaction of Z with a 30 bp region containing an AP-1 consensus sequence. EBV also activates transcription from the HIV-1 LTR.

	EBNA-1 (strain B95-8)	EBNA-2 (strain B95-8)	LMP-1 (strain B95-8)
Mass (kDa): predicted	56	52.5	42
expressed	p80	p82	p58

Cellular location

EBNA1: nucleus; free in nucleoplasm; some association with chromatin but little with the nuclear matrix. EBNA2: Nuclear matrix. LMP1: Transmembrane; localized in patches.

PROTEIN FUNCTION

Cancer

EBV causes infectious mononucleosis (glandular fever) and is associated with Burkitt's lymphoma (BL), nasopharyngeal carcinoma (NPC) and Hodgkin's lymphoma. The endemic (African) form of BL is usually associated with Epstein–Barr virus whereas the sporadic form is normally EBV⁻.

All BL tumours express only the EBNA1 EBV gene. High titres of antibodies directed against viral proteins precede the appearance of tumours by several months. The fully malignant phenotype requires the development of a BL clone and a chromosome translocation involving *MYC* (see *MYC*). NPCs always express EBNA1 and some (~65%) express LMP1 [5].

EBV infection of primary B cells *in vitro* causes little or no virus production but gives rise to an immortal lymphoblastoid cell line (LCL) that is not tumorigenic. LCL cells express six EBNAs, LMP1, LMP2A and LMP2B, two small RNAs (EBERs) and two terminal proteins (TP1 and TP2). LCLs are good targets for lysis by T cells, in contrast to BL cells (see below).

EBNA1

EBNA1 does not have transforming capacity but is a *trans*-activating factor required for replication from the latency origin of replication (*oriP*) which is also an EBNA1-dependent enhancer. EBNA1 thus maintains replication of the EBV episome in the latent cycle. EBNA1 protein is inadequately processed for MHC class I recognition and thus escapes immune surveillance.

EBNA2

EBNA2 is a transcription factor involved in the latent cycle that binds p105^{RB1} and is phosphorylated by casein kinase II. It is one of the first genes expressed after primary B cell infection *in vitro* and it *trans*-activates LMP1, LMP2A, LMP2B and a lymphoid-specific enhancer in the *Bam*H1 C promoter of EBV [6]. EBNA2 also regulates *CD23*, *CD21* [7] and *FGR* [8].

EBNA2 is essential for EBV immortalisation of human B cells and regulates transcription from several viral and cellular promoters. It has a region of partial homology with the p105^{RB1}-binding domain of Ad5 E1A, SV40 T Ag and HPV-16 E7 [9]. Ser469 in EBNA2 corresponds to those in E7 and T Ag that are phosphorylated by casein kinase II.

Evidence that EBNA2 is required for transformation: (i) deletion of EBNA2 in the P3HR-1 or Daudi EBV genome is associated with the unique inability of these viruses to transform B cells, (ii) transformation-competent recombinants between P3HR-1 and another EBV genome have a restored EBNA2 coding region and (iii) EBNA2 confers the ability of Rat-1 cells to grow in media with low serum concentration [10].

LMP1

LMP1 is a transforming protein that reduces serum dependency, contact inhibition and anchorage-dependent growth and increases tumorigenicity in rodent fibroblasts [11,12]. LMP1 expression is *trans*-activated by EBNA2 via a 142 bp *cis*-acting element [13]. The short half-life of the protein (2–5 h), its localized distribution on the cell surface and association with the cytoskeleton are necessary for its transforming function [14]. EBV transformation causes a major reorganization of intermediate filaments and microtubules and LMP1 appears in secondary lysosomes together with ubiquitin–protein conjugates and HSP70 [15]. Transient expression of LMP1 causes upregulation of *CD21*, *CD23*, *ICAM1* and *LFA1* and induces DNA synthesis in human B cells [16].

Human B cells are protected from apoptosis by the expression of LMP1 which activates transcription of *BCL2*. BCL2 protein is 25% identical to a 149 amino acid region of the EBV immediate early *BHRF1* gene [17]. *BHRF1* is abundantly expressed early in the lytic life cycle but is not required for EBV-induced transformation of B lymphocytes *in vitro*. However, BHRF1 may be essential for infected cell survival when *BCL2* is not induced by LMP1. In BL cells the *BCL2* and *BHRF1* gene products are equally effective in rescuing the cells from apoptosis [18].

LMP1 and LMP2A associate in the plasma membrane. LMP2A is phosphorylated and, in EBV-transformed B lymphocytes, forms a complex with the LYN tyrosine kinase [19].

The cumulative effect of the expression of the latent EBV proteins appears to be to activate growth-regulating pathways involved in normal B cell stimulation [20], including the expression of a variety of surface antigens (the EBV receptor (C3d or CR2 (*CD21*)), *CD23*, LFA-1β (*CD18*) and LFA-3 (*CD58*)).

Fusion of BL cells and non-tumorigenic EBV-immortalized B-lymphoblastoid cells suppresses the malignant phenotype of the BL cell line, despite the fact that the hybrid cells contain EBV and express deregulated *MYC* [21]. These observations may reflect the action of tumour necrosis factor (TNF) or a related protein. The synthesis of TNF by tumour cells correlates with reduced tumorigenicity and invasiveness [22]. A TNF-like gene may be disrupted in BL with complementation occurring in the hybrid cells.

SEQUENCE OF EBNA1

```
  1   MSDEGPGTGP  GNGLGEKGDT  SGPEGSGGSG  PQRRGGDNHG  RGRGRGRGRG
 51   GGRPGAPGGS  GSGPRHRDGV  RRPQKRPSCI  GCKGTHGGTG  AGAGAGGAGA
101   GGAGAGGGAG  AGGGAGGAGG  AGGAGAGGGA  GAGGGAGGAG  GAGAGGGAGA
151   GGGAGGAGAG  GGAGGAGGAG  AGGGAGAGGG  AGGAGAGGGA  GGAGGAGAGG
201   GAGAGGAGGA  GGAGAGGAGA  GGGAGGAGGA  GAGGAGAGGA  GAGGAGAGGA
251   GGAGAGGAGG  AGAGGAGGAG  AGGGAGGAGA  GGGAGGAGAG  GAGGAGAGGA
301   GGAGAGGAGG  AGAGGGAGAG  GAGAGGGGRG  RGGSGGRGRG  GSGGRGRGGS
351   GGRRGRGRER  ARGGSRERAR  GRGRGRGEKR  PRSPSSQSSS  SGSPPRRPPP
401   GRRPFFHPVG  EADYFEYHQE  GGPDGEPDVP  PGAIEQGPAD  DPGEGPSTGP
451   RGQGDGGRRK  KGGWFGKHRG  QGGSNPKFEN  IAEGLRALLA  RSHVERTTDE
501   GTWVAGVFVY  GGSKTSLYNL  RRGTALAIPQ  CRLTPLSRLP  FGMAPGPGPQ
551   PGPLRESIVC  YFMVFLQTHI  FAEVLKDAIK  DLVMTKPAPT  CNIRVTVCSF
601   DDGVDLPPWF  PPMVEGAAAE  GDDGDDGDEG  GDGDEGEEGQ  E (641)
```

Domain structure

87–352   Glycine/alanine-rich region

SEQUENCE OF EBNA2

```
  1   MPTFYLALHG GQTYHLIVDT DSLGNPSLSV IPSNPYQEQL SDTPLIPLTI
 51   FVGENTGVPP PLPPPPPPPP PPPPPPPPPP PPPPPPPPSP PPPPPPPPPP
101   QRRDAWTQEP SPLDRDPLGY DVGHGPLASA MRMLWMANYI VRQSRGDRGL
151   ILPQGPQTAP QARLVQPHVP PLRPTAPTIL SPLSQPRLTP PQPLMMPPRP
201   TPPTPLPPAT LTVPPRPTRP TTLPPTPLLT VLQRPTELQP TPSPPRMHLP
251   VLHVPDQSMH PLTHQSTPND PDSPEPRSPT VFYNIPPMPL PPSQLPPPAA
301   PAQPPPGVIN DQQLHHLPSG PPWWPPICDP PQPSKTQGQS RGQSRGRGRG
351   RGRGRGKGKS RDKQRKPGGP WRPEPNTSSP SMPELSPVLG LHQGQGAGDS
401   PTPGPSNAAP VCRNSHTATP NVSPIHEPES HNSPEAPILF PDDWYPPSID
451   PADLDESWDY IFETTESPSS DEDYVEGPSK RPRPSIQ (487)
```

Domain structure

59–100   Poly-proline region

458–474   p105^{RB1} and casein kinase II recognition region, homologous to those in HPV E7, adenovirus E1a and SV40 T antigen (underlined)

SEQUENCE OF LMP1

```
  1   MEHDLERGPP GPRRPPRGPP LSSSLGLALL LLLLALLFWL YIVMSDWTGG
 51   ALLVLYSFAL MLIIIILIIF IFRRDLLCPL GALCILLLMI TLLLIALWNL
101   HGQALFLGIV LFIFGCLLVL GIWIYLLEML WRLGATIWQL LAFFLAFFLD
151   LILLIIALYL QQNWWTLLVD LLWLLLFLAI LIWMYYHGQR HSDEHHHDDS
201   LPHPQQATDD SGHESDSNSN EGRHHLLVSG AGDGPPLCSQ NLGAPGGGPD
251   NGPQDPDNTD DNGPQDPDNT DDNGPHDPLP QDPDNTDDNG PQDPDNTDDN
301   GPHDPLPHSP SDSAGNDGGP PQLTEEVENK GGDQGPPLMT DGGGGHSHDS
351   GHGGGDPHLP TLLLGSSGSG GDDDDPHGPV QLSYYD (386)
```

Domain structure

1–24 and 187–386   Cytoplasmic domains

25–44, 52–72, 77–97, 105–125,   Six potential transmembrane domains
139–159, 166–186   (underlined)

242–386   P25 peptide

SEQUENCE OF LMP2A/LMP2B

```
  1   MGSLEMVPMG AGPPSPGGDP DGYDGGNNSQ YPSASGSSGN TPTPPNDEER
 51   ESNEEPPPPY EDPYWGNGDR HSDYQPLGTQ DQSLYLGLQH DGNDGLPPPP
101   YSPRDDSSQH IYEEAGRGSM NPVCLPVIVA PYLFWLAAIA ASCFTASVST
151   VVTATGLALS LLLLAAVASS YAAAQRKLLT PVTVLTAVVT FFAICLTWRI
201   EDPPFNSLLF ALLAAAGGLQ GIYVLVMLVL LILAYRRRWR RLTVCGGIMF
251   LACVLVLIVD AVLQLSPLLG AVTVVSMTLL LLAFVLWLSS PGGLGTLGAA
301   LLTLAAALAL LASLILGTLN LTTMFLLMLL WTLVVLLICS SCSSCPLSKI
351   LLARLFLYAL ALLLLASALI AGGSILQTNF KSLSSTEFIP NLFCMLLLIV
401   AGILFILAIL TEWGSGNRTY GPVFMCLGGL LTMVAGAVWL TVMSNTLLSA
451   WILTAGFLIF LIGFALFGVI RCCRYCCYYC LTLESEERPP TPYRNTV (497)
```

Domain structure

1–497	Membrane protein LMP2A.
120–497	Membrane protein LMP2B. Separate mRNAs are transcribed to give rise to two proteins, the shorter of which (LMP2B) lacks 119 N-terminal amino acids [23].
122–141, 150–168, 178–198, 208–235, 242–259, 267–288, 300–316, 321–339, 355–373, 392–411, 419–443, 450–470	Eleven potential transmembrane domains (underlined)

DATABASE ACCESSION NUMBERS

	PIR	SWISSPROT	EMBL/GENBANK	REFERENCES
EBNA1	A03773	P03211	V01555	[24]
			M13941, M13180	[23, 25]
EBNA2		P12978	L11366	[24, 25]
LMP1 (B95-8)	A03794	P03230	X01995	[24–26]
LMP1 (Raji)	C28918	P13198	M80488	[27]
LMP2A/2B	A30178	P13285	M24212, Y00835	[23, 28]

References
1 Chee, M. and Barrell, B. (1990) Trends Genet. 6, 86–91.
2 Middleton, T. et al. (1991) Adv. Virus Res. 40, 19–55.
3 Kouzarides, T. et al. (1991) Oncogene 6, 195–204.
4 Kenney, S.C. et al. (1992) Mol. Cell. Biol. 12, 136–146.
5 Rowe, M. et al. (1987) EMBO J. 6, 2743–2751.
6 Abbot, S.D. et al. (1990) J. Virol. 64, 2126–2134.
7 Wang, F. et al. (1990) J. Virol. 64, 2309–2318.
8 Knutson, J.C. (1990) J. Virol. 64, 2530–2536.
9 Inoue, N. et al. (1991) Virology 182, 84–93.
10 Sample, J. et al. (1986) Proc. Natl Acad. Sci. USA 83, 5096–5100.
11 Wang, D. et al. (1988) J. Virol. 62, 2337–2346.

[12] Baichwal, V.R. and Sugden, B. (1988) Oncogene 2, 461–467.

[13] Tsang, S.-F. et al. (1991) J. Virol. 65, 6765–6771.

[14] Martin, J. and Sugden, B. (1991) J. Virol. 65, 3246–3258.

[15] Laszlo, L. et al. (1991) J. Pathol. 164, 203–214.

[16] Peng, M. and Lundgren, E. (1992) Oncogene 7, 1775–1782.

[17] Marchini, A. et al. (1991) J. Virol. 65, 5991–6000.

[18] Henderson, S. et al. (1993) Proc. Natl Acad. Sci. USA 90, 8479–8483.

[19] Burkhardt, A.L. et al. (1992) J. Virol. 66, 5161–5167.

[20] Calender, A. et al. (1990) Int. J. Cancer 46, 658–663.

[21] Wolf, J. et al. (1990) Cancer Res. 50, 3095–3100.

[22] Vanhaesebroeck, B. et al. (1991) Cancer Res. 51, 2229–2238.

[23] Sample, J. et al. (1989) J. Virol. 63, 933–937.

[24] Baer, R. et al. (1984) Nature 310, 207–211.

[25] Petti, L. et al. (1990) Virology 176, 563–574.

[26] Moorthy, R. and Thorley-Lawson, D.A. (1990) J. Virol. 64, 829–837.

[27] Hatfull, G. (1988) Virology 164, 334–340.

[28] Laux, G. et al. (1988) EMBO J. 7, 769–774.

Index